WHY IS MY DOCTOR SO DUMB?

WILLIAM B. FERRIL, MD

The Bridge Medical Publishers
Whitefish, Montana

For Mckenna, Conner, Hayes, and Billy

The Bridge Medical Publishers

© 2004 William Ferril

All rights reserved. No part of this book may be reproduced or transmitted in any form or by any means, electronic or mechanical, including photocopying, recording, or by any information storage and retrieval system without permission in writing from the publisher.

Published by The Bridge Medical Publishers
P.O. Box 324
Whitefish, Montana 59937

ISBN 0-9725825-2-5
Printed in the United States of America

Cover Design by Philip Senart

Author photo by Mike Potter

10 9 8 7 6 5 4 3 2

Printed by Satori
200 ½ Wisconsin Ave.
Whitefish, MT 59937
406 862-8289

Acknowledgments

To my patients, who always point the way to better methods.

To the holistic mental giants that laid the clues for this book: Robert Atkins M.D.; Richard Bernstein M.D.; Jeffery Bland, Ph.D.; Depok Copra M.D.; Alan Gaby M.D.; William McKenzie Jefferies M.D.; John Lee M.D.; Carolyn Myss, PhD.; Uzzi Reiss M.D.; Norman Shealy, M.D.; Diana Schwarzbein M.D.; Andrew Weil M.D.; and Jonathan Wright M.D.

To my wife, Brenda, who loves me in a way that facilitates my passion for holistic healing.

To my editor Hannah Plumb, I am thankful for her patience and guidance.

To Ginny Wilcox, as usual, for helping to do the final details at Sartori Publishing.

Special thankfulness extends to Rick Nagle, Esq., for his professional instruction in regards to format for some of the earlier versions of this material.

Perpetual thankfulness goes to Steven Small Salmon who patiently instructed me about the futility of being seduced into the negative emotions.

To Patty Perigo for her kind heart and genius

Disclaimer

This book is intended as an educational tool to acquaint the reader with alternative methods of understanding, preventing, and treating some common middle age diseases. The Bridge Medical Publishers hopes that this book will enable the reader to improve their wellbeing, and to better understand, assess, and choose the appropriate course of treatment. Because some of the methods described in this book are alternative in nature, by definition some of them have not been investigated and/or approved by any government or regulatory agency.

The information contained within *Why is My Doctor so Dumb?* is not intended as a substitute for the advice and/or medical care of a physician. Nor is the content of this book intended to discourage or dissuade the reader from following the advice of his or her physician. The contents of this book are for informational purposes only and are not intended to diagnose or treat illness. The diagnosis and treatment of illness requires a specific exam, tests, history, and an appreciation for each individual's uniqueness of presentation. For those, the reader is advised to seek the counsel of a competent holistic physician. Individuals who desire weight loss, improved health or healing from chronic disease need close supervision and follow-up from their physician.

If the reader has any questions concerning the information contained in this text, or its application to his/her particular medical profile, or if the reader has unusual medical or nutritional needs or constraints that conflict with the advice in this book, he or she should consult his or her physician before embarking on any medical treatments advised in this text. Pregnant or nursing readers should consult their physicians before embarking on the nutrition and lifestyle programs suggested in this text. The reader should not stop taking prescription medications without the advice and guidance of their personal physician.

Table of Contents

The Scope of the Problem Test... vii

Introduction..xvii

SECTION 1: Thinking Outside the Box 22

Chapter 1: Intelligent Energy Fields 23

Chapter 2: Introduction to Syndrome X....................... 34

Chapter 3: Why do people shrink as they age? 37

SECTION 2: Nutrition Imbalance-caused Disease..... 45

Chapter 4: Nutritional Solutions for High Blood Pressure 46

Chapter 5: Nutritional Deficiency and Brain Dysfunction 82

Chapter 6: Attention Deficit Hyperactivity Disorder and Other Childhood Disordered Brain Function Pathologies 137

SECTION 3: Skinny on Fat 141

Chapter 7: The Real Reason Americans get Fatter Each Year is a Secret 142

Chapter 8: The "Torture Chamber" Diet: 187

Chapter 9: A Deeper Understanding of Syndrome X: a deadly form of obesity... 211

SECTION 4: Medical Myths That Promote Suffering 224

Chapter 10: Diminished Adrenal Reserve Caused Disease 225

Chapter 11: Hormone Replacement Therapy in America 241

Chapter 12: Information Carried in the Bloodstream 260

Chapter 13: Follow the Blood Fuel, and you will Understand Diabetes and Heart Disease 290

Chapter 14: Inflammation and Heart disease: The Second Part of the Secret 316

Chapter 15: The Glandular Failure Epidemic 331

Chapter 16: Nutritional Deficiency Caused Fuel Burning Problems 335

SECTION 5: Methods for Dumbing Down Doctors. 343

APPENDICES 405

BIBLIOGRAPHY 432

INDEX... 455

The Scope of the Problem Test

Dear Doctor, four years ago I could not answer correctly the majority of these questions. I have had four years to study and read about the other side of the story, which science has revealed, but I believe ignores because of profit. This book is not about putting other doctors down. Rather, it covers the disparity of what is taught versus' what is known. Further, it exposes the disorganization, half-truths, fear tactics and crummy article techniques used to manipulate doctors into believing in a largely fictional treatment strategy for middle age diseases. I believe that these fictional treatment strategies are designed to perpetuate the medical industrial economy. Almost all the answers to these medical questions are found within this text. A few are only found in *The Body Heals*. Space limitations and the scope of this manual made their inclusion impractical. The few of these that occur are marked with an asterisk (*).

Space limitations also prevented answering these questions directly. However, there is an additional reason: Without reading the text doctors prove rather tenacious for stasis within our professional training paradigm. Our patients provide us with clues that something very important is missing from our educations. I believe reading this text finishes us off and pushes us over the hump into a new world where we again become the healers that we set out to be.

Critical Information Test for Doctors

1. Please describe seven central roles that adequate potassium intake plays in the maintenance of health but curiously remains absent in today's textbooks
2. Please describe how sufficient magnesium intake benefits three common diseases (asthma, high blood pressure, and heart disease).
3. What stomach factor determines the ability for magnesium to absorb into the body?
4. Please describe three crucial health roles that zinc levels determine?
5. Please describe the consistent trend that undermines health resulting from mineral imbalance that food from a box, can or bag provides (processed food).
6. What factor determines whether or not the body can absorb zinc found in the diet?
7. Which organ always receives the highest (pancreas secretion related) insulin message content?
8. Can you tell me three other names for IGF-1 in the scientific literature?
9. Please explain how two of these names describe additional important roles for IGF-1 not openly discussed within the mainstream medical writings of today.
10. Can you describe three diseases that are radically affected because doctors are not taught about the other alias names for IGF-1, meaning the same thing?
11. What does IGF-1 do in the body Doctor?
12. Why do you insist that fake hormones are better than real hormones?
13. What class of molecules turns the genes off and on Doctor?
14. In what important way does the name Vitamin A mislead towards understanding its health effects within the body?
15. Describe your level of competence for interpreting the results of a 24-hour urine test for steroids.

16. What three types of molecular class structure types turn on and off the DNA programs?
17. Healthy people have the proper amount of these three types of informational substances and unhealthy people do not, name them.
18. When was the last time you thoroughly evaluated for all of them in an unhealthy patient?
19. Describe common pitfalls of blood testing for thyroid hormones, adrenal and gonad steroids
20. Please describe the basic nutrients needed in the following body synthesis projects:
    A. Brain neurotransmitters need what basic nutrients for each of their manufacture?
    B. Adrenals need what nutrients to make epinephrine?
    C. Steroid synthesis needs what nutrients and determiners?
    D. DNA needs what basic nutritional stability factor that depletes within the body at one billion times a second?
    E. A major nutrient in the skin and GI tract that is critical for epithelial cell maturation (retards tumor growth here)
21. What nutrients are needed to burn fat aerobically Doctor?
22. What nutrients are needed to burn sugar aerobically and avoid lactic acid build up?
23. Where is the highest concentration of Vitamin C in the body?
24. What health consequences commonly occur when a body lacks the nutrients to change norepinephrine into epinephrine?
25. What substance elevates in the blood stream when nor-epinephrine's conversion into epinephrine becomes nutritionally compromised?
26. Describe the mechanisms for how imbalances connected with each of the below causes high blood pressure.
    A. Potassium deficiency
    B. Magnesium deficiency

C. Insulin excess
   D. Methyl donor deficiency
   E. Stiff red blood cells (appendix A)
   F. Nitric oxide deficiency
   G. Syndrome X
   H. Sodium excess (they all know this one)
   I. Type A personality other than catecholamines
27. Why do people shrink as they age Doctor?
28. What class of informational substance determines the repair rate within the body Doctor?
29. Explain how high levels of cortisol leads to more body fat?
30. How is dietary fat and cholesterol absorbed into the body doctor?
31. Why don't lymph vessels plug up with fat then?
32. Explain the difference between the type of fat and cholesterol that lymph vessels encounter and those that the arteries encounter.
33. What hormone turns on cholesterol synthesis within the liver?
34. What hormone turns down cholesterol synthesis within the liver?
35. Which hormone do the statin drugs impair in its ability to deliver message content to the liver?
36. Explain the likely mechanism for how statin drugs decrease arterial inflammation.
37. What logical health consequences follow from this mechanism?
38. Describe two holistic strategies that decrease arterial inflammation but avoid the health consequences of the statin drugs.
39. What opposes gravity trying to squish my cells flat Doctor?
40. What is Thimerosal, Doctor?
41. Doctor, what are the acute phase reactants and why do they elevate?
42. By what mechanism does an elevated acute phase reactant level tie into increased insulin need?

43. What type of personality or chronic life situation promotes elevated acute phase reactants?
44. How does understanding and negating this fact help to heal most heart disease risk?
45. Describe the mechanisms for how these, when deficient, cause heart failure
    A. Carnitine deficiency
    B. Co enzyme Q10 deficiency
    C. Histamine deficiency
    D. Epinephrine deficiency
    E. Testosterone deficiency
46. Which ones of the five above molecules depletes while taking cholesterol-lowering medication?
47. Describe the molecular similarities between testosterone and digitalis-like medications that creates a common message content (they both strengthen the force of the heart's contraction).*
48. What hormonal conversion process occurs that leads to gynecomastia with taking either digoxin or testosterone treatments?*
49. What nutrient's presence retards this process?
50. Can you tell me ten additional hormone aberrations that cause diabetes but are not emphasized in clinical practice?
51. When was the last time you checked for any of them?
52. Can you describe the mechanism for how liver injury promotes beta cell burnout?
53. Can you describe the mechanism by which healing the liver causes insulin sensitivity to improve?
54. Doctor, explain why ACE inhibitors, given for high blood pressure, often cause a dry cough?
55. Doctor, can you explain why people with autoimmune disease can get worse while taking ACE inhibitors for their high blood pressure?
56. Describe three additional ways that ACE inhibitors lower blood pressure but are not commonly acknowledged.

57. Doctor, explain why people taking cholesterol-lowering drugs have an increased risk of their muscle cells tearing apart from one another?*
58. List the nutrients that make up the methyl donor system, which the body needs at the rate of one billion times a second.
59. Doctor, what nutrients are needed to keep the liver healthy and deactivate toxins? (Appendix C)
60. Describe the mechanism by which acetaminophen can irreversibly injure hemoglobin (Appendix A).
61. Describe the mechanism by which sulfa drugs can irreversibly injure hemoglobin (Appendix A).
62. What important role does reduced sulfur play in body health?
63. What major hormone keeps the blood sugar adequate between meals, fasting, and during exercise in healthy people?
64. What two things are different about this hormone compared to the other three hormones that predominantly elevate the blood sugar between meals in unhealthy people?
65. What is so important about keeping the protein content in the tissues adequate?
66. What molecular class of body structure components burns up calories?
67. Which three hormones keep the blood sugar adequate between meals, while fasting, and during exercise in unhealthy people?
68. Why would the predominance of the above hormones be harmful to body structure?
69. Name two common reasons that cause unhealthy bodies to have the need to elevate insulin in the fasting state (insulin resistance)?
70. Explain why insulin elevation, in the fasting state of unhealthy people, needs to occur even though it sets up competing message content at the level of the liver in order to stay alive.

71. Explain why healthy bodies need essentially no insulin in the fasting state.
72. Name nine hormones that cause or promote or protect from obesity (these nine have a proven relationship to gaining body fat and their optimization leads to weight loss)? These are not inclusive of the theoretically important hormones, like adiponectin, graelin, and leptin.
73. What body process burns the lion's share of calories while at rest?
74. Does the brain have more fat weight or nerve weight?
75. What type of nutrients deplete when one fails to obtain adequate fats in their diet?
76. How many causes for increased insulin need (insulin resistance) can you name?
77. Name five central reasons that cause growth hormone secretion rates to diminish.
78. Name four reasons that prolactin secretion rates increase.
79. Name one big consequence to health when prolactin elevates without a placenta being present?
80. Describe a hormonal pathway and its consequences, other than increased epinephrine, for why Type A personalities develop heart disease.
81. Describe a more holistic explanation for why C reactive protein elevates in the context of modern society?
82. Provide two likely holistic hormonal explanations for how statin drugs lower inflammation that are not openly discussed with doctors.
83. Describe why an elevation of the acute phase reactants logically extends to the increased angiogenesis tendency observed with insulin resistance.
84. Name as many acute phase reactants as you can, Doctor?
85. For which ones is there accumulating evidence that when they increase they directly contribute to blood vessel injury?
86. How does this knowledge shed light for a possible benefit of chelation therapy?

87. Why do rheumatoid arthritis, asthma, allergies, colitis, Crohn disease, and lupus all tend to have elevated eosinophils and a right shift in their WBC differential?
88. Why does each of the above diseases also worsen with stressful situations?
89. What three situations cause aldosterone to release from the adrenal?
90. Which steroid's amount determines the manufacture rate of all other steroids?
91. What other steroids secrete from the adrenal along with cortisol and why is this ratio significant?
92. Explain how, by only replacing cortisol-like message content the other important adrenal steroids further imbalance.
93. Which has the higher affinity for the kidney enzyme, 11B-hydroxysteroid dehydrogenase, cortisol or aldosterone?
94. Why will stress during or before the blood draw for thyroid function assessments falsely elevate the thyroid hormone test and depress the TSH?
95. When was the last time that you considered this in a patient who clinically appeared hypothyroid?
96. What nutrient proves necessary for the thyroid message to be heard at the DNA level?
97. What nutrient proves necessary for T4 to convert to T3 (T3 is eight times more powerful than T4)
98. What hormone deficiency commonly causes the anemia of chronic disease?
99. What steroid hormone concentrates by a factor of five to six within the brain compared to the blood steam?
100. Why is this significant in the prevention of Alzheimer's disease?
101. What steroid hormone powerfully proves trophic to Schwann cells in the brain (the cells that deteriorate in Multiple Sclerosis sufferers)?
102. Why do you insist that growth hormone is diabetogenic?

103. By what mechanism does an increased serotonin within the pituitary lower gonad steroid production?
104. Why is the prescribing of growth hormone without a liver function, thyroid, adrenal and gonad assessment risky?
105. Describe the difference between the fat particles that the lymph vessels encounter and those found in the arteries.
106. Explain the hormonal cascade for how high estrogen levels lead to elevated triglycerides and LDL cholesterol.
107. Describe an additional hormone elevation that results when estrogen levels are high and a placenta is absent that also promotes obesity.
108. Name two hormone types that decrease as estrogen amounts reach high levels when a placenta is absent (birth control pills)?
109. How do the combined answers to the last two questions describe why these women have an increased insulin need (insulin resistance)?
110. What hormonal situations cause sex hormone binding globulin levels to deviate widely?
111. Explain how health consequences occur when a patient's doctor fails to ascertain this value.
112. Describe the hormonal cascade; manufactured within the placenta, that mitigates increased insulin need in the healthy pregnant state.
113. Describe the most likely mechanism that SSRI-like medications lead to sexual dysfunction.
114. Describe the most likely mechanism that SSRI-like medications can cause weight gain.
115. What atomic element is the most powerful oxidizing agent when unpaired?
116. Name some commonly prescribed prescription drugs that contain this element.
117. Which class of drugs contains brands that penetrate the mind and contain this element?

118. Name the only molecule that the mitochondria can burn aerobically.
119. Which hormone excess powerfully promotes the growth of fatty arterial blockages in both the obese diabetic and the typical heart disease sufferer?
120. What hormone excess powerfully revs up the activity level of the liver enzyme HMG Co A reductase?
121. When was the last time that you counseled your patients about this fact?
122. Explain how a high IGF-1 level lowers the insulin needs of the body?
123. Name three inconsistent details that promote suspicion about mainstream medicine adherent's belief in the supposed association with increased IGF-1 levels and tumor growth.
124. Name four inconsistent details that cast suspicion on mainstream medicine adherent's belief in the supposed association about growth hormone promoting cancer.
125. What popular diabetic medication that is touted as raising insulin sensitivity, in all likelihood really acts by raising growth hormone secretion rates and consequently IGF-1?
126. By what mechanism does the above medications causing lactic acidosis support this belief?
127. What health consequences predictably occur in the blood vessels when medication continuously creates lactic acidosis?
128. By what mechanism does increased blood heparin lower serum cholesterol?
129. What caution is in order about giving heparin to lower cholesterol?
130. What common nutritional deficiency explains why garlic has a blood pressure lowering effect?

Introduction

Healing has but one side effect, its negative impact on profit from within the medical industrial complex. Somewhere between the suffering patient and the hysteria to make more money the science about how the body heals collects dust. Sound holistic healing principles are not taught in their congruent whole in medical school. The textbooks contain most of these facts but they present in ways designed to groom the doctor's mind in a way favorable to the complex.

Power complexes historically begin to falter before their particular elite realizes that the oppressed are organizing. Czarist Russian elitists did not fully appreciate the formidable force created by organized peasants. The French revolutionaries similarly surprised their oppressors by the magnitude of underground support for a new way of doing things. The uprising against the dominant medical industrial complex has the same old slumbering elitist components.

While the elitists smugly continue pandering symptom-control methods, which always have side effects, a better way continues to gather momentum. Slowly, but surely, the downplayed art of healing has been rediscovered and is increasingly practiced within the growing holistic community. More Western humans with each passing day leave the dominant medical treatment model. Often their departure centers on a sense that something very important is missing from mainstream medicine's approach to health versus disease.

The medical industry is a profit-oriented system. Logically, these multi-conglomerates exist to make money. What is for sale is therefore sensationalized through the media. However, the downside (the side effects and toxicities) remains minimized. The pursuit of maximum profit provides the disincentive for sharing more effective healing strategies.

Along these lines, it remains consistent that a profit-driven medical system would stoop to conduct various disinformation campaigns. The media has advertising revenue to consider, and consequently, often become all too happy to promote these half-truths, which propagate fear in those who seek alternative counsel. Common methods include the results of a poorly run study against various alternative modalities, the professional opinion of 'certified' experts and the mantra about the lack of scientific data when they know all along that they control which data is collected. Dr. John Lee mentions in the introduction of his book, **Some Things Your Doctor May not Tell you about Menopause,** that his reputation initially suffered at the hands of the complex. However, he adds that the complex underestimated the power of the international women's network regarding what works.

An insight into the consequences of a medical system run by the profit interests of the complex is analogous to junk food. Although junk food taste like real food, it will harm the body if it is continuously ingested. American owners are bombarded by clever advertising schemes that encourage the consumption of these injurious ingredients. Most owners now know that these processed foods are harmful, but until recently everyone seemed to eat them. Slowly, but surely, more owners have become aware that processed foods, which are altered by chemicals, hormone mimics, and nutrient depletions-will injure the body. The food industries' media campaign still touts the latest clever come on, but there are less vulnerable owners with each passing year. Similarly, the emerging health care revolution cultivates awareness for the consequences from following the profitable dictums of mainstream medicine.

Part of the success for perpetuating the dominant medicine paradigm arises by incompletely educating physicians on what science has revealed. I, too, was a victim of my complex funded education. Without realizing it, I became a believer in the corrupted mainstream view of the medical universe. I have been unintentionally guilty of prescribing treatments that were not in my patients' best interest. I believed in a system of health care where side effects and toxicities were treated with more medications and procedures. I regretfully remember discouraging patients from continuing or seeking alternative treatment modalities. However, I thank several of my doggedly stubborn patients who continually pointed out to me the inconsistencies of my educational paradigm. To my credit, I kept mulling over in my head the unexplainable outcomes toward patient healing when they adhered to fringe advice. As the years ticked by, I continued to collect inconsistencies that were unexplainable by the mainstream view of health versus disease.

A major breakthrough occurred when I married my wife, Brenda, about eleven years ago. Brenda is a chiropractor. Initially, I humored myself by offering her space in my office. I still remember with humility witnessing what two hands accomplish compared to my medical training for a variety of afflictions. My wife also began to instruct me about the importance of medicinal herbs, colon health, and nutritional supplements.

Over the last several years I have had time to heal myself, study newer versions of my medical textbooks and contemplate what is missing from these books. Sometimes it is not missing but it presents in a disorganized format or as isolated 'pearls' that are not indexed. Tedium describes the hours of detective work needed to uncover and weave together a more holistic perspective for what happens to the body around middle age.

The middle-aged body wants to heal itself. Around middle age there are seven interrelated principles of health that tend to falter. Unless all are attended to the chronic degenerative diseases of middle age begin to insidiously propagate their deterioration on the body form. Common examples of these imbalances which arise from one or more faltering principles of health include: obesity, high blood pressure, heart disease, asthma, arthritis, hormone imbalance, and diabetes. Each of these common diseases can be healed without side effects when all seven principles of health rebalance. **The achievement of balance requires the afflicted owner's active participation.** When this first requirement continues to be ignored symptom-control medicine remains the only treatment possibility. However, in owners who are willing to take an active role in their disease solution there are many cases where the above diseases heal or at least stabilize.

The seven interrelated principles are:

1. Prevent rust formation within the tissues
2. Prevent hardening processes within the blood vessels
3. The hormones giveth and the hormones taketh away
4. You become what you supply and absorb
5. Take out your cellular trash water
6. Avoid "low voltage cell syndrome"
7. Maximize the ratio between the energies that heal contrasted against the energies that maim the body tissues

Each of these principles of health is explained in my earlier book, ***The Body Heals.*** Although these principles are touched upon in this book the focus here will be to help the reader understand the missing educational content that allows the perpetration of symptom-control medicine. Doctors, in general, possess an innate and keen intelligence. This creates a formidable ongoing challenge to keep them dumbed down. The revolution in health care emerging today seeks to recall what science already knows about how the body heals.

The revolution in health care choices begins with principle seven. Principle seven concerns the quality of the life energies' integrity. Mainstream medicine almost completely ignores this important consideration always operating within a diseased body. This dominant approach can be likened to the slab of meat approach. The slab of meat is all that is left when the mysterious life energies are removed from consideration. Fortunately, these important energies form a common denominator between many alternative-healing modalities. Chiropractic, homeopathy, acupuncture, massage, yoga, meditative prayer, and chakra energy work all, each in their own way, reinvigorates the life energy field. The life energy field improves because these modalities have in common that they facilitate a release of the chaotic energies while facilitating the rhythmical energies.

Neglecting to consider the rhythmical energies describes one consequence of living within a profit driven health care system. The fallout of this makes important scientific information largely inaccessible in its congruent whole. Profit considerations influence which universities receive the pharmaceutical companies' research funds. This financial reality in turn influences the way medical schools educate physicians to think about disease. Of course physicians like myself have very little reason to doubt our educations until our patients begin providing living inconsistencies about how the body heals. Some physicians become tired and invested in the complex's way of doing things. I am living proof of how kind and informed patients can point the way to better methods. One of the better methods involves the rhythmical life energies.

A re-inclusion of the rhythmical life energies pulsating within each body cell bridges a common denominator between many alternative-healing modalities. The health care revolution bears the burden of educating those who are unaware. Like other times of exponential change, the dominant power elitists are largely unaware of the strength and conviction within the holistic health care movement. Other than the first chapter, the remainder of this book discusses and explores the other side of what science has revealed but continues to ignore. A little woo woo before all the hard science helps to balance the scientific discussion of health against the mystery of the unfathomable.

SECTION 1: Thinking Outside the Box

Chapter 1: Intelligent Energy Fields

Health is a Question of Balance

The reoccurring body theme of balance forms a prerequisite for true health. Balance reverberates all the way down to the opposing molecules that are interacting within a cell. Western medicine often ignores this because of the reductionism logic on which it is founded.

The science exists to unite these holistic principles into a comprehensive assessment of the tendency towards health or disease. Reductionism of the logistical and detailed investigations into the biochemical reactions of life has merit. However, at some point it becomes devoid of the common interwoven theme of energetic balance. When science becomes more unified it brings people to the realization that life is based on balance between opposing energetic forces. Wherever there is imbalance, deterioration and disease eventually result.

Other medical scientific theories embrace the energetic understandings of balance. For example, traditional Chinese medical theory has the life energies quality at its foundation. The foundation of their energy science uses the concepts of Yin energy that directly opposes Yang energy in a harmonious way. The harmony between these two energetic entities proves as a prerequisite for health.

Conversely, the western system ignores the dynamic forces between yin energy and yang energy. These forces are mysterious energies that oppose one another. Thousands of years of accumulated evidence show that balance is necessary for health. Yin energy can be thought of as quiet, calm, contemplative, reflective, cool, deep, patient, and content.

Whereas Yang energy can be thought of as loud, rushed, hurried, hot, shallow, and explosive, on-the-move, action and impatient.

Evidence has been accumulating for more than 60 years that the life force exists as an intelligent energy grid that permeates every cell. Every cell in the body depends on this organizing energy until death. The evidence seems to indicate that when this life force energy evenly distributes and occurs at the right vibration frequency all is well within the body.

In contrast, as stated earlier, the western medical approach can best be described as the "slab of meat approach". The slab of meat is all that is left when the mysterious energies that organize the human form are ignored. The western scientific paradigm ignores the qualities of the life force. When life energy imbalances are the cause of disease, owners in these situations will continue to suffer. The western medical complex fails to consider energy aberrations that can cause a disease process. The Chinese are not the only group with a medical theory that includes the life force energy.

Eastern Indian scientific theory has long understood the flow of optimal life giving energy through chakras in healthy individuals. Recently there have been some interesting applications of these imbalanced energy states, and how they correlate with disease. This evidence involves the other side of the story of what science has revealed but remains ignored. In this chapter, the ignored evidence will be reintroduced. The trouble with re-including it in the mainstream medical discussion, of health versus disease, is that many of the mainstream approaches and explanations of the inner-workings of the universe begin to look inconsistent and incomplete.

Conversely, this information about many of the alternative treatment modalities makes more mechanistic sense and often appears less superstitious. Life field enhancement forms a common denominator for the proven effectiveness of acupuncture, chiropractic, yoga, prayer, herbal therapies, massage therapy and homeopathy. Each of these therapies, each in their own way, benefits the life field's harmony.

Down through the ages many wise men have contemplated the human condition. Dr. Paul Brand, MD, author of the book 'Fearfully and Wonderfully Made', points out that knowledge has been lost. He says that the Egyptian physicians of thousands of years ago could perform surgeries that cannot even be contemplated today. High technology solutions can only go so far before one confronts the ignored energy of life. The life force needs to be considered and appreciated in order to carry healing over the 'bridge' that unites the mainstream with the alternative modalities.

The Unseen Intelligent Energy

The body contains approximately one hundred trillion cells. The 46 chromosomes that contain the DNA within most cells are in some ways analogous to a computer encryption code. Without an intelligent operator the encryption code hides useful information. Something is missing at the encryption (DNA) level. Something else is needed to explain the precise and ordered unraveling and repair of DNA. The replication of DNA and RNA is superbly directed by some, as yet unseen, guiding principle. In addition, the RNA directed protein synthesis, which results in elaborate and unique protein architecture, needs direction.

The direction of the construction of cell architecture involves many types of fat and specialized sugar groups. What directs how these all fit precisely together is not explained by the genetic code contained within the DNA. The DNA only contains the sequencing information for the construction of the amino acid sequence, which make up all proteins. It does not contain information, which regards the synthesis of the many different types of fat and modified sugars added onto certain proteins. These also need to be precisely arranged in three-dimensional space for life to continue. A plausible explanation for what directs these complex processes is currently beyond western scientific understanding.

Interesting research exists, regarding the nature of the force that intelligently directs the DNA. In the early 1920's the scientific pioreer Dr. Harold Saxon Burr, a long time researcher at Yale University, began documenting the electromagnetic field properties, found to occur in all living things. Dr. Burr later named this electromagnetic field, the life field. He pointed out that if one hadn't seen his or her friend in over six months, new molecules during the intervening time period would have replaced every molecule in his or her friend's face.

The fact that the body replaces all soft tissue molecules frequently is secondary to the body's ongoing cellular rejuvenation program. The cellular rejuvenation program occurs throughout life at varying degrees of efficiency. Dr. Burr's research led him to conclude that it was the life field that served as an organizing template. He theorized that the electromagnetic field, which he measured, was the organizer of the structure contained within living things. He concluded that the electromagnetic 'template' preserves the pattern in the friend's face. The underlying energetic template reproduces a consistent appearance, even though the molecules themselves are different. He extended this concept to explain the mystery of embryological cells, knowing how to organize, divide and differentiate into fetal form.

Mainstream science remains unable to explain these two fundamental life processes because they ignore theories like Dr. Burr's. No mainstream explanation exists for why one's face stays recognizable after the molecules are replaced. In addition, mainstream science remains baffled about the process of embryogenesis. Embryogenesis denotes the organized process of cell differentiation, spatial arrangement and orientation of the embryo's development.

In his book, ***The Body Electric***, Robert Becker MD, elaborated on this research. Dr. Becker comments, "Embryo genesis is as if a pile of bricks were to spontaneously rearrange itself into a building, becoming not only walls but windows, light sockets, steel beams and furniture in the process." Later on he summarized this mystery that led to his life research," As I contemplated their findings and all of biology's unsolved problems, I grew convinced that life was more complex than we suspected. I felt that those who reduced life to a mechanical interaction of molecules were living in a cold, gray, dead world, which despite its drabness, was a fantasy. I didn't think electricity would turn out to be any élan vital in the old sense, but I had a hunch it would be closer to the secret than the smells of the biochemistry lab or the dissecting rooms preserved organs."

Drs. Burr and Becker are in good company. Another scientist agrees with their line of thinking in regards to solving the mystery of an organizing energy field. Dr. Albert Szent Gyorgyi won the Nobel Prize for his work on tissue oxidation and the elucidation of the molecular structure of Vitamin C.

According to Dr. Becker, when he addressed the Budapest Academy of Science on March 21, 1941, Dr. Gyorgyi pointed out that as scientists broke living things down into constituent parts, life slipped through their fingers and they found themselves working with dead matter. Dr. Gyorgyi emphasized, "It looks as if some basic fact about life is still missing, without which any real understanding is impossible." For the missing basic, fact Dr. Gyorgyi proposed putting electricity back into science's investigation of living things. More than 60 years later, mainstream science is still trying to explain life within the limitation of molecular matter while ignoring the evidence for organizing energy.

The continued omission of the life force has altered medical treatment decisions. Some of the consequent treatment decisions have associated toxicities. Some of these toxicities are avoidable. In contrast, the alternative treatment modalities, mentioned above, address the importance of an owner's life force quality. This fact has resulted in these alternative-healing disciplines growing success.

The life force quality forms a powerful common denominator between many of the alternative methods of healing. Some holistic physicians feel that the common denominator regards their common practice of improving, maintaining, and cleansing this life field. The alternative therapies practitioners believe that the life force functions more efficiently during health than in disease.

Some call the life force energy, measured years ago by Dr. Burr, intelligent energy. Intelligent energy denotes the property of the life force to organize molecules into complex arrangements which life requires. This fundamental requirement of living things violates the science of physics' third law of thermodynamics. The third law of thermodynamics states that molecular arrangements will tend to move in a random fashion toward more disorder. Again, mainstream medicine remains unable to explain how living things violate this basic physical law of the nonliving components of the universe.

Some newer mathematical theories predict that the life force swirls around at speeds faster than the speed of light. The faster-than-the speed-of-light requirement has merit because when energy moves this fast the math predicts it to behave with an organizational intelligence. Dr. Richard Gerber in his book, '*Vibrational Medicine*' explains quite well the math pioneered by Carl Muses. In his work on hyper numbers, Carl Muses proposed that when energy moves faster than the speed of light organizational consequences occur. Dr. William Tiller of Stanford University expounded on these mathematical consequences and described this type of energy as difficult to measure within the dimension of the physical world, except that it would create a weak magnetic field. All living things studied, to date, create a magnetic field until death occurs.

The faster-than-speed-of-light property would help explain the above-mentioned long-standing physics' conundrum. Specifically, the third law of thermodynamics in physics states that energy naturally moves in a direction of more and more randomness (increased entropy). Life's complexly created molecules, which precisely arrange so that life may continue, violate this basic tenant of physics. However, if one limits the third law of thermodynamics to a description of energy's behavior when energy travels at speeds equal to, or less than the speed of light, it remains consistent. Until very recently no mathematician or scientist had really thought about the consequences of energy moving at speeds greater than the speed of light.

Understanding the conundrum regarding life energy violating physic's thermodynamic law is best grasped by considering the chicken egg. If one dropped a million eggs on the floor, breaking each of the eggs, there would be a mess. There would be no chick formed. The physicist would say that the third law of thermodynamics was consistent in this case. However, it is only consistent because the act of breaking open the shell kills the life contained inside of it. Contrast this to successfully incubating any one of the eggs through its gestation time. The live chick would be formed. The baby chick is an example of increasing complexity, which is created from uncomplicated molecules inside the chicken egg. What was just a gooey mess inside the egg was energetically organized into the complex multi-organ and multi-cellular baby chick. What is the nature of this intelligent energy that violates the laws of physics? The theory of energy moving faster than the speed of light and behaving with an organizational intelligence provides a viable explanation for how the life force may organize matter like the gooey chicken egg into a baby chick.

Drs. Muses and Tiller were some of the first mathematicians to look into how energy behaves moving faster than the speed of light. They theorized that when energy travels faster than the speed of light it would behave with an organizational intelligence with only a weakly measurable magnetic field. They thought of the physical world, for which owners have sensory apparatus to experience, as the speeds equal to or less than light dimension. They further predicted that at speeds greater than light the measurement of the electrical properties of this type of energy would exceed today's technological capabilities. The one predicted exception being the ability to detect a weakly measurable magnetic field. This theory remains consistent with the measurability of a weak bodily magnetic field, which changes in strength and polarization during different levels of activity and consciousness. These facts provide evidence, which would help explain life's mysterious energetic properties more completely yet it routinely remains ignored in the mainstream world of medicine.

The life energy can best be thought of as moving within another dimension than the physical world. Current technologies cannot detect energy moving faster than the speed of light. In fact, this becomes the basis for claiming that it does not exist. The mathematical theory of matter moving faster than the speed of light, which predicts that it would create a weak but measurable magnetic field, tends to be ignored.

Interestingly, research looking into the organization of the body's magnetic field, has found an unvarying energy grid, corresponding to the ancient Chinese system of acupuncture meridian lines (see ***The Body Electric***).

Science has come a long way in eloquently explaining cellular biochemical reactions. Science has advanced its understanding about the contents of the DNA program. However, the DNA programs (the genes) only explain the protein component of the human body composition. The DNA program does not explain spacial orientation of the complex cell components. Nor does it explain the complex fats and modified sugar building blocks manufacture and their spacial orientation. The mystery for how life organizes simple molecules into complex cellular and multicellular structures, with precise organization, remains unexplainable by the mainstream.

Scientific theory, going back thousands of years in India and China, recognizes the importance of living things containing an optimal energy flow. The Indians call the life energy prana and the Chinese call it Chi. In both scientific systems the attention to the overall quality and integrity contained within the life energy field proves fundamental to health. In addition, the Chinese realized the quality of energy penetrating the body's trunk organs could be palpated in the peripheral pulse. This system quantitates the amount of Chi contained within the various organs and is called pulse diagnosis. Pulse diagnosis was developed over the last several thousand years. Pulse diagnosis allows an elaborate understanding of the consequences of energetic excess or deficiency within each organ.

The electromagnetic lines, known as the acupuncture meridian lines, were painstakingly developed with their corresponding organ effects noted. Out of this several thousand years of observation, there developed an understanding of ways to increase or decrease the energetic meridian tone depending on what was needed. The energetic energy tone is composed of the opposing energies, Yin and Yang. When Yin and Yang imbalance the recipient organ system develops dysfunction.

The Chinese scientific theory regards Chi as organizing life energy. This energy concept is worthy of some consideration. This theory predicts that Chi needs to be balanced by the forces of yin and yang within any organ system in the body or disease occurs. Investigations into Chi energy could solve the mystery about the missing mainstream explanation for how life creates complexity.

In other words, the alternative idea of the existence of intelligent energy serving as the ultimate director of the cellular biochemical reactions of life has healing possibilities. Healing possibilities could be realized when the Chi energy improves. Improvement in the Chi energy will improve the quality of the hormones secreted in a rhythmic and harmonious way. These alternative theories predict that the areas of body breakdown result from the Chi energetic deficiency or excess. Chi is the Chinese description of intelligent energy, the life force, or prana.

The merging of energy theory and what is known about the biochemical reactions of life incorporates the intermediary step of the hormones and neurotransmitters. The hormones deliver the message, which was stimulated by the intelligent energy. The quality of the intelligent energy, within the body, becomes a determinant of how an organ functions. If the intelligent energy distribution and quality proves favorable, this communicates to the body's cells by the informational substances.

The informational substances include the hormones and neurotransmitters. The Chinese theory regarding Chi predicts that practices, which facilitate the life energy, will promote health by way of the informational substances. Any practice that injures the quality of the intelligent energy will promote aging and eventually disease. Western science can measure the diminished quality of informational substances. However, western science does not specifically appreciate or acknowledge the possibility of the life force energy being a determinant of these informational substances.

The Chinese and East Indians have developed theories that explain the life force energy. Western medical thought begins its treatment decisions at the level of the informational substances. Often times even this level of inquiry becomes less than adequate.

The theory of intelligent energy can best be thought of as the organizational template which directs the overall living body processes. The quality and completeness of this life energy determines which informational substances secrete. Quality informational substances depend on a highly functioning intelligent energy field. This belief has long ago been appreciated and incorporated into Chinese and East Indian scientific medical thought. The belief that these energies move faster than the speed of light provides an explanation for why they prove difficult to detect by conventional technological means. Similarly, before the understanding of television and radio waves, the presence of these wave energies in the natural environment largely went unnoticed until technology developed that measured their existence. The key to understanding this possibility regards an appreciation of the fact that television and radio waves existed down through the ages. Their properties of existence were not affected because humans were unaware of their presence. Today the upper limits of scientific study concerns energies which move slower than or equal to the speed of light. However, the evolution of mathematics considers the consequences of what energy would behave like when moving greater than the speed of light. Part of these consequences includes the possibility that would explain how life organizes matter into complex arrangements. If an owner can be open to this possibility, then a mechanistic explanation for how alternative therapies improve owner vitality becomes possible.

Chapter 2: Introduction to Syndrome X

Syndrome X denotes owners who exist on an accelerated path to not only an old body but heart disease as well. Truncal obesity proves to be the most reliable red flag that warrants a deeper inquiry. Fat that accumulates here signals excess insulin secretion rates occurring within.

Insulin is one body hormone. Hormones carry information within the blood steam that directs how the body's cells spend their energy. Insulin's message concerns energy storage. Most body energy stores as fat. Fat storage proves impossible without insulin. Only 500 grams of sugar can store as glycogen within the liver and muscles. Above this limit the extra sugar converts into fat and cholesterol. Cholesterol is just one type of body fat. By calling it cholesterol, doctors and patients alike become confused about the consequences of insulin levels increasing within a body.

Mainstream physicians are not taught about the simple relationship between increased insulin and the rise in activity level of the enzyme in the liver that converts sugar into cholesterol. They are also not taught how in certain high insulin owners their elevated blood pressure often results from their elevated insulin levels, as well (chapter 4). Even more disturbing concerns the common practice of prescribing insulin-raising medications to already obese diabetics. Obese diabetics develop heart disease for the same reasons as the typical syndrome X patient. They both grow fat within their arteries because excess insulin message content exaggerates the amount of LDL cholesterol that the liver secretes into the blood stream. The excess LDL cholesterol accumulates within the macrophages in places like the coronary arteries inside surfaces. The chronically over fed, mentally stressed and sedentary state provides the ideal situation that allows these fat accumulations to enlarge slowly but surely. Typically, some external event destabilizes the plaque's surface and a blood clot forms closing off the already fatty narrowed area. Alternatively, chronic reversed minerals intake, common to the processed food diet, predispose the coronary arteries to spasm. In both cases, a heart attack follows.

The difference, the blood sugar level, between the obese diabetic and the typical heart disease owner receives the advertising dollar and the lion's share of clinical attention. Preoccupation with blood sugar control has merit but failing to realize the killer side effects of continually increasing insulin message content to normalize the blood sugar has grave consequences in the form of arterial fatty growths. Insulin contains the fat-maker message. The other hormone aberrations that cause increased insulin need, when corrected, allow the blood sugar to come down naturally (chapter 7). It should be emphasized that a minority of adult onset diabetics derive from often overlooked other hormone abnormalities and again the mainstream doctor receives little training for how to recognize these cases. Chapter 13 describes these cases and how to identify them

The mainstream doctor is then taught to prescribe cholesterol-lowering drugs that mostly become necessary when insulin levels rise within the liver. These drugs poison the ability of the liver to listen to the increased insulin message content. Rather than simply educate physicians about this basic physiologic fact, these medicines remain the standard of care. Deviating from the standard of care alienates a physician into a medical malpractice risk. The above example is the first of many where healing science remains ignored through legal intimidation and peripheral science, in the interest of corporate profits, receives the approval of the herd.

Cholesterol lowering drugs have many side effects such as: liver injury, muscle injury, and heart failure. These medications promote heart failure because a critical heart nutrient, Co enzyme Q10, requires this same liver enzyme that makes cholesterol for its manufacturel (they also are likely to promote heart failure by their emerging effects on decreasing inflammation through a less realized side effect, explained in the physicians side bar in chapter 14). Again mainstream physicians are not taught about these physiological facts. Equally disturbing is the fact that this same enzyme within the liver makes what are called dolichols. Dolichols hold cells under tension together. Muscle cells exemplify the need to hold together under tension. Because the statin drugs inhibit these molecules manufacture rate leaking muscle enzymes become more understandable. Re-including this detail sheds light on the side effect of muscle enzyme elevation, secondary to leaking cells, so common with these prescriptions.

So far, the Syndrome X and diabetes common symptoms of excess body fat, unfavorable cholesterol profile, frequent blood pressure elevation and accelerated heart disease risk have been introduced. The only difference in the obese diabetic concerns their blood sugar elevation. Increased insulin need drives both disease processes. Most of these owners develop increased blood sugars because their insulin need exceeds their pancreas' ability to maintain it (chapter 13). Also introduced was the fact that by correcting other hormone abnormalities the insulin needs comes down naturally and so do the blood pressure, cholesterol and blood sugar (chapter 7).

Chapter 3: Why do people shrink as they age?

Consistently present among the cells, but beyond the view of the electron microscope, there exists an important anti-aging architectural framework. This sub-microscopic architecture solves the problem of internal cell pressure. Inside the cell, neighboring cells that are stacked on top of and around every cell create pressure. Gravitational pressure desires to squish the cells flat. Healthy owners have a high integrity framework operating inside and around each cell that opposes the force of gravity. Gravity is opposed because the architectural framework of the body possesses an electrical charge. This fact prevents the gravitational forces from expressing cellular fluid.

One of the reasons owners age involves the fact that this sub-microscopic framework becomes compromised under certain conditions. When the electrically charged framework of a cell crumbles, cellular collapse appears clinically as the shrinkage of old age. As water squeezes out, the framework of the cell begins to collapse and everything becomes smaller. Physicians dating back to antiquity noted that aging involves a drying out process within the body.

The architectural framework attracts sufficient water by the amount of its electrical charge. When a sufficient electrical charge exists in the framework, water sucks inward to further inflate this framework creating wrinkle free cells.

Overly ripe fruit wrinkles for the same reasons that body cells shrink and wrinkle. In both cases, it involves the loss of the electrically charged and water-sucking framework within. The difference concerns that the healthy body continually recreates new electrically charged framework. Adequate framework, which possesses sufficient electrical charges, powerfully sucks water into a body area. In contrast, its deficiency allows the gravitational forces to squeeze water from the cells.

Processes that accelerate this sub-microscopic framework's deterioration also accelerate the shrinkage into old age. Conversely, processes that re-enforce this framework's continued rejuvenation maintain a prolonged youthful vitality. The cartilage cells serve as an excellent example for how this electrically charged architecture keeps itself in repair. The ongoing repair process exemplifies the importance of adequate electrically charged architectural framework.

The Cartilage within the Joints

Many things can go wrong when the integrity of the sub-microscopic framework becomes compromised and cellular collapse begins. Once the framework begins to give way, re-inflating the cell becomes difficult. Understanding ways to slow down deflationary cellular forces is most effective early in the aging process.

The same electrically charged architecture that is responsible for keeping the majority of the cells inflated also applies to the joint cells. The difference concerns the amount of reinforcement-architecture needed because of the environmental variations that the different cell types experience. The spaces surrounding joint cells require the most electrically charged grid because gravitational forces concentrate here.

Healthy joints need a few basic molecular building parts supplied on a regular basis (see list below). Joint cells also need adequately equipped cellular factories. Cellular factories must be able to manufacture new framework structures during the entire life of the cell. Cell factories need informational direction that can only be given by contact with high quality hormones. Joints are on a path to deterioration unless these three elements remain present.

In one-way or an other, inflammation follows from the repair rate not keeping up with the injury rate. It seems rather counter intuitive at first that prevailing shrinking forces lead into swelling and pain. It helps to think about the disruption to a cell's function when its anatomy alters. Part of the altered anatomy change concerns the loss of a formidable barrier to the penetration of harmful molecules always lurking outside the cell. Not only do the electrically charged architectural framework molecules attract water but they also form a selective barrier to harmful molecules. Also, if water escapes from inside the cell it collects outside of it leading to swelling. Swelling is one component of inflammation. Swelling tissues cause pain.

Mainstream physicians receive very little educational emphasis about how one continues to possess an optimal electrical water-sucking grid throughout an owner's body. This fact becomes quite disturbing when one realizes how this architectural framework associates in many important body locations. Some examples are: inflates the inside of all body cells, connects and supports the outside of all body cells, lines the inside surfaces of all blood vessels, lines the respiratory tract, lines the entire length of the digestive tube and is the substance that inflates skin cells so that they remain wrinkle free. Awareness of these facts explains why many diseases have a component of causality in the disruption of this electrical water-sucking grid. Some common electrical water sucking grid associated diseases are: colitis, heart disease, asthma, arthritis, and diabetes. This fact becomes more believable when one realizes each of the above diseases operates with a component of inflammation.

Part of the mainstream medical confusion about the extensive involvement of this grid in so many diseases concerns the additional disturbing fact about the many disjointed alias names that they use to describe them. In order to appreciate that the above listed body locals all contain and rely on this electrical architectural water-sucking meshwork, a physician would need to know that the following alias descriptors mean basically the same thing: glycosaminoglycans, cytoskeleton, ground substance, basal lamina, mucopolysaccharides, extra cellular matrix, cell coat, cell wall, cartilage, and mucous layer, to name a few.

Ignorance further propagates because the molecular makeup of these many ways to name the same substance largely remains ignored. The most accurate chemical descriptor for the above alias names is glycosaminoglycans (GAG). GAG is made from the molecular building blocks, glucosamine and galactosamine. These basic building blocks string together to form chains and crisscrossed chains thousands of molecules long. In addition, it is the addition of various amounts of sulfate and acetate to each glucosamine and galactosamine that powerfully attracts and retains water. This property results from the fact that these two molecular additions are electrically charged and therefore attract water. Only when galactosamines and glucosamines contain the proper electrical charge additions will water content remain adequate.

Many practitioners achieve benefits by supplementing with glucosamine and galactosamine. However, there are additional determiners for how much of this electrical water sucking grid a body manufactures. The central more important determiners involve increasing the repair rate while slowing the injury rate. The injury rate concerns harmful toxins within one's blood stream that penetrate a cell's protective barrier. Part of the injury rate can be slowed with methods that digest or neutralize toxins within the digestive tract (see below). The repair rate concerns three factors: 1) the nutritional completeness to provide molecular replacement parts, 2) the amount of antioxidants and anti-inflammatory molecules within a cell that serve to neutralize harmful invaders, 3) the quality of one's repair hormones within.

Before discussing these three determinants of properly inflated and un-inflamed cells, the contrast of mainstream medicine's treatments needs mention. More people probably die from complications of aspirin-like medication in one week than have ever died of ephedra. Yet, millions of dollars continually channel into various media outlets expounding on the wonders of these related drugs. In contrast, media campaigns continually expound on the severe dangers of ephedra consumption. A healthy level of skepticism for these tactics evolves with each passing year. Owners increasingly employ healing strategies instead of the mainstream symptom-control solution pandered by the complex. Symptom-control measures always have side effects and toxicities. **Healing has one side effect, the impact to the complex's bottom line.**

Nutritional molecules necessary for the formation of new electrically charged architectural framework:

**Magnesium
Zinc
Potassium
Selenium
Glucosamine and galactosamine
Sulfur containing compounds like MSM**

Antioxidants that prevent cell damage

**Quercitin
Milk thistle
Oregon grape root
Stinging nettle extract
Tocotrienols extract
Resveratrol
Bioflavanoids
Vitamin C**

Nature's anti-inflammatories

**Tumeric
Ginger
Ashwagandha
Quercitin
Chinese skullcap root
Feverfew
White willow bark
Rosemary**

Substances that help digest and neutralize toxins

Super oxide dismutase

Bromelain

Hormones that increase the repair rate of body tissues

Testosterone
DHEA
IGF-1
Growth hormone
Aldosterone
(Note: These hormones are all interrelated and see chapter 7 for more info)

    Around middl-age many owners begin to suffer the consequences of diminished hormone secretion quality. Hormones deliver messages to cells that tell them what to do. The many different types of body cells are faithful servants that only do as the messages delivered by the hormones direct. Here lies the middle-aged problem: Deficiency of hormone rejuvenation message content leads cells into disrepair. One of the consequences of disrepair concerns the diminished amount of new electrical water-sucking grid molecules manufactured.

    The quality of the GAG layer, like other body tissue components, depends on specific hormones that direct its manufacture rate. Again, the major reason that many physicians do not understand this concept concerns the way these facts are organized within the textbooks. Additional confusion arises because of the many alias names given to a single important hormone for forming fully charged GAG throughout the body.

    Currently medical literature calls this important GAG manufacture rate-determining hormone, insulin-like growth factor type one (IGF-1). Older literature describes this same hormone as: sulfation factor, somatomedin C, and the non-suppressible insulin-like activity of the blood stream. Some holistic physicians feel that by disconnecting important hormones, like IGF-1, by renaming and separating it from the other literature perpetuates physicians practicing in the dumbed down state. The dumbed down state of practice results when doctors are not taught simple holistic facts about how the body heals. Everyone suffers from the dumbed down state except the industrial medical complex.

The sulfation factor name for IGF-1 describes its critical rate-determining role in the formation of fully electrically charged GAG. GAG that does not fully charge possesses diminished ability to retain water.

Diminished water content leads to wrinkled cells and the shrinkage of old age. In fact, beyond the hysteria to avoid the sun and sell sun blockers this major determiner for youthful skin remains ignored. Skin wrinkles result from the same reason that over ripe fruit wrinkles. This truism extends to other body cells as well. The amount of GAG in an apple or a body cell type largely determines its ability to hold onto water. Human cells require adequate IGF-1 to re-synthesize GAG as it deteriorates. Because ripened fruit lacks hormones they rot and wrinkle as their GAG content diminishes.

It now becomes important not to confuse the IGF-1 released by the liver into the blood stream with that inside the body cells. Healthy people possess 100 times IGF-1 levels compared to insulin within their blood streams. IGF-1 helps the cells outside the liver and fat cells in their procurement of body fuel (sugar, fat and amino acids). IGF-1 and insulin are best thought of as the body's ""fuel nozzle" hormones". Just as filling a car fuel tank with fuel requires a nozzle, similarly the body cells require a "fuel nozzle", which these two hormones provide (chapter 7).

In contrast, IGF-1 within cells delivers a message of cell rejuvenation and repair. Part of rejuvenation and repair concerns the manufacture of fully charged GAG. Only sufficient and fully charged GAG prevents the shrinkage into old age. One of the major reasons that young people have fewer wrinkles involves their greatly increased IGF-1 levels.

Around middle age IGF-1 begins to fall off and this results in less GAG formation. The lower the GAG level and its electrical charge the more water leaks out of the body tissues (the drying out process of old age). Skin wrinkles exemplify one example of this process. Other diseases for the same reason have a component of causality from diminished GAG content and its electrical charge in their area of pathology. For example: the thick mucous of the asthmatic, the copious mucous in the colitis patient occurring when GAG fails to form properly, breaking down at an accelerated rate into mucous, the decreased GAG content in the osteoarthritis afflicted joint causing it to dry out and become brittle, the decreased GAG in the blood vessels of some diabetics, and the decreased GAG in the blood vessels of some heart disease patients.

While the above diseases severity cannot be entirely explained by GAG deficiency, in each case there is a profound contribution to the course of these diseases arising from their association with diminished GAG. Since the above diseases cause so much suffering and are part of the shrinkage into old age, the determinants of IGF-1 level deserves attention (chapter 9). This sadly is not yet the case.

Remember, inflammation within the body arises from the repair rate not keeping up with the injury rate. Anti-oxidant levels, nutritional status and the amount and quality of the repair hormones determine the repair rate. The injury rate subdues by limiting environmental toxin exposure, avoiding inflammatory fat consumption, and supplementing with digestive enzymes. One can observe the glaring reality that the medical industrial complex fails to advise in all the above considerations. In its place are the symptom-control measures. Symptom-control measures always have side effects and toxicities and have little to do with how the body heals. Thus, the health care revolution continues to grow.

SECTION 2: Nutrition Imbalance-caused Disease

Chapter 4: Nutritional Solutions for High Blood Pressure

Part One

Mainstream medical textbooks claim that more than ninety percent of all high blood pressure originates from unknown causes. They label these cases as essential hypertension. The implication usually leads doctors and patients to believe it is largely genetically determined. It is, as if, whenever the genetics get blamed the next step becomes how clever science is about their symptom-control approaches.

At the same time there is very little discussion of how the survival of the fittest led to the aberrant genes being selected down through the ages. Healing paths open up when one begins to look at the outdated survival advantages, operating in owners who possessed these genetic tendencies. The examples of insulin production and sodium conservation are both obsolete survival advantages carried over from the ancestors of primitive times. Mineral deficiencies contribution to high blood pressure follows and then the interrelation between these factors is reviewed. The case of insulin will be discussed at an introductory level here (and is more completely discussed later in the chapter). The case of sodium retention will also only be introduced (chapter 8).

The ancestor who could make insulin during times of plenty was at a big advantage during times of scarcity. A survival advantage occurred because insulin caused both a behavioral effect and a metabolic effect. Insulin stimulated within the owner a behavioral pre-occupation with food. This behavioral preoccupation focused the owner on feeding. Insulin message content creates a preoccupation with the next feeding event. However, today food scarcity rarely comes and owners with this survival trait tend to become fat and have high blood pressure, as well (see below). The continued exposure to high insulin message content directs the liver to make fat and cholesterol. Insulin is the body hormone that carries the fat-maker message. Cholesterol is one type of body fat. The more insulin, the more body fat. Insulin needs increase with carbohydrate intake and prolonged mental stress.

The old survival advantage has become a curse in today's world of high carbohydrate foods and mental stress. This curse occurs in today's world because the owner who can make more insulin than the next owner will make extra fat, as well. Increased body fat associates with high blood pressure. High insulin levels also contribute to other hormonal and mineral aberrations. In turn these aberrations elevate the blood pressure. Owners can heal their insulin caused high blood pressure problem when they are motivated and understand a way to heal. The insulin connection with blood pressure is more thoroughly discussed later in this chapter and throughout the text. For now it is only important to realize that the modern literature calls these high insulin-producing hypertensives Syndrome X (also known as metabolic syndrome or insulin resistance syndrome).

The second outdated genetic trait concerns the ability to retain sodium better than the next owner. Sodium and potassium are both minerals. In prehistoric times, sodium was rare. Natural food has many more times potassium than sodium. The owner during times of low sodium availability, who could conserve body sodium, possessed a survival advantage. Today, it causes the curse of high blood pressure because processed food has a reversed mineral content compared to that of natural food.

Natural food contains high potassium and low sodium. Processed food contains very high sodium and much lower potassium content (see mineral table below). Processed food is any food that comes in a can, box, and bag or from a fast food restaurant. Processed food provides reversed mineral content that deviates from body design. Natural food constitutes any food that the heavenly father made before it has its mineral makeup altered to extend its shelf life (see mineral tables where natural foods are fairly obvious or see chapter 8)

Mental stress that is so prevalent in modern times causes the stress response to activate. Part of the primitive survival stress response involves sodium conservation. Sodium conservation allows water retention. This provided a survival advantage in prehistoric times when most stress was physical. Examples of physical stress are: blood loss from combat or animal bites, and running for long periods in the heat. The trouble today arises because most stress is mental and not physical. The body cannot discern whether the stress is real or imagined. The body responds the same to all stress whether it is physical or mental in nature. Here lies the causality for the blood pressure problem of many owners living in the modern world.

Many prehistorically equipped 'survival machines' have stress and eat reversed minerals year after year. The fluid retention that follows elevates blood pressure. Rather than educate doctors about the importance of correct mineral ratios intake provided for in the natural foods diet (unprocessed food) phisicians are schooled to give vague advice about the desirability of a low sodium diet. This has merit, but unfortunately very few doctors understand the consequences of chronically reversed minerals intake that occurs from food processing. Blood pressure lowers when the correct minerals ratios are added back into the diet (between calcium, magnesium, potassium and sodium). Just as it took years to deplete the body of its optimal mineral ratios, it also takes up to six months to correct through proper mineral intake.

Processed food, among other depletions, contains low amounts of several mineral nutrients. One mineral aberration contained in processed food concerns its unnaturally high sodium content. The food industry adds sodium to prolong the shelf life of these processed products. Shelf life prolongs because bacteria have just as hard a time flourishing with high sodium content, as do other cells. Sometimes, processed foods contain only relatively low magnesium and potassium content because of all the sodium that has been added. The mineral content of processed food has been significantly diminished from the natural state. Health becomes compromised when an owner eats these processed foods and experiences chronic stress. Stress hormones alter the ability to remove extra sodium from the body causing fluid retention. Stress hormones also increase the loss of magnesium and potassium from the tissues creating further health consequences.

As a general rule, 4,000 mg of potassium, 1000 mg sodium, 300 mg of magnesium, and 500 mg of calcium are needed every day. Most Americans consume the reverse ratio between sodium and potassium (see mineral table below). The ideal mineral intake ratio applies only when one has normal kidneys and adrenals. Perpetually thin people and those with low blood pressure usually need more sodium then overweight people because they usually have adrenal defects. Defective adrenal secretions lead to a diminished salt-retentive hormone secretion rates (an altered stress response). Extremes of environmental heat or exercise habits increase sodium requirements. Individual variation occurs on the optimal amounts of minerals needed. This general reference will put most owners back on the path to adequate cellular charge.

When one consumes food that confers these mineral ratios, the body can effectively charge its trillions of "cell batteries". This remains true even when an owner experiences stress. If the kidneys have not been damaged from the processed food diet, blood pressure should drop. This will be especially true when a concomitant effort to diminish insulin production and obtain optimal vitamin status occurs.

Mineral Table

All mineral amounts are in milligrams below

Breads, Rolls, Etc	Amount	sodium	potass.	calories	mag.	calcium
White Bread	1 slice	142	29	76	0	32
Rye Bread	1 slice	139	36	61	0	20
Whole Wheat Bread	1 slice	132	68	61	0	20
Biscuit	1 (2"dia.)	185	18	104	0	0
Cornbread	2 1/2 sq.	263	61	178	0	133
Pancake	1 (6" dia.)	412	112	164	16	60
Waffle	1 (7" dia.)	515	146	206	13	143
Graham Cracker	2(2 1/2" sq.)	95	55	55	14	12
Brown Rice	1 c + salt	550	137	236	86	20
White Rice	1 c + salt	767	57	223	26	24
Bran Flakes	1 cup	207	137	106	108	26
Corn Flakes	1 cup	251	30	92	16	6
Oatmeal	1 c (cooked)	523	146	132	57	22.5
Pufffed Rice	1 cup	148	33	140	0	10
Wheat Flakes	1 cup	310	81	106	108	100
Wheat Flour	1 cup	130	0	499	0	0
*Egg Noodles	1 cup	3	70	200	31	19
*Macaroni	1 cup	1	103	192	20	8
*Spaghetti	1 cup	1	103	192	0	0

Beverages	Amount	sodium	potass.	calories	mag.	calcium
Coffee, Instant	1 Tblspn	3	87	3	*80	*50
Coffee, Regular	1 cup	2	65	2	10	3
Beer	12 oz	25	90	150	46	36
Gin, Rum, Vodka	1 oz (80 proof)	0	1	65	0	0

Sweets	Amount	sodium	potass.	calories	mag.	calcium

		sodium	potass.	calories	mag.	calcium
Angel Food Cake	1/6 cake	340	106	322	0	88
Brownie	small	50	38	97	0	0
Chocolate Bittersweet	1 oz	1	174	135	30	6
Chocolate, cupcake	1 piece	74	35	92	0	0
Chocolate chip cookies	10 (2.5" dia.)	421	141	495	0	32
Chocolate Syrup	1 oz	20	106	92	24	3
Gelatin, sweet	3 oz	270	0	315	0	1
Honey	1 Tblspn	1	11	64	0	1
Jelly	1 Tblspn	3	14	49	trace	4
Sherbert, Orange	1 cup	19	42	259	16	104
Sponge Cake	1/6 cake	220	114	196	0	42
Sugar, Brown	1 cup	44	499	541	0	187
Sugar, White	1 cup	2	6	770	trace	trace
Sugar, powdered	1 cup	1	4	462	trace	0

Fruits	**Amount**	**sodium**	**potass.**	**calories**	**mag.**	**calcium**
Apple	1 (2 1/2" dia.)	1	116	61	6	10
Apricots, Fresh	3 medium	1	301	55	8	15
Apricots, Dried	5 lg halves	6	235	62	11	10
Banana	1 medium	1	440	101	33	7
Blackberries	1cup	1	245	84	28	46
Cantalope	1/2 (5" dia.)	33	682	82	28	28
Cherries, Sweet	10 count	1	129	47	8	10
Dates	10 count	1	518	219	29	27
Figs	1 piece	1	126	52	8	18
Grapefruit	Half	1	132	40	10	13
Grapes	1 cup	3	160	70	3	9
Honeydew Melon	half (6 1/2" dia.)	90	1881	247	9	8
Orange	1 medium	1	290	66	15	56
Peach	1 (2 3/4" dia.)	2	308	58	6	5
Pear	1 (2 1/2" dia.)	3	213	100	5	10
Pineapple	1 cup	2	226	81	22	12
Plum	1 (1"dia.)	0	30	7	<1	1
Prune, Dried	10 medium	5	448	164	51	58

Raisins	1 tablespoon	2	69	26	3	5
Raspberries	1 cup	1	267	98	22	28
Strawberries	1 cup	1	244	55	16	22
Tangerine	1 (2 3/8" dia.)	2	108	39	10	12
Watermelon	1 cup	2	160	42	18	14
Avocado	1 medium	21	1097	324	70	19

Fresh Vegetables	**Amount**	**sodium**	**potass.**	**calories**	**mag.**	**calcium**
Asparagus	1 cup	3	375	35	22	30
Beans, Lima	1 cup	3	1008	191	126	54
Beets	1 cup	81	452	58	28	22
Broccoli	1 cup	34	868	72	38	72
Carrot	1 medium	34	246	30	11	19
Celery	1 stalk	50	136	7	4	16
Corn, Sweet (no butter, no salt)	1 ear	0	131	70	34	2
Cucumber	1 large	18	481	45	33	42
Eggplant	1 cup	2	300	38	10	30
Lettuce, iceberg	1 head (6" dia.)	48	943	70	48	102
Onion	1 cup	17	267	65	16	32
Peas	1 cup	3	458	122	34	62
Potato, Baked	1 medium	6	782	145	55	20
Potato, Boiled	1 medium	4	556	104	30	7
Radishes	10 large	15	261	14	4	9
Spinach	1 cup	39	259	14	158	244
Sweet Potato	1 medium	15	367	272	32	70
Tomato	1 medium	4	300	27	13	6
Watercress	1 cup	18	99	7	8	40

Canned Vegetables	**Amount**	**sodium**	**potass.**	**calories**	**mag.**	**calcium**
Asparagus	14 1/2 oz can	970	682	74	22	34
Beans, Green	8 oz can	536	216	41	18	36

	Amount	sodium	potas.	calories	mag	calcium
Beans, Lima	8 oz can	1070	1007	322	94	50
Beets	8 oz can	535	379	77	40	34
Carrots	8 oz can	535	272	64	22	62
Corn, Creamed	8 oz can	585	241	203	44	8
Peas	8 oz can	569	231	159	22	44
Spinach	8 oz can	519	550	42	132	144
Tomatoes	8 oz can	540	300	88	13	6

Dairy Products

	Amount	sodium	potas.	calories	mag	calcium
American Cheese	1 oz.	322	23	105	6	124
Blue Cheese Dressing	1 Tblspn	164	6	76	0	0
Cheddar Cheese	1 oz.	147	17	84	8	204
Cream Cheese	1 oz.	80	25	110	2	23
Cottage Cheese	1 cup	580	144	172	14	154
Parmesan Cheese	1 oz.	208	42	111	14	390
Swiss Cheese	1 oz.	70	29	105	10	272
Butter (salted)	1 stick	1119	26	812	2	27
Butter (unsalted)	1 stick	<1	<1	812	2	27
Buttermilk (cultured)	1 cup	319	343	*88	27	285
Skim Milk	1 cup	127	355	*88	28	302
Whole Milk	1 cup	122	351	159	33	291
Evaporated Milk	1 cup	297	764	345	60	658
Heavy Cream	1 Tblspn	5	13	53	1	10
Ice Cream (no salt)	1 cup	84	241	257	9	88
Hot Chocolate	1 cup	120	370	238	24	93
Hot Cocoa	1 cup	128	363	243	0	0
Egg Yolk	1 medium	8	15	52	1	23
Egg white	1 medium	42	40	15	4	2
Egg Broiled	1 medium	54	57	72	5	25
Yogurt, Plain	1 cup	115	323	152	26	274

Meat and Poultry	Amount	sodium	potas.	calories	mag.	calcium

(Beef)

Corned Beef Hash	1 cup	1188	440	398	14	9
Frankfurter	1 medium	627	125	176	6	7
Heart	1 oz	29	66	53	0	0
Hamburger	2.9 oz	49	221	235	5	2
Liver	3 oz	156	323	195	0	0
Rib Roast	6-9 ribs	149	680	1342	22	11
Flank Steak	3 oz	45	207	167	26	7
Porterhouse Steak	11 oz	155	680	1400	28	9
Sirloin Steak	11 oz	173	793	1192	32	12
T-Bone Steak	11 oz	152	660	1431	28	9
(Lamb)						
Chop	1 medium	51	234	341	27	28
Roast	3 oz	60	273	158	36	16
(Pork)						
Bacon	1 slice	123	29	72	<2	<1
Chops	3 oz	47	214	300	15	6
Ham, baked	3 oz	770	241	159	18	5
Roast	3 oz	698	218	281	0	0
Spareribs	2 pieces	65	299	792	0	0
(Veal)						
Loin cut	3 oz	60	570	220	9	10
Roast	3 oz	57	259	229	21	23
(Chicken)						
Broiled	4 oz	75	310	154	28	19
*Light Meat	4 oz	60	240	120	25	18
*Dark Meat	4 oz	45	100	180	27	19
(Turkey)						
White Meat	4 oz	70	349	150	29	29

Dark Meat	4 oz	42	169	87	26	26
(Fresh, Fish & Seafood)						
Bass, striped	3 oz	0	0	168	69	27
Clams	4 clams	144	218	56	52	12
Cod	3 oz	93	345	144	16	36
Crab	1 cup	0	0	144	78	0
Flounder	3 oz	201	498	171	15	27
Haddock	3 oz	150	297	141	27	33
Halibut	3 oz	114	447	144	37	72
Lobster	1 cup	305	261	138	138	80
Mackerel	3 oz	0	0	201	9	63
Oysters	3 small	21	34	19	39	45
Salmon	3 oz	99	378	156	180	29
Shrimp	3 oz	159	195	192	45	30

Mineral Imbalance caused High Blood Pressure

The larger problem of mineral imbalance is caused by a processed food diet. Processed foods have drastically altered mineral composition when compared to real food. Real food tends to be high in magnesium and potassium and intermediate in calcium content. Real food is usually low in sodium. Processed food has reversed mineral content compared to real food.

The body is energized by an electrical system that maintains itself by potential differences across trillions of cell membranes in the body. The body requires specific mineral proportions in order to accomplish an optimal cell charge. A real food diet supplies these and a processed food diet does not. Around middle age cells begin to lose their electrical pizzazz. It is a miracle that the body can tolerate reversed minerals ratios intake for as long as it does before it begins to fail.

The car batteries' mineral composition provides an analogy that demonstrates the effect of mineral imbalance. Like the body cells that charge themselves by concentration differences around cell membranes, so to it is with car batteries. Car batteries maximally charge only when the different minerals are at extreme differences across the membrane. For this to occur, the battery manufacturer adds the proper minerals into the battery fluid. The chronic consumption of processed food is analogous to dumping battery fluid on the ground and replacing it with a reversed proportion of minerals. Most owners would see this behavior as foolish. Yet, this is what they are doing every time they eat processed food. Around middle age the 'battery fluid' in the body begins to alter despite the best effort of the kidneys to compensate for the reversed ratio of mineral intake. This process describes the origin of many disease processes. One common disease that results from this imbalance is high blood pressure.

As stated previously, most owners need about 4000 mg of potassium, 1000 mg of sodium, 500 mg of calcium and 300 mg of magnesium every day. Profuse sweating increases sodium needs. Altered kidney and adrenal function will also alter these amounts. Most Americans obtain about 6000 mg of sodium a day and much less potassium and magnesium than they need.

Around middle age, the cells have usually sacrificed much of their potassium to maintain the blood potassium level. One consequence to health when potassium escapes from cells concerns a decreased energy charge within the cells. This means that the afflicted cells perform less work because of fatigue. Early fatigue often serves as a sign of aging.

98% of body potassium sequesters inside the cells. This larger tank sacrifices its potassium to the 2% tank in the blood stream. Many owners are misled when they have their blood drawn and their potassium result comes back normal. Their normal blood test result says nothing about the state of potassium content in their cells. Only when the 98% percent tank contained within the body cells outside of the blood stream severely depletes will the blood stream amount begin to fall off. At this point, the heart rhythm irregularities that follow create a real medical emergency.

The overall point is that owners who desire optimum health past middle age must consume the proper mineral ratios consistent with body design. The only diet that provides the proper ratios is the real food diet. Real foods are fairly obvious in the above mineral table. The fairly consistent trend concerns the fact that these foods are in their natural state. In other words, they are not generally processed into a box, can and bag or found in a fast food restaurant.

The above introductory discussion on healing blood pressure discussed three interrelated nutritional aberrations that elevate the blood pressure. They are: potassium deficiency, magnesium deficiency, and sodium excess. In addition, the contribution of insulin excess was introduced.

Total subsistence on a real food diet sometimes becomes impossible. In these instances, it makes sense to consider mineral supplements that will offset the imbalances. In all cases of high blood pressure, the sodium content within the diet must be dramatically reduced. Failure to reduce sodium necessitates symptom-control medicine's paradigms with all its side effects and toxicities. In addition, when stress occurs, exercise needs to occur. Exercise, for reasons beyond this discussion, lowers the insulin needed when mental stress occurs. Less insulin in the body translates into lower blood pressure and weight loss. Part Two of nutritionally healing blood pressure will build on these introductory factors that cause hypertension.

Part Two

High Blood Pressure and Nutritional Remedies,

This subsection continues the discussion for the causes of high blood pressure, and some simple supplements and methods that can be used to heal the problem. The owner who uses these methods suggested may avoid the need for prescription medications and their unavoidable side effects. The earlier in the disease process that nutritional intervention is implemented the higher the success rate for blood pressure reduction. When the owner addresses the nutritional cause of their elevated blood pressure, the need for prescription medication will decrease and further damage to their organs will diminish.

The last chapter described three common imbalances that cause an elevation of blood pressure (magnesium, sodium and potassium). The hormone insulin's introductory role for blood pressure elevation was also mentioned. This subsection will describe other nutritional events that contribute to elevated blood pressure. The goal is to provide some additional insight for ways to heal high blood pressure. The ways one can heal is the goal instead of the acceptance of symptom-control medicine's paradigms. Symptom-control always leads to side effects and toxicities. Symptom-control contributes nothing to how one heals.

When the adrenals exist with deficient molecular parts blood pressure will rise

Specific deficiencies in the adrenal gland can initiate the hypertension disease process. The owner using nutritional strategies can successfully treat these deficiencies. These nutritional strategies can reduce the owner's blood pressure and lower the owner's heart disease risk profiles, as well.

This first adrenal deficiency arises out of the methyl donor deficiency syndrome (explained below). Deficiency caused diseases of the various components of the important methyl donor system includes both high blood pressure and heart disease states.

Differences in the message content between epinephrine and nor-epinephrine (both are known as catecholamines) exist. Alternatively these are called adrenaline and noradrenaline, respectively. When certain nutritional deficiencies develop epinephrine decreases first and concurrently more norepinephrine production occurs within the adrenal gland. This situation leads to significant physiological consequences within the blood vessel. High blood pressure provides one example of the differences in message content between norepinephrine and epinephrine (see below). The altered blood vessel performance then increases the risk for heart disease from the resulting high blood pressure.

The adrenal gland divides into two components: the cortex and medulla. Both parts of the adrenal gland secretions message content concern the survival of stress. The better the secretion function within both adrenal compartments, the better an owner survives the stresses of life without physiologic consequences. High blood pressure provides one example of the physiologic consequences when the adrenal secretion quality diminishes.

Biological, emotional, and environmental stresses are hard on both compartments of one's adrenal gland. Stress constantly triggers the steroid producing outer section of the adrenal gland. This causes cortisol to be secreted (among other steroids). Only when sufficient cortisol circulates in the blood stream can the cell receptors recognize epinephrine and nor-epinephrine message content. Epinephrine and nor-epinephrine secrete from the adrenal medulla with stressful stimuli. The dependence of the adrenal medulla for adequate cortisol from the adrenal cortex proves important. Without cortisol preparing the manufacture of the receptors for these adrenal medulla hormones (epinephrine and nor-epinephrine), their message content will go unrecognized (chapter 7). This subsection will only address the nutritionally induced imbalance between epinephrine and nor-epinephrine secreted by the adrenal medulla.

Normally, the adrenal medulla secretes 90% epinephrine and only 10% nor-epinephrine. Epinephrine is preferred because it opens up the blood supply to the heart, skeletal muscles, and the liver. In contrast, nor-epinephrine does not do this. All other blood vessels (except the brain where blood flow is kept constant in the healthful state) are directed to clamp down when nor-epinephrine provides the message (hormones contain message content). In contrast, the net effect of epinephrine message content (because the muscle and liver blood vessels percentage of total body blood vessels are so large) results in a lowered peripheral vascular resistance. This effect leads to a lower diastolic blood pressure. Epinephrine has this effect within the body even when the epinephrine level within the blood stream reaches relatively high levels. Epinephrine also increases cardiac performance, which may result in a slight rise in systolic blood pressure.

The effects of epinephrine within the heart, liver and skeletal muscle vessels directly contrast with the message that norepinephrine delivers to these same blood vessels. Norepinephrine message content directs the vessels to clamp down on everything except the blood supply to the brain. When blood vessels constrict without a corresponding dilation somewhere else, blood pressure elevates. Healthy owner's adrenal medulla's (inner adrenal layer) manufacture and secrete 90% epinephrine and only 10% norepinephrine. However, when the adrenal medulla experiences deficiencies in certain vitamins and cofactors, this ratio changes for the worse. **A nutritionally caused inability to make epinephrine will tend to raise blood pressure when norepinephrine secretes instead of epinephrine**.

Both of these hormones act rapidly and effectively for the redistribution of blood flow. This effect causes the blood stream to maintain an adequate flow of blood within the brain during normal body movement. Sufficient epinephrine or norepinephrine needs to secrete or unconsciousness results. For example, when an owner gets out of bed the forces of gravity cause the blood pressure to suddenly drop. Healthy owner's adrenal medullas make epinephrine in sufficient quantities to deliver a smooth machine that goes from lying flat to standing upright with grace and ease. Normally these hormones have a lifespan of about 2 minutes within the blood stream. Because these hormones have very short life spans there arises a constant need for these hormones when one either stands upright or experiences stress.

An additional process occurs during body movement that affects the blood pressure level. When an owner stands up or perceives stress, the sympathetic nerves discharge out of their endings. The endings of these nerves imbed in the blood vessels.

These nerves release norepinephrine only, onto the motor end plate of the smooth muscles of the blood vessels. The release of norepinephrine causes these muscles to contract and thereby constrict the recipient blood vessels.

Norepinephrine released from the sympathetic nerves directly affects the blood vessel muscles' contractile state. Concurrently nor-epinephrine released from the adrenal medulla into the blood stream diffuses towards the same muscular layer but from the other direction. The additive effect between the sympathetic nerve activation that releases nor-epinephrine into the blood stream and the adrenal-secreted norepinephrine powerfully elevates blood pressure. The moderator of high blood pressure, in these situations, proves to be epinephrine. Epinephrine increases blood flow to the heart, muscles, and liver. Blood flow increases when blood vessels expand. Adequate epinephrine release, therefore, proves to be one cornerstone for the prevention of high blood pressure.

Normally, this results in a tug-of-war between the full contraction and full relaxation of the blood vessel. Where a blood vessel ends up on the continuum is determined by the sum of the informational substances within the blood stream and the nervous tone instructions that reach this blood vessel. When a sub-optimal or unbalanced release of adrenal medulla derived epinephrine occurs, an increase in blood pressure becomes likely.

Awareness for this process allows for a nutritional strategy that may be implemented to reduce blood pressure and the exacerbations of the symptoms of heart disease. After all, part of the heart disease experience concerns the diminished blood flow within the coronary arteries that a diminished epinephrine allows. Diseased coronary arteries are narrowed and hence need all the expansion they can receive from the help of epinephrine's message.

In order to obtain epinephrine the adequate molecular building parts and all of the nutritional cofactors must be present within the adrenal gland (discussed specifically below). These factors form a necessary pre-condition for the biosynthesis of epinephrine within the adrenal gland. Epinephrine and norepinephrine derive from adequate supplies of the amino acid tyrosine. Tyrosine can be obtained from the amino acid phenylalanine.

The adrenal gland cannot convert tyrosine to epinephrine unless all of the nutritional cofactors exist within the adrenal medulla (see below). Each step of the assembly line that eventually leads to the end product of epinephrine has a scientifically validated cofactor that must be present. If any one of these nutritional cofactors are missing, assembly stops and epinephrine synthesis becomes impossible.

The most common adrenal medulla deficiency involves the methyl donor system (explained below). The methyl donor system proves necessary for the conversion of norepinephrine to epinephrine. The last step in the assembly process involves the conversion of norepinephrine to epinephrine. This last step cannot occur without a particular cofactor that disintegrates with each epinephrine molecule made.

Scientists call this cofactor S-Adenosyl methionine (SAMe for short). SAMe is part of the methyl donor system. The SAMe cofactor donates its one methyl group to make one new epinephrine molecule from one norepinephrine. This spent cofactor needs to be recharged. Failure to recharge into SAMe causes S-adenosyl homocysteine to form. This deactivated molecule will further degrade into adenosine and homocysteine within the blood stream.

Unless adequate SAMe remains available in the body, adequate epinephrine biosynthesis cannot occur. Insufficient epinephrine biosynthesis leads to an increased biosynthesis of norepinephrine. Increased release of norepinephrine will raise the blood pressure. An additional exacerbating factor for blood pressure elevation exists when SAMe proves deficient.

When SAMe levels deplete, a marked decrease in the body's ability to clear both epinephrine and norepinephrine from the blood stream arises. Not only do these bodies have the wrong hormone being secreted, norepinephrine, because of the SAMe deficiency, but because of this same deficiency there occurs the decreased ability to remove norepinephrine from the blood stream!

These hormones clear from the body when other SAMe within the blood stream methylates them. The difference between norepinephrine and epinephrine is that the later contains a methyl group, which SAMe donates. However, both hormones require additional methyl additions for their deactivation and removal from the body. When norepinephrine and epinephrine receive these types of methyl additions, they become inactive. Once inactivated they readily secrete from the kidney into the urine.

The SAMe deficient owner can become trapped in a vicious cycle of high blood pressure because their bodies possess a diminished ability to manufacture epinephrine and from the decreased clearance of the sub-optimal norepinephrine. Without inactivation from other SAMe in the circulation this hormone remains free to continue spreading its contraction message.

SAMe disintegrates within the body to homocysteine at the rate of one billion times a second (Cooney '96). The many other roles SAMe plays within healthy owners will be explained later. For now, realize that nutritional attention for the ways to recharge one's methyl donor system (SAMe is one of the members in this group) often has the ability to heal the epinephrine deficiency and the norepinephrine excess. The correction of epinephrine deficiency proves important because only epinephrine can oppose the clamping down of the sympathetic nerves during stressful times (as was previously explained). Deficient epinephrine output during adrenal medulla activation allows the blood pressure to rise dramatically.

The blood pressure rises dramatically because all information occurs as contraction information at the blood vessel level. This result occurs because only epinephrine moderates the contractile response. Epinephrine can do this because it contains message content, which directs the liver, heart and skeletal muscles blood vessels to dilate. Conversely, norepinephrine cannot do this because it contains all contractile message content. All blood vessels in the body, except the brain, are being directed to contract, therefore, the blood pressure rises dramatically. The same deficiency that diminishes synthesis of epinephrine also causes the diminished breakdown of elevated nor-epinephrine (see above). This added insult occurs because SAMe proves necessary to inactivate norepinephrine.

Only epinephrine contains the special message content for opening up the blood vessels within the heart, skeletal muscle, and liver. Sufficient epinephrine within the body directs blood into the above important areas and this fact prevents the dramatic rise in blood pressure. Blood pressure does not rise dramatically because the increased blood flow within these areas offsets the decreased blood flow elsewhere within the body. Within the rest of the body (excluding the brain) epinephrine directs the clamping down of blood vessels (constriction raises the pressure). The net effect usually evidences as a slight rise in the upper blood pressure value (systolic) and a slight lowering of the lower blood pressure reading (diastolic). Medical writings describe this as a widened pulse pressure. A widened pulse pressure indicates an increased cardiac output. In contrast, the stress response directed from the sympathetic nerves directs the constriction of all blood vessels except the brain. Adequate epinephrine release proves crucial in times of stress to prevent the sky rocketing of the blood pressure. Sky rocketing blood pressure means that blood flow delivery to heart, muscle and liver decreases. The sympathetic nerve activation coupled with the constriction effects of norepinephrine from the adrenal medulla will increase blood pressure abnormally, without adequate epinephrine.

The below listed cofactors are well documented in basic biochemistry textbooks as all being necessary for epinephrine to be manufactured. Basic medical physiology textbooks point out the marked difference between the effects on blood flow patterns and blood pressure between epinephrine and norepinephrine.

The synthetic sequence of catecholamines is: tyrosin>dopa>dopamine>norepinephrine>epinephrine. The necessary cofactors that are needed in the synthesis sequence of tyrosine to the end product epinephrine are: tetrahydrobiopterin (made from folate), pyridoxal phosphate (Vitamin B6), Vitamin C, and SAMe.

Many additional cofactors and vitamins prove necessary for the recharging of SAMe. These cofactors and vitamins needed to recharge SAMe are called the methyl donor system. The molecules that make up the methyl donor system are: methionine, serine, Vitamin B6, Vitamin B12 and folate. These additional factors allow the remanufacture of SAMe once it has been degraded to S-adenosyl homocysteine. The methyl group, contained in SAMe, transfers to convert nor-epinephrine to epinephrine.

As stated previously, all of these cofactors involved in recreating SAMe, are known collectively as the methyl donor system. Depletion of this system has predictable consequences but paradoxically has been largely ignored by mainstream medicine in the clinical setting. It should be emphasized that the consumption of extra methionine or SAMe without proper attention to the adequacy of the other methyl donors will lead to elevated blood homocysteine levels because each one is needed to recharge SAMe after creating each epinephrine. This will occur at the rate of one billion times a second when severe deficiency exists.

Summary of vitamins and cofactors needed to convert tyrosine into epinephrine

Tetrahydrobiopterin (made from folate)
Vitamin C
Vitamin B6
SAMe

A real food diet provides most of these cofactors and the methyl donor group, especially if one eats eggs. Eggs are rich in methionine. However, a processed food diet will likely lack one or more of these vitamins and cofactors. Many B-vitamin formulations are often deficient in folate content. Without adequate folate the methyl donor system will not function. All members of the methyl donor system need to be present or SAMe levels fall and homocysteine levels will rise.

The rise of blood homocysteine levels has been documented to signal a powerful risk factor for blood vessel disease. However, if one applies basic biochemical principles to the analysis for a homocysteine role in the development of heart disease it reveals it to be an unlikely agent in the direct injury of blood vessels. Rather, it is more probable that it provides a biochemical red flag that nutritionally something is wrong. When blood homocysteine rises, epinephrine synthesis will decrease proportionately. Later, it will be explained how methyl also proves necessary for repair, brain fat manufacture, neurotransmitter formation, DNA stabilization and detoxification processes throughout the body. Remember that the body uses methyl at the rate of one billion times a second.

Elevated homocysteine levels denote a malfunction within the methyl donor system that leads to decreased epinephrine production and increased norepinephrine production. Elevated blood homocysteine levels may reflect a convenient biochemical marker to identify a depleted methyl donor system. One of the pathologies of a depleted methyl donor system is that it often causes high blood pressure to develop, among other things. Elevated blood pressure and diminished blood flow to the heart muscle will result whenever norepinephrine occurs in the blood stream in higher than normal amounts compared to epinephrine. Natruopath, Dr. Steven Gordon, points out that finding an elevated blood homocysteine level may provide high blood pressure's etiology and it's solution as well.

It needs to be acknowledged that a group of owners exists who have high homocysteine levels without elevated blood pressure. Some of these owners maintain a normal blood pressure because their bodies lower their anabolic and aldosterone steroids production. This compensation produces other aging effects (discussed in **The Body Heals**). Other owner's hearts produce high levels of the hormone, atrial natruretic peptide. This hormone overrides blood pressure elevation tendencies that other adrenal hormones promote. Both of these types of owners are found in the minority and hence blood pressure elevation occurring around middle age occurs in the majority.

When one appreciates the fundamental role that both a highly functional and interrelated methyl donor system plays in body health, a way to treat blood pressure becomes possible.

When one considers these facts in their disease prevention strategies it begins to make sense why the adrenal medulla nutritional state proves important.

This brings up the beauty of healing paths versus symptom-control medicine. Prescriptions are all about symptom-control and contain all their inevitable side effects as well. Healing does not have negative side effects. This truism results because once a problems cause resolves it occurs no more.

None of these cofactors is more risky than if one takes a multiple vitamin (not very risky). Each of the above listed cofactors has proven biochemical necessity in the synthesis of the epinephrine hormone. Healing involves working with the body to correct unbalanced states. Healthy owner's adrenals predictably contain optimal amounts of each of these cofactors and produce adequate epinephrine to maximize bodily function.

The caution is to avoid allergic reactions (very rare), which some owners have to the fillers and trace contaminants in certain brands of nutritional supplements. In general, one should choose the best brand and quality (pharmaceutical grade). Once in a while there will be an owner who is allergic to Vitamin C. Obtain the advice of a competent physician who will work on natural healing of the adrenal's function and reduce the blood pressure naturally.

It turns out that the sympathetic tone often increases in hypertensives and this central nervous system effect contributes greatly to the observed increase in blood pressure. The neurotransmitter involved in this case is norepinephrine. What is often under appreciated with regard to blood pressure is the tug of war between the sum of the hormones' message content within the blood stream and the message content delivered by the central nervous system. This dynamic equilibrium provides insight into the consequences of epinephrine deficiency.

Norepinephrine delivers a more powerful messenger (has more effect) when delivered within the nerves to the blood vessel (these nerves end in the muscular layer and when active direct contraction here) than when it acts within the blood stream. Here, norepinephrine has more ability to raise blood pressure at a given concentration of secretion (within the nerves) than it does when it secretes into the blood stream. This fact describes a subtle but important point. Epinephrine deficiency can cause blood pressure elevation merely because insufficient counter balance to the powerful nerve message contained in the presence of norepinephrine occurs.

Epinephrine, within the blood vessels, has powerful effects starting at 50pg/ml, but nor-epinephrine doesn't exert its vasoconstrictor effects within the blood stream until 1500pg/ml. The norepinephrine ability to raise blood pressure derives mainly through its effect as a neurotransmitter within the sympathetic nervous system. Sufficient epinephrine message content as a counter response to the sympathetic nervous system's tendency to raise blood pressure proves fundamental to normal blood pressure.

Another Deficiency Syndrome that Leads to High Blood Pressure

Insufficient nitric oxide causes a second nutritional deficiency syndrome, often overlooked in many owners that suffer from high blood pressure. The lack of nitric oxide gas in certain situations can raise blood pressure. The inner blood vessel lining cells manufacture nitric oxide. This gas proves a powerful artery and vein relaxant. Healthy owners produce nitric oxide in the right amounts and locations. This needs to happen to keep the blood flow optimal.

A deficiency in the production of this powerful and locally acting messenger gives the green light to many nasty blood pressure raising substances. Otherwise these troublesome blood pressure raising substances in the presence of adequate nitric oxide would not be manufactured within the blood vessel lining cell. Nitric oxide powerfully relaxes blood vessel walls. Nitric oxide also powerfully suppresses the insulin-induced manufacture of the blood pressure raising hormone, endothelin. Both nitric oxide and endothelin are informational substances that act only near the site of their release. The enzyme, nitric oxide synthase, which makes nitric oxide gas from the amino acid arginine, needs four cofactors or it cannot perform this task. The absence of any one of these cofactors causes a nitric oxide deficiency and the blood pressure rises.

Scientists call the enzyme that makes nitric oxide, nitric oxide synthase. It needs the presence of the cofactors arginine, thiol, tetrahydrobiopterin (made from folate), flavin mononucleotide (FMN), and flavin dinucleotide (FAD) in order to produce nitric oxide. FMN and FAD are made from riboflavin (Vitamin B2). A deficiency of any one of these cofactors, within the numerous cells that line the body's waterways, causes diminished nitric oxide production. Diminished production tips the antique weight scale in the direction of unopposed blood pressure elevation.

One of the cofactors required for the production of nitric oxide elucidates one of the reasons that garlic lowers blood pressure Garlic contains thiol, which prove as one of the cofactors necessary for the production of nitric oxide. The other four cofactors are also obtained from nutritional sources. One obtains tetrahydrobiopterin by consuming royal bee jelly or the body manufactures it from folate. FAD and FMN derive by ingesting adequate riboflavin (Vitamin B2) in the diet. Lastly, arginine, an amino acid, needs to be adequately consumed in the diet or made from Krebs cycle intermediates. Krebs cycle intermediates exist mostly within the mitochondria of cells (note to non-medical readers do not worry about Krebs cycle intermediates).

In some instances oral replacement proves inadequate for these types of deficiencies. Some cases occur where certain owners, for one reason or another, lack the ability to absorb optimal vitamin nutrition orally. In these cases, it warrants the extra precaution of intravenous or intra-muscular vitamin replacement therapy (such as chelation therapy).

Conventional chelation protocols contain most of the above vitamins and cofactors. Perhaps this fact partially explains their continued devotees in the face of the ongoing mainstream medicine criticism. The addition of thiol would complete the supplementation of the above necessary cofactors needed by nitric oxide synthase. In the case of methyl donor deficiency, mentioned in the previous subsection, the addition of folate, methionine and serine would possibly prove of benefit in the chelation setting.

The Secret: Prescription Medications that Raise Nitric Oxide Levels

An additional insight now occurs about nitric oxide production and it's relationship to a popular blood pressure lowering medication called the angiotensin converting enzyme inhibitors (ACE inhibitors). These types of medications additionally effect the histamin- like content of the body, which also powerfully lowers blood pressure. The mainstream textbooks say very little about this powerful association. Instead, they discuss in great detail the blood pressure lowering effects as being the result of lowered angiotensin two levels.

It is really quite a shock to most physicians when they begin to see evidence that the touted mechanism for a drug's action fails to describe their major effects on the body. The ACE inhibitors provide such an example. The drug literature focuses almost exclusively on the supposed powerful role that angiotensin plays in tightening up the blood vessels directly. However, very little of this literature discusses the well-documented fact that inhibition of this very same enzyme raises the total body content of a histamine like substance, bradykinin.

Normally, the lung contains this enzyme and its activity here keeps bradykinin levels, a histamine-like substance, normal. Extra histamine-like substance promotes swelling. This explains why a dry nagging cough is these drugs number one side effect. In addition, while increased bradykinin lowers blood pressure, increased leakiness of the capillaries in areas like the lungs and kidney describes the price paid. Maybe there was a marketing problem if this mechanism was related to an increased histamine like substance content within the body. No one will probably ever know for sure. Nonetheless, it is instructive to see a possible bigger problem with other drugs in how the physician gets 'groomed' into thinking about how these drugs work.

Because these drugs increase bradykinin within the body they also increase nitric oxide production, as well. Increased bradykinin powerfully stimulates the turning on of the nitric oxide synthesis enzymatic machinery within the endothelial cells lining the arteries. Bradykinin and histamine share the same receptors in the body. They also act in a similar manner. They contain similar message content. Once bradykinin becomes elevated it tends to stimulate the mast cells to release histamine, as well.

The other touted benefit of these angiotensin converting enzyme inhibitors (ACE inhibitors), concerns their documented benefit in the preservation of kidney function. To understand that this benefit occurs as both a circuitous and expensive solution in many cases one needs to recall four things. First, ACE inhibitors conserve body potassium and this has a known kidney protective effect on the tendency to become potassium deficient. Second, this medication then lowers blood pressure despite the elevated sodium in the body by the less realized mechanism of increased bradykinin within the body. Third, bradykinin increased presence also lowers blood pressure by being a powerful stimulus for nitric oxide production.

Parenthetically, if a given patient was correctly counseled about a real food diet instead of a processed food diet, before kidney damage occurs from chronically low potassium intake, blood pressure medication, in this case, would no longer be needed.

The fourth fact to understand about the consequences of decreased angiotensin two production concerns its effects on the adrenal glands (non medical readers do not need to worry about angiotensin type two details). Rather than get lost in the inconsistent evidence that these ACE inhibitors have on aldosterone levels it becomes more instructive to look at the consistent evidence. The evidence proves consistent that decreased angiotensin two will directly correlate with a decreased ACTH output. A decreased ACTH output will decrease stimulation to the adrenal glands release of aldosterone, cortisol and DHEA. This little detail has powerful implications for describing yet another mechanism for how these medications lower blood pressure. It also has powerful implications as to why diseases like autoimmune disease are made worse when owners take these types of medications.

Owners are made worse with autoimmune disease because they already have a wounded adrenal system (chapter 10). The addition of an ACE inhibitor will only exaggerate the diminished adrenal function, which operates in these diseases. This also provides a clue as to why these same types of owners will be at increased risk for neutropenia and lymphocytosis (chapter 10).

Now it is time to turn the analysis on its head. The biggest roadblock, mentally, concerns the realization that people who consume high potassium and magnesium diets relative to total sodium intake tend towards a high aldosterone production rate (an increased potassium intake will powerfully stimulate aldosterone release). However, in these cases a diuresis (water loss) will ensue because total body sodium is not excessive. Stress (ACTH) alone tends to raise aldosterone and cortisol levels and in the situation of a high sodium diet, this is inappropriate. When this happens, blood pressure will rise (remember that prehistorically, most stress was physical and most food had a low sodium content). The point to consider is that perhaps a little effort spent counseling early hypertensives on how to change their mineral intake ratios by eating 'real foods' (chapter 8) would have some merit before condemning them to medication with all it's side effects.

ACE inhibitors have been shown to improve a patient's clinical situation while in heart failure. What is not said is that histamine-like substances have a powerful strengthening action on heart muscle. This effect is obviously one benefit of these medications. The increased histamine-like content within the blood stream, as well, will reduce the effort of the heart in getting the blood pumped with each beat. ACE inhibitors effect multiple organ systems in the body.

Steroids Have a Role in Blood Pressure

Certain steroids increase the calcium concentrations within the cells and therefore alter cell functions. The trigger to synthesize nitric oxide within the cells lining the blood vessels is the increase of calcium concentrations within these cells, the endothelium. Low insulin levels, high bradykinin levels, and high levels of certain steroids all lead to increased calcium within the cells that line the arteries, the endothelial cell.

Parenthetically, calcium salts accumulates in some owners' arteries along with their fatty growths. One consideration about why these occur involves nitric oxide nutritional deficiency that results from missing cofactors needed for nitric oxide gas creation. Could it be that owners that have Vitamin B2, folate, thiol, and/or arginine deficiencies pump abnormal amounts of calcium into their endothelium where it precipitates like gravel because the desired chemical reaction has become nutritionally defunct?

The ability of certain steroids like progesterone to increase cell calcium content is well documented. When sperm encounters the progesterone molecule, within the cervical mucus, this promptly triggers the rise in intracellular calcium. High intracellular calcium will disable a sperm. This fact describes one of the reasons that high progesterone levels prevent pregnancy.

This routinely occurs within the central nervous system, as well. Progesterone effects the nerve cell's intracellular calcium concentration and also changes the neural cell's operational properties. In fact, progesterone, at very high levels produces anesthesia. At more physiologic levels there is a calming effect. Nerves become calm when they can charge up their membrane (increase the voltage about the membrane). Generally, nerves are less irritable when their membrane voltage increases.

DHEA floats around at the highest concentration of any steroid within the blood vessels in the body. Because certain steroids increase cellular calcium it becomes possible to speculate that they are also one of the triggers that increase calcium concentrations within the endothelial cell. No one has specifically studied which steroid does this within the blood stream. However, reasoning strongly suggests it to be progesterone or DHEA.

That the messages of DHEA or some other steroid direct an increase in the cell calcium content is believed to be non-genomic. Non-genomic mechanisms mean that these steroids act outside of generally accepted steroid message delivery methods. They occur without interacting with cellular DNA programs. The non-genomic method is an additional ability to the other methods for how steroids control cell function (turning off and on different DNA programs within a given cell).

The emerging data suggests that steroids play an important role in blood vessel health. The effect that certain steroids have on cellular calcium concentrations will probably turn out to be another way that the body controls blood pressure. The ability of steroids like progesterone or DHEA to encourage nitric oxide formation could be a powerful determinant in blood vessel longevity. If the data proves to be accurate, it will provide another method for encouraging blood pressure back to optimal levels.

Syndrome X is One Cause of High Blood Pressure

Gerald Reaven, MD, of Stanford University, coined the term, Syndrome X. This term describes those owners who have embarked on an accelerated path to old age. These owner types age because their blood vessels 'rust' and then go on to develop consequent blockages. Dr. Reaven believes that Syndrome X results from having high blood insulin. He explains the clinical signs of this syndrome as the result of the high insulin state as: increased abdominal fat, **high blood pressure**, increased blood triglyceride level, elevated LDL cholesterol, increased skin tag growths on the neck and under the arms, increased blood clotting tendency and an accelerated rusting (oxidation) rate within the blood vessels.

The author of this book feels that the signs of high blood pressure, increased blood clotting tendency and increased rusting rate are better explained by three additional factors. The first concerns the chronically elevated production of cortisol caused by a mental stress-filled lifestyle. The second involves the fact that these owners tend to consume a processed food diet. The third factor, and perhaps more central to the underlying cause of this syndrome, is the fact that they have a diminished IGF-1 level, which exaggerates insulin need (insulin resistance).

There are only two hormones that allow the cell fuel tanks to fill up. It helps to think of these two hormones as **"fuel nozzle" hormones**. Just as in filling a car with fuel, a "fuel nozzle" is necessary, so it is with most body cells, a molecular 'nozzle' is necessary to fill the 'tanks' of the cells with the fuel circulating in the blood stream.

The two '"fuel nozzle"' hormones are insulin and insulin-like growth factor type 1 (IGF-1). Healthy people have at least 100 times more IGF-1 than insulin in their blood streams. Each of these two "fuel nozzle" hormones has a preference for the cell types it prefers to fill up. Because there are roughly 100 times more cells that prefer IGF-1, it makes sense that healthy people have at least 100 times this hormone as insulin. Only when the body becomes unhealthy and IGF-1 levels consequently fall off, will the body attempt to raise insulin hormone production rates keep the total amount of "fuel nozzle" hormones constant. Hungry cells result when "fuel nozzle" hormones become scarce.

However, the insulin hormone contains message content that the IGF-1 hormone does not share. Insulin contains the fat-maker message. Overweight people have a problem with too much fat-maker message. Until the fat-maker message decreases they will continue to gain weight year after year.

Whatever the secretion rate of insulin from the pancreas, the liver always receives the highest message content concentration. This is true because the pancreas secretes its hormones into the portal vein that leads straight into the liver. Greatly increasing the effect concerns the fact that fat and liver cells have the highest pure insulin-type receptor concentration of all body cells, occurring at 200,000 per cell. In healthy people, very little insulin ever makes it outside of the liver, because of this anatomical fact. However, unhealthy people need excessive insulin to make up for a fall off in their IGF-1 levels.

The pancreas is little and the liver is large. The large liver, while healthy, easily secretes 100 times IGF-1 compared to the pancreas-secreted insulin. However, when the liver begins to falter, the little pancreas is forced to pick up the slack (commonly called insulin resistance). The pancreas strains itself to make enough insulin that spills over into the general circulation beyond the liver. In this way, these sickly bodies still have a way for their cells to procure nutrition but there are complications from this desperate approach.

When IGF-1 levels remain high, the body cells, outside of the liver and fat, procure an increased proportion of blood fuel following meals. Because of the anatomical location of the pancreas dumping insulin directly into the portal vein, the liver always receives the highest amount of insulin message content. A falling IGF-1 level tips the advantage to the liver procuring more fuel for the manufacture of cholesterol and fat. **Fact: the higher the insulin and the lower the glucagon level within the liver, the more active HMG CoA reductase. HMG CoA reductase is the enzyme, which makes cholesterol in the body. This detail explains how the high insulin states like adult onset diabetes and Syndrome X develop abnormal cholesterol profiles**.

Once again, instead of the medical industrial complex revealing this simple scientific relationship, the more lucrative cholesterol lowering drugs fill media advertising space. How one heals from Syndrome X involves an emphasis on the methods that will increase one's IGF-1. Improvement here leads to an improved cholesterol profile without side effects or toxicities.

Syndrome X owners exist on an accelerated track to an old body. Their fundamental defect concerns their elevated insulin levels, which become necessary because of their falling IGF-1 levels. This syndrome worsens in a setting of increased stress. Increased stress will accelerate potassium loss, as well.

Low potassium and low magnesium diets with elevated sodium intake will increase the disease process (chapter 8).

In many ways, a high stress hormone output could help explain how Syndrome X patients age so quickly and have high blood pressure as well. This is better illustrated by the fact that chronically elevated cortisol tells the body that an emergency situation chronically exists. During the emergency situation, whether real or imagined, the body retains salt and water and this leads to **blood pressure elevation**. Also, when the body perceives an emergency (real or imagined) the body's energy gets redirected into survival pathways (catabolic instead of anabolic). In syndrome X owners, the survival pathway becomes the norm instead of rejuvenation activities.

When body energy chronically directs into survival pathways, wear and tear changes will become more likely. **Wear and tear changes within the body cells manifest clinically as an old appearing and feeling body.** Wear and tear changes become more likely secondary to the lack of cellular repair activities. Additionally, the elevated blood pressure increases the injury rate as well. Cellular repair and rejuvenation activities cannot occur unless sufficient anabolic message content reaches the cells. This helps to explain why Syndrome X owners tend to age so quickly. Not only do they tend to have high insulin derived disease but high cortisol derived disease, as well. Cortisol directs body energy into catabolic pathways. Increased catabolism means that body consumes its structure to increase the blood fuel level and repair activities delay. Anabolic means that the body uses fuel to build up (repair) the body, the opposite effect of catabolic. Too much catabolism within the blood vessels leads to wear and tear changes.

In one way or another, the initial blood vessel lesion (rust) grabs hold when the blood vessel repair processes fail to keep up with the injury rate (excess iron or fluoride ions). The degree of anabolism determines the repair rate. Conversely, the amount of catabolism puts repair on hold and survival pathways activate instead.

The severity of the Syndrome X exacerbates from the consumption of processed foods. This fact is explained later but for now remember that processed foods contain reversed mineral proportions compared with body design. Reversed minerals intake, stress, and high insulin, combine in ways that greatly accelerate the injury rate to these owner's blood vessels.

Dr. Reaven correctly attributes increased insulin as having some role in the blood pressure elevation of these owner types. One of the reasons that elevated insulin raises blood pressure concerns the fact that it powerfully stimulates the blood vessel lining cell's production of endothelin. When endothelin production increases, blood pressure rises. High insulin levels also diminish the ability of the blood vessel lining cells to produce nitric oxide. The diminished production of nitric oxide further reduces the body's ability to maintain an appropriate blood pressure level.

Large amounts of insulin within the blood stream require large amounts of cortisol to effectively counter insulin's behavior of moving every last sugar molecule out of the blood stream. Remember abnormal insulin need occurs most often when IGF-1 levels fall. Almost always, the fall in IGF-1 levels has a component of causality in a diminished growth hormone secretion. Bodies that cannot produce sufficient growth hormone need increased insulin and increased cortisol in order to maintain their cells nutrition and blood sugars respectively between meals (see the stress response discussion in chapter 7).

Cortisol counters the effect of insulin by increasing the blood sugar levels. Cortisol, however, directs body energy and molecular building parts into survival pathways and out of repair and rejuvenation pathways. Anti-oxidant synthesis and blood vessel repair defer with a chronically high cortisol levels. Cortisol also powerfully retains sodium and water, which elevates the blood pressure.

The Typical Path that Leads to Syndrome X

Troubles start around middle-age in sedentary and stressed owners. These two lifestyle traits combine to diminish IGF-1 levels. A lower IGF-1 level means that insulin secretion must rise to abnormally high levels in order to attempt to offset the decrease in IGF-1 levels (thus keeping the total amount of "fuel nozzle" hormones constant).

This detail explains why Syndrome X types present with elevated fasting insulin and/or C-peptide levels. Healthy owners have essentially no insulin in the fasting state. Most mainstream labs allow some insulin in the fasting state before they consider it too high. However, this belief proves inconsistent with what role insulin serves when one remains healthy.

The body is smart and consistent. Insulin's design helps to store fuel in the liver following meals so there will be enough fuel released from the liver between meals to keep the blood fuel constant. However, a rise in IGF-1 facilitates the uptake of nutrition between meals that growth hormone release directs, while sparing body proteins' usage for fuel. Remember, growth hormone release also directs the liver to simultaneously release sugar and fat that was stored in the liver following the last meal under insulin's direction, into the blood stream.

The healthy body relies on sufficient insulin following meals to store adequate fuel for the between meals state. In the between meals state, sufficient growth hormone release tells the healthy liver to release the stored sugar, fat and IGF-1. In this way, the healthy body's cells have access to sufficient blood fuel at all times while protecting their protein content from combustion for usage as fuel. Sufficient IGF-1 negates the need for insulin in the between meal state.

In contrast, unhealthy people do not release sufficient growth hormone. Instead, they release cortisol, glucagon and epinephrine between meals in order to stay alive (keep their blood fuel adequate). Unhealthy people have processes operating in their lives that prevent sufficient growth hormone release and hence IGF-1 levels fall and insulin needs rise. Body protein now becomes fair game for fuel usage and because levels of IGF-1 fall off, more insulin needs to be secreted between meals. Insulin secretion in the between meals state is abnormal. It only becomes necessary when IGF-1 levels have fallen.

> (Side bar for physicians) Why would a healthy body instruct the liver to draw down the blood sugar further in the between meal state? Unhealthy bodies do this only because they exist with a lack of "fuel nozzle" hormones (a fallen IGF-1 level) for the cells, as in muscle and organs. In order to keep alive, they accept the complications of increasing insulin output enough to spill over into the general circulation and allow these cells their "fuel nozzle". The major complication results from the fact that whatever the insulin secretion rate, because of the pancreas-portal vein connection to the liver, the liver receives the highest concentration of its message content before the other body cells can get any 'insulin "fuel nozzle"s'. This means a contradictory message occurs within the unhealthy body's liver during the fasting state.
>
> The contradictory message within the unhealthy body results from the fact that insulin causes opposite effects within the liver compared to other body cells between meals (fasting state). Remember, the liver and fat cells have the highest pure insulin-type receptor concentration per cell at about 200,000. A high insulin release rate becomes necessary to spill some insulin beyond the liver and out into the general circulation but this also excessively stimulates the cholesterol and fat-making machinery.
>
> This fact leads to the liver performing counter productive tasks during the fasting state. Some liver cells, under the influence of insulin, begin sucking sugar out of the blood stream while the body is in the fasting state, and thus worsen the falling blood sugar. Other liver cells under the influence of the counter hormones like cortisol, glucagon and epinephrine tell other liver cells to dismantle protein (gluconeogenesis) to make sugar and release it into the blood stream. The end result accelerates protein degradation and increases the manufacture rate of fat and cholesterol. These side effects occur just to keep the unhealthy body's blood sugar sufficient between meals.
>
> Remember that normally, between meals, the healthy liver responds to growth hormone's release by simultaneously

> releasing IGF-1, sugar and fat into the blood stream. Growth hormone's release also protects body protein content between meals. Between meals (fasting state) healthy bodies avoid competing messages at the level of the liver and conserve organ and muscle protein stores, as well.

Insulin has a half-life of five to ten minutes. IGF-1 has a half-life of about four days (half life eauals the time for half to be gone). For the reasons mentioned above, measurable insulin in the fasting state should raise the suspicion about Syndrome X. Fasting insulin and C-peptide provides a fairly good marker for diminished IGF-1 levels (excluding diabetics). The primary health effects when IGF-1 levels fall and insulin levels rise concerns pancreas strain, high blood pressure and the activation of the fat and cholesterol-making machinery within the liver. In addition, these owners combust their body protein content for fuel needs. Not only are these owners becoming fat-making machines, they work their pancreases to death and dismantle their muscles and organs, as well.

Chapter 5: Nutritional Deficiency and Brain Dysfunction

Part One

Nutritional Deficiency Caused Mental Illness

The Physical Health of the Brain and Nerves

The brain has a unique protection system that is commonly known as the blood brain barrier. The blood vessel lining cells (the 'tiles' discussed in the blood vessel chapter in ***The Body Heals***) within the brain form a tightly interconnected surface that forms a barrier. This barrier selectivity allows what passes in or out of the brain blood vessel. This barrier proves complete except in a few areas deep within the central underside of the brain. Scientists call these four small areas where the blood brain barrier doesn't exist the circum-ventricular organs. These small areas provide a window for the brain to more directly interact with the body environment. It also allows an area of vulnerability for unwanted substances.

Physicians treating for possible brain infections constantly keep in mind that only a few antibiotics can penetrate beyond the blood brain barrier. This creates a problem when attempting to medicate brain function. Illnesses like Parkinson's disease improve when more dopamine makes its way into the injured neurons responsible for its manufacture. However, dopamine cannot cross the blood brain barrier. Scientists circumvent this fact by providing a synthetic dopamine precursor, L-dopa that is able to penetrate the blood brain barrier. Once it penetrates the blood brain barrier, L-dopa converts to dopamine.

The blood brain barrier creates a challenge for the brain cells. The challenge for brain cells involves their continued procurement of all the needed molecular building blocks. The brain needs more molecular building parts because it comprises an area of high metabolic activity. High metabolic activity means that molecular parts wear out and need replacement more quickly. All this active replacement requires the use of lots of fuel and oxygen. The combustion of fuels and oxygen necessitates an increased need for efficient waste removal and rust prevention. In addition, only some of the most powerful body hormones can gain access to the entire brain. This fact has powerful repercussions when one wants to know how to keep the brain functional.

Keeping in mind the physical blood brain barrier will facilitate the understanding of nine determinants of physical brain health. These are: 1) availability and completeness of neurotransmitters within the brain, 2) availability and direction for the use of molecular building parts, 3) adequate fuel delivery unique to the brain, 4) blood vessel health within the brain, 5) informational directions regarding cell architecture and rejuvenation activities, 6) anti-oxidant versus oxidant activity peculiar to the brain, 7) toxin accumulation, 8) the quality of the force field that the individual nerve cells generate 9) status of the energies that heal contrasted to the energies that maim (discussed in *The Body Heals*). An enhanced ability to make better choices in the day-to-day little decisions promotes brain health.

THE DETERMINANTS OF BRAIN HEALTH

1. The Neurotransmitters

The many different neurotransmitters within the mind convey specific information to the neighboring nerves. A discussion of the numerous different neurotransmitters can become complicated. Some of the most basic considerations will help to avoid gullibility about the medical business complex. It becomes important to acquire an overall feel for the different types of neurotransmitters. Neurotransmitter's availability depends on certain nutritional and biochemical factors. These nutritional and biochemical factors need to be present in order for a healthier and more efficient brain function.

The first group of neurotransmitters is called the biogenic amines. These same neurotransmitter molecules (epinephrine, norepinephrine, dopamine, histamine and serotonin), when they occur within the blood stream, are known as hormones. A large proportion of this group of informational substances has blood vessel effects on tone when acting as hormones. Thus, the terms neurotransmitter and hormone are thought of as a distinction of where in the body their action occurs and not as different molecules.

The bioactive amines exist in both the nervous system and blood stream. These same molecules are called hormones when they act within the blood stream and neurotransmitters when secreted within the nervous system. Some physicians have proposed the simplified and unifying term, informational substance, in place of this confusing and arbitrary semantics drama between hormone and neurotransmitter. Until that far off day, one needs to grasp this duplicity of ways to say the same thing in as complicated a way as possible.

Examples of the precursors, which form the biogenic amine types of neurotransmitters, are the amino acids: tyrosine, tryptophan, and histidine. Tyrosine can be manufactured into epinephrine (adrenaline), nor-epinephrine and dopamine. Tryptophan can be manufactured into serotonin and melatonin.

Finally, histidine can be manufactured into histamine. A few others exist but these will be discussed later in the chapter in order to keep the initial discussion less burdensome.

The biosynthesis of these neurotransmitters depends, to varying degrees, on a number of nutritional cofactors (synthesis facilitators). Without sufficient cofactors, these neurotransmitter's manufacture becomes impossible. When was the last time anyone heard of a mainstream physician inquiring about the nutritional adequacy of a given owner's ability to manufacture these essential neurotransmitters? This provides yet another example of how the educational emphasis within medical schools proves deficient when compared to the holism of what science has revealed.

The conversion of tyrosine into the above neurotransmitters occurs in an orderly fashion. Each step of the progression requires certain molecular cofactors. The assembly line order of progression, for each neurotransmitter, depends on adequate molecular replacement parts for each step of its manufacture. Health consequences follow when any one of these parts becomes deficient. Tyrosine first converts to dopa, then into dopamine, then into nor-epinephrine and finally into epinephrine.

An exciting youth conserving mechanism culminates this process. When one understands the simple cofactors that the brain needs in order to make proper amounts of each one of these neurotransmitters, one can step on to the brain functioning advantage track that leads to vitality.

In order of need in the above listed assembly line progressions of neurotransmitter manufacture are: tetrahydrobiopterin (made from folate), Vitamin C, Vitamin B6, and finally S-adenosylmethionine (SAMe). These molecules comprise the basic cofactors needed for synthesis along the assembly line from tyrosine to epinephrine. Insuffcient amounts, of any single nutrient, causes synthesis to come to a halt.

It should be emphasized that for each one of these types of neurotransmitter molecules made: one to two Vitamin C's degrade, one tetrahydrobiopterin unloads, and in the case of epinephrine, one SAMe unloads (only epinephrine requires

SAMe). Unless a highly functional molecular re-supply system operates, these cofactors rapidly deplete. In addition, SAMe can only recharge when adequate folate, Vitamin B6, Vitamin B12, and the amino acid, serine, remains available (these are the nutrients of the methyl donor system). Recognize that as each SAMe unloads it needs one molecule of folate, Vitamin B6, Vitamin B12, and one serine available or recharging SAMe becomes impossible.

The demands for newly manufactured bioactive amines are much greater within the blood stream. The blood stream needs more bioactive amines because these informational substances only exist for about 2 minutes in this body location. Once released into the circulation, these informational substances have two minutes to convey their message, before being deactivated and then eliminated within the urine. This fact contrasts with their ability, within nerves, to be released and recycled many times once they have been manufactured.

When owners decline mentally, the cause could be from one or more of the above nutritional deficiencies. SAMe and the molecules which recharge it each time it donates a methyl group is called collectively, the **methyl donor system**. The methyl donor system depletes at the rate of one billion times per second (Cooney). An owner is only as good as the least present nutrient within his or her methyl donor system.

Serotonin

One of the most likely bioactive amines to deplete comes from the amino acid, tryptophan. The unique reason for this will be explained shortly. This amino acid exists in high concentrations in eggs, dairy products, and turkey.

Serotonin deficiency becomes more likely, compared to the other bioactive amines, because some of it converts into melatonin each day. In contrast, the other neurotransmitters more efficiently recycle each time they release into the synapse. Serotonin, within the brain, concerns itself with arousal. Deficiency in the arousal state leads to one of the types of clinical depression. This fact provides a business opportunity that has been well realized with the skyrocketing sales of drugs like Zoloft, Paxil, and Prozac. These drugs keep the serotonin that releases between nerves around for a longer time in the active little space between nerves called the synapse.

These prescriptions poison the enzymatic machine, which pulls serotonin out of the active little space occurring between nerves, the synapse. Without these enzyme machines being poisoned every day, the serotonin would only effect arousal for a normal time per excretion of it into this little space. However, with the advent of these drugs that penetrate beyond the blood brain barrier, this enzymatic machine becomes incapacitated for a while.

The serotonin in this little space between the arousal nerves sends the arousal message for a longer time. It should be mentioned that two of the three most popular drugs in this class contain the most powerful oxidizing element on the planet (stronger than the oxygen radical). This cannot be good when it penetrates the blood brain barrier by being attached to the carrier molecule (explained below). How much of this breaks down within one's brain setting off a frenzy of rust production? The most powerful oxidizing element of all is fluorine and will be discussed later in this chapter. Fluorine's oxidizing properties are introduced here to help facilitate learning in regards to the other side of the scientific story: The potential down side of what the complex sells.

Here come the protest and rationalizations about how these types of antidepressant drugs saved Uncle Albert, whom no one could help before. What isn't being said regards the rate-limiting step for serotonin manufacture: The amount of tryptophan delivered into the blood stream. Science long ago revealed that serotonin levels within the brain prove directly related to three factors. First, the amount of tryptophan consumed in the diet. Second, the ability of the digestive tract to absorb the tryptophan presented to it. Third, Vitamin B6 is needed to convert tryptophan into serotonin. This means that supplementing with tryptophan and Vitamin B6 in the diet, and making sure that the digestive process operates correctly, will do what these expensive prescriptions will do.

The reason tryptophan currently remains relatively unavailable in America today results from suspect policies occurring within the FDA. How convenient, right when these new serotonin uptake poisons were to become the depression drugs of the nineties, a single source of a contaminated batch of tryptophan was discovered. Later it was found that the only reason that this batch caused severe muscle toxicity was that a single Japanese company tried to save money by changing the standard protocol by which it was traditionally made (Wright, 1998). Since the FDA answers to no one, they have used this excuse into the present time and thus limit effective strength tryptophan to prescription only. The prescription only designation makes this natural treatment much more expensive.

Serotonin depletion occurs because of two general processes. First, within the pineal gland there arises the daily need to manufacture melatonin from available serotonin. Second, depletion occurs when cofactors diminish or dietary derived tryptophan present within the brain and the pineal gland deplete. The Vitamin B6 cofactor converts tryptophan to serotonin within a specific enzyme machine. The essential cofactor, for melatonin synthesis, is SAMe. SAMe forms part of the methyl donor system, mentioned above, which depletes within the body at the rate of one billion molecules a second.

The previous discussion mentioned the need for Vitamin B12, folate and serine to recharge SAMe. SAMe needs to recharge each time it makes a new melatonin molecule from serotonin. When healthy owners go to bed, serotonin release slows within their brain. Conversely, melatonin made during the day and stored within the pineal gland releases into the blood stream with the onset of sleep. Young children release much higher amounts and this gradually decreases until melatonin release becomes quite diminished in old age.

Adequate melatonin provides a cornerstone for a good nights sleep. The high levels of melatonin that occur as children sleep may explain its soundness (difficulty awakening them). The above process describes the daily drain off of serotonin within the brain in order to make new melatonin each day. This fact explains the first reason why serotonin deficiency remains more likely than other neurotransmitter deficiencies.

The second mechanism for brain serotonin depletion occurs when inadequate tryptophan becomes available to satisfy the body's serotonin and melatonin needs. Serotonin deficiency can occur from either poor dietary choices or a decreased ability of the digestive tract to properly dismantle proteins. The dietary deficiency of niacin (Vitamin B3) will accelerate the body's need for tryptophan. Tryptophan usage accelerates because it can be used to make niacin. Niacin deficiency eventually causes the disease pellagra.

Melatonin releases into the blood stream from the pineal gland, during sleep and this depletes brain stores of this substance. Melatonin escapes each night when it rhythmically releases into the blood stream, from the pineal gland, and performs its mysterious sleep-enhancing activity. The melatonin released eventually degrades and the kidneys remove it. The continual drain off of melatonin from the brain causes the continual need for new sources of tryptophan. Tryptophan continuously depletes and therefore needs to be replaced by the diet.

In contrast, the other biogenic amine neurotransmitters operate under a theme of a highly effective recycling system. The other biogenic amines recycle more efficiently because they exist without a drain off for other uses within the blood stream. The other neurotransmitters release and recycle into the little spaces between nerves, the synapse. Here, they deliver a message that each of their unique shapes imparts. Shortly after message delivery they recycle back to where they originated, the nerve ending. Because of this recycling system, the same rate of depletion fails to occur with the other biogenic amine-derived neurotransmitters.

The majority of serotonin in the body, occurs outside the brain. The platelets and digestive tract contain the majority of serotonin. Within the digestive tract's blood stream, it serves as a hormone that instructs this tube how it should behave. The serotonin message contained within the blood platelets involves the orchestration of clotting parameters. In addition, it encourages blood vessel spasm (vasoconstriction).

The three above additional serotonin purposes utilize greater than 90% of total body serotonin content. Therefore, when owners take drugs that keep serotonin around longer, a percentage of the effect occurs within these areas! This fact explains the common experience of increased gastrointestinal distress while taking these drugs. For the scientific reader, it should be acknowledged that there are 7 different types of serotonin receptors. The drug companies research findings, which sell SSRI-like drugs, documents that the highest affinity for these drugs occurs within the limbic system in the brain. The limbic system contains only type 6 and 7 receptors.

Serotonin levels affect the amount of the hormone prolactin released from the pituitary. A higher prolactin level leads to inhibition of gonad function. A cognizance of this little detail helps explain the high rate of sexual dysfunction that commonly occurs when owners take these prescriptions.

This does not mean that serotonin reuptake inhibitors are never warranted. In fact, once someone begins his or her prescription it becomes a pretty tricky business to safely navigate its discontinuation. However, the risk of decreased gonad function underscores the need to consider nutritional deficiencies early in the depression presentation. No side effects occur when one heals.

While an owner takes these types of medications he or she should monitor his or her prolactin levels. If sexual dysfunction occurs, a well-run 24-hour urine study should be obtained and analyzed by a competent physician. If the gonad steroids prove to be low and continued serotonin reuptake inhibitors are still warranted, real sex hormone replacement therapy could be considered.

Histamine

The next neurotransmitter in the bioactive amines class, to be discussed, is histamine. Histamine manufacture occurs from the amino acid histidine. This molecule proves as an important neurotransmitter and hormone. The role of this important informational substance largely remains ignored. Histamine likely remains ignored because there is a lot of money at stake, which revolves around the popular drugs known as the anti-histamines. This has far reaching implications on how physicians and owners are groomed in their thinking patterns.

Histamine secreting nerve cells (neurons) have their center (cell body's) within the tuberomammillary nucleus of the posterior hypothalamus (in the central brain area). From here, the neuron cell body sends projections (axons) into all parts of the brain and spinal cord. The axons carry the nervous impulse to the next nerve synapse where histamine releases. This small group of histamine secreting neurons, which connects to all parts of the nervous system, has a broad scope of influence. Some examples of histamine secreting nerves influence are: consciousness, blood pressure, pituitary hormone secretion, thirst, and sexual behavior.

Mast cells are one type of immune system cell that tend to concentrate within the pituitary gland. Mast cells contain histamine. This proves important because the pituitary gland is commonly known as the master hormone gland. Under the direction of the higher brain structures the pituitary secretes powerful hormones that control the activity of the gonads, adrenals, thyroid, pancreas, placenta, and thymus. Adequate histamine within the pituitary modifies the release of many of these master gland's hormones release rates (ACTH, FSH, LH, prolactin, TSH and GH). In addition to histamine, dopamine and serotonin within the pituitary, also exert a modifying effect on how the pituitary responds to commands from the higher brain centers. The textbooks imply that interplay occurs between these three neurotransmitters, which influence the response of the master hormone gland to higher brain commands.

The bigger picture for histamine's role within the brain includes consciousness level, sexual behavior, regulation of body secretions, regulation of the release of the pituitary hormones, blood pressure regulation, drinking fluids behavior, and in pain thresholds. Histamine proves especially important in activating the sleep center within what scientists call, the diencephalic sleep zone.

This doesn't mean that the popular anti-histamines are of low value in some medical conditions. Rather the implication is that the public deserves a better understanding for the consequences of chronically consuming a substance that affects powerful nervous system activities. Anti-histamines become unnecessary when one corrects the cause of the problem. For example, the use of DGL licorice root for gastritis and heartburn has proved effective. The ways to evaluate the adrenal deficiency, which causes allergies, autoimmune disease, and some asthma, are discussed in chapter 10.

Epinephrine

The neurotransmitter, epinephrine, conveys a sense of alertness within one's mind. Sufficient epinephrine signifies the crowning glory of what can only be manufactured when all the above listed biochemical cofactors remain present (the methyl donor system plus Vitamin C, Vitamin B6 and tetrahydrobiopterin). Epinephrine contains unique message properties that remain largely unrecognized. In its place, a tendency exists to lump the actions of epinephrine into those of nor-epinephrine and dopamine. Add to this, the biochemical sloppiness that regards the common practice of trying to explain these above three bioactive amines in a complicated and arbitrary system of different types of receptors. Commonly these are referred to as: alpha 1, Beta 1, and Beta 2 receptors. This method limits the discussion that regards each of the above three neurotransmitter actions. This arbitrary nomenclature keeps many a well-meaning physician confused.

Sometimes it helps to ignore the discussion of these arbitrary methods of 'pigeon holing' these informational substance's receptors. In its place, one can begin to glean an overall picture of why the body would prefer one of these neurotransmitters to the other. One complication of ignoring the interplay between the different neurotransmitters regards the over prescribing of anti-histamines when the real problem is diminished epinephrine production.

Most allergies occur by a peripheral action of histamine acting as a hormone and not as a neurotransmitter. When owners take many of the anti-histamines, they potentially affect both the neurotransmitter availability and the peripheral-acting histamine that produces allergies (among other things). This symptom treating approach always leads to side effects because of the central role that histamine plays within the brain (discussed above). Often, as previously discussed, it is safer to take epinephrine like medicines for allergy control than the anti-histamines so commonly utilized.

The mantra about blood pressure elevation resulting from herbs like ephedra becomes largely the hype of clever little sound bytes of disinformation when the other side of what science has revealed is included (**see Methods for Dumbing Down Doctors section**). Never the less, when taking powerful medicinal herbs like ephedra, it remains wise to be followed closely by a physician just in case there exists the slightest chance that one's blood pressure could become elevated. In addition to epinephrine like medication for the short-term control of allergies it is always a good idea to check these owners' adrenal glands function (chapter 10).

Perspective widens when one realizes that more people die from the complications of aspirin-like medication in one week than have ever died of ephedrine or epinephrine allergy treatments. Another possible role for epinephrine-like medication involves the treatment of depressive illness. Many ephedra users for weight loss notice a marked improvement in their mood. Epinephrine proves safer than norepinephrine because it does not raise the blood pressure as avidly. This explains why many patented pharmaceuticals for asthma possess epinephrine-like molecular structure instead of norepinephrine molecular structure. Blood pressure side effects prove bad for the bottom line and the drug companies realize the difference. However, before this possibility can be realized there needs to be adequate studies performed.

Norepinephrine and Epinephrine

In regard to the neurotransmitter role of epinephrine and nor-epinephrine, these substances can only be manufactured when the previously mentioned cofactors remain available. Briefly, these are: tetrahydrobiopterin, Vitamin C, Vitamin B6 and SAMe. SAMe degrades at the rate of one billion times a second within the body. Without re-forming it degrades further into homocysteine. Cognizance elucidates the fact that elevated homocysteine levels signify more than blood vessel disease risk. SAMe needs folate, Vitamin B6, Vitamin B12 and serine to recharge it each time it donates a methyl to convert nor-epinephrine into epinephrine. Because nor-epinephrine and epinephrine are some of the major neurotransmitters, these facts involve an important consideration. When one realizes the extent of the continual need for the above nutritional cofactors it helps one to be open to yet another cause of some cases of clinical depression. Depression often results from a nutritional deficiency. These deficiencies affect the ability for these parts of the brain to manufacture these important molecules (see nutritionally caused depression later in this chapter).

Dopamine

For now, dopamine is the last, of the bioactive amines needing to be discussed. Dopamine can be generalized to be involved with pleasure and fine motor coordination. When the part of the brain stem concerned with fine motor coordination fails in its production and release of dopamine, Parkinson's disease begins. Cocaine usage is generally felt to result in the increased presence of dopamine within the pleasure centers of the brain. This is believed to happen because cocaine poisons this brain areas ability to reuptake dopamine within these little spaces between the pleasure nerves (synapses). Therefore, more dopamine remains in these spaces. The higher the dopamine level within the synapse, the more messages conveyed for the pleasure message.

An additional important role for dopamine exists as a neurotransmitter within the brain that was briefly alluded to above. This regards dopamine's effects on pituitary hormones when its level increases. Like serotonin and histamine, dopamine also effects the pituitary responsiveness from higher brain centers. Dopamine levels increase within the pituitary gland when the nerve endings within the hypothalamus release it. The hypothalamus is the area of the brain immediately above the pituitary, which controls the pituitary secretions. In turn, higher brain centers control the hypothalamus. As dopamine increases within the pituitary, growth hormone release enhances and prolactin release retards. Conversely, as serotonin increases within the pituitary, prolactin release enhances and growth hormone release retards.

A pivotal point in the understanding of how one keeps younger far longer than his numerous peers now occurs. To better understand why, one needs to recall two things. First, increased prolactin levels directly correlate with decreased gonad function (except when a placenta exists). Decreased gonad function means a lowered "steroid tone" and pressure will occur (chapter 7). When "steroid tone" and pressure lower the wear and tear changes inflicted by life fail to repair properly. Failed repair accelerates the aging process. The second point is more completely explained in the Follow the Fuel and You Will Understand Diabetes chapter. However, briefly stated growth hormone has many youth conserving properties. As owners age, growth hormone levels gradually decline to low levels and become really low just before death. Processes that increase growth hormone levels, androgens and a healthy liver will tend to increase cellular rejuvenation activities (explained in the following sections of this manual).

Part Two
Physical Health of the Brain and Nerves
Applying Biochemistry to Longevity

Millions of Americans' depression symptoms are treated with serotonin reuptake inhibitors (SSRI). SSRI raises the level of serotonin within the brain. Increased serotonin within the brain has the potential to raise prolactin and decrease growth hormone. It's instructive now to return to the consequences of an increased prolactin secretion and decreased growth hormone secretion within the pituitary. This situation results when serotonin levels increase in the brain. The aberrations in growth hormone and prolactin levels can injure certain body tissues. Heart valve tissue provides one example of potentially vulnerable body tissue secondary to these types of hormone imbalances.

Cardiac heart valves derive from specialized cartilage tissue. As was discussed earlier in the Why We Shrink as We Age chapter, a big part of the continued health of cartilage relies on the quality of the message content it receives. When high quality message content occurs these types of cells receive instruction to invest appropriate energy in rejuvenation activities. The big players in this regard prove to be adequate androgen and growth hormone. When these two hormone groups reach these cell types rejuvenation activity becomes possible.

A few years ago, certain pharmaceutical companies expressed great surprise and remorse when it became obvious that some owners who took the popular diet drug, fenfluramine (commonly known as the fen-phen diet of which fenfluramine was one of the components), developed heart valve damage. A common denominator for how these owners' heart valves were injured emerges if one applies the previous discussion regarding increased serotonin levels within the pituitary gland. Drugs like fenfluramine raise pituitary levels of serotonin. It becomes more alarming when one realizes that the popular antidepressants Prozac, Paxil and Zoloft are all structurally related, to varying degrees at the molecular level, to that of fenfluramine. These types of drugs also tend to raise pituitary serotonin levels.

Recall that higher serotonin levels, within the pituitary, have been noted to raise prolactin levels and decrease growth hormone levels. Now apply the above discussion, which regards the role of increased prolactin and decreased growth hormone on the tissues like heart valves. First, the increased pituitary serotonin causes increased prolactin release and this increase inhibits gonad function. The inhibition includes androgen release and production from the gonads. Second, when decreased growth hormone and androgen message content reach cardiac valve tissue, a diminished message to instruct these cells to rejuvenate occurs. The heart valve cells need instruction to invest appropriate energy into repair and rejuvenation activities. With low growth hormone and high prolactin in operation some owners' heart valves will succumb to disrepair. This scenario provides a likely mechanism of injury for these patients' heart valves when these types of medications are taken.

The Physcians Desk Reference (PDR) does not group fenfluramine as a serotonin reuptake inhibitor like the other antidepressants, which have a similar molecular structure. However, if one examines their molecular structures and active sites it becomes probable that the PDR division is arbitrary. The PDR and other pharmaceutical textbooks discuss the possibility of growth hormone secretion depression for all of these substances including fenfluramine. In addition, the basic medical physiology text link increased pituitary serotonin levels to an increase in prolactin secretion and to a decrease in growth hormone secretion. It is important to point out that because fenfluramine has been known to damage heart valves, this drug probably raises pituitary serotonin levels more than the others do.

Very few doctors or patients understand these potential dangers. Some of the confusion occurs because of the likely arbitrary divisions in classification between fenfluramine and the other types of SSRI. These risks would be unnecessary if the public still had affordable access to tryptophan. Owners who need these medications should be followed for elevated prolactin and decreased growth hormone levels. In addition, they should have their steroid status monitored. These same owners should also have their heart valve function checked until the actual risks are quantitated. When either of these tests results become abnormal, supplementation could be considered to correct the deficiencies of either androgen and/or growth hormone.

A Comment on a Possible Safer Way toTreat Depression with Medication

Certain anti-depression medication works by raising brain dopamine levels. Increasing dopamine levels within the brain will decrease prolactin and raise growth hormone levels. The downside to this medication is the slight risk for seizure while taking this drug. The additional need exists to monitor thyroid status while on this medication (see below).

The benefit from raising growth hormone levels and suppressing prolactin levels concerns the youth conserving properties with these two types of hormones relative relationships. Specifically these hormones relative balance increase the tendency for appropriate message content delivery to the body's cells to invest in rejuvenation activities. The scientific name for this medication is burprion (Wellbutrin). Stopping short of abusing cocaine, with all its predictable sad consequences, this route describes one method for raising brain dopamine content. Another likely method would be to take L-dopa but this method needs clinical testing before its endorsement.

Dopamine is the neurotransmitter responsible for pleasure. Owners that choose the Wellbutrin route of treatmen need to have their thyroid monitored. Thyroid monitoring becomes necessary because whenever dopamine levels rise within the pituitary, thyroid function may become depressed. When this medication causes a depressed thyroid function, the conventional test for low thyroid function, the TSH test, will be unreliable as a measure of thyroid function. The axillary (armpit) body temperature provides a supportive step, but a 24-hour urine test for thyroid function, will be even more helpful.

The important point here concerns the fact that Wellbutrin has potential advantages in the treatment of depression, when one understands its side effect profile. Monitoring patients for possible thyroid dysfunction will avoid missing thyroid dysfunction caused by this medication. Thyroid dysfunction is more easily treated than when the gonads and growth hormones status become compromised. Until dietary tryptophan again becomes available, the Wellbutrin method of treating depression is less risky to one's health than the available forms of SSRI. In addition, a group of owners exist who will dramatically respond to nutritional supplementation for the manufacture of the needed neurotransmitters previously discussed above.

2. The Brain's Molecular Building Parts Replacement Program

Brain molecular building parts include unique components. **Some of the need for unique brain molecular components arises because the brain is composed of more fat than nerve in its makeup.** In turn, the fats, which make up one's brain, are constructed with unique components. The brain needs unique components because fat serves as insulation to prevent electrical cross firing between the different nerve cells. The brain also needs adequate molecular supplies to rebuild the brain structures that wear out. A continuous need exists to replace the nerve cell enzymatic machines that begin to breakdown. The high metabolic rate of the brain increases the rate at which molecular parts become defective. Because the brain burns about 25% of the oxygen within the body, at normal basal conditions, it remains more vulnerable to 'rusting' (oxidation damage). As stated above, the brain contains more fat than nerve by weight and this fact increases the rust vulnerability many times. The increase in vulnerability results from the rusting processes creating rancid fats within the brain.

It is accurate to describe the brain as a fatty bag that contains well-connected neurons (Pert, 96). The bag releases hormones and neurotransmitters. In health, the fatty bag releases these in a rhythmical manner. This causes the appropriate amount of informational substances between the various nerves (the neurotransmitters). Concurrently, a rhythmical release occurs, from the brain, of other informational substances into the blood stream (the hormones). The rhythm of the brain's release of information breaks down when a failure arises to provide it with ongoing replacement parts as the old ones wear out. This subsection concerns what the brain needs to regenerate. Since fats comprise the number one component, which makes up one's brain an emphasis for its procurement occurs next.

Fat is the Major Building Block that Makes up One's Mind

As mentioned above, the brain exists as a bag of fat. Brain fat has well-connected nerve cells within it. Within the fat are some specialized areas that secrete powerful informational substances into the blood stream. Therefore, the quality of this fat proves pivotal to intelligence.

Some owners make the procurement of molecular replacement parts for their fat bag a difficult process. No one counsels these owners about how all the brain fat needs to be kept in the right condition. In addition, they usually have not a clue about how to take out the fat trash that begins to stink. Everyone knows that when fat rots, it begins to smell rancid. Fat within the brain serves as a support and cushion for its delicate connections. In addition, fat keeps the electrical activity confined by its effective insulating abilities. Because the fat in the brain has so much to accomplish, it makes sense that these fats are special. Because brain fats are special, they have unique needs in order to keep them from rotting.

Myelinated nerves serve as examples of how fat's integrity within one's brain rests on the continued replacement of myelin fats, which have rotted. Scientific writings frequently mention myelinated nerves and their importance for optimal brain and nerve functioning. In fact, the disease of multiple sclerosis (MS) describes a disease process, which results from injury and breakdown of the myelin coating around these nerves.

Myelin serves as an example of one of the specialized fats occurring within the nervous system. Certain important nutritional factors need to occur in order for myelin fat to remain healthy. Additional informational substances need to be around in adequate amounts in order for optimal myelin synthesis to be maintained. For example, adequate myelin sheath formation (explained below) depends on sufficient progesterone. In one way or the other, the greater the disease injury rate (myelin sheath injury), the greater the repair rate needs to be. Progesterone sufficiency in the brain increases the repair rate. Yet, mainstream physicians often neglect inquiring into his/her MS patient's progesterone status.

Another example of the unique needs of the brain for its ongoing molecular replacement program is the neurotransmitter, acetylcholine (a new neurotransmitter added to the discussion). The choline half is a specialized fat component needed in large quantities within the brain for its neurotransmitter formation and specialized fat formation, including myelin sheath formation. The need for choline is underscored by its role in the synthesis of the neurotransmitter acetylcholine. This use of choline occurs in addition to the important, already mentioned, synthesis of the myelin sheath.

Now that the discussion centers on the fat, which builds one's brain, it becomes important to include the neurotransmitter, acetylcholine. The choline half provides a component of the specialized fat for the structural and insulating properties within the brain. Ample supplies of choline are also necessary for acetylcholine biosynthesis. Acetylcholine is the major neurotransmitter of the brain and nerves of the body. Ample supplies of choline are easily obtained with a high fat diet.

Conversely, owners on a low fat diet make their nervous systems acquirement of choline difficult and draining to other body systems. For example, in order to make one choline molecule from scratch it uses up three SAMe molecules plus all the recharging cofactors (explained below). In contrast, owners who regularly ingest quality sources of choline need less SAMe. Eggs and fish provide really good sources for this important brain constituent. Another important molecular building block for structural brain fats is called phosphatidylcholine. Lay people commonly call phosphatidylcholine, lecithin. Significantly, all brains and nerves in the body need a continuous and adequate supply of this essential building block or neurological efficiency becomes compromised.

The nervous system continually needs new sources of choline for its building block role. It uses choline for many construction processes. Because these processes are so numerous within the brain, to not include this in one's diet could eventually deplete the methyl donor system (SAMe, Vitamin B6, Vitamin B12, folate, serine, and methionine). The methyl donor system depletes at the rate of one billion times a second. **When was the last time a western trained physician counseled a middle aged patient, who was concerned about brain function, about this basic scientific fact?** Again, it is probably not a mean-spirited conspiracy but rather a result of yet another evisceration from the mainstream medical education in regard to the importance of basic preventative and nutritional advice.

How one makes more intelligent choices on how to obtain their brain fats from the highest quality sources forms the topic of this subsection. In general terms, regular consumption of olive oil is a start. The essential fatty acids found in wild fish and green algae supplemented chicken eggs are important. In addition the lecithin found in eggs is important. Finally, the vitamins that make up the methyl donor system are fundamental, as well, in order to preserve or regain mental function.

Brain structure as well as maintenance has particular and unique molecular building parts needs. Owners who make it easier on their brains to acquire these basic essentials have an advantage for brain longevity. This information occurs within basic medical textbooks in a scattered and confusing way. The time has come for a re-inclusion of these basic scientific facts in a way that physicians and patients can understand.

3. Fuel Delivery to Brain Cells is Crucial

The uniqueness of the fuel delivery requirements for brain function further explains how the brain becomes vulnerable when its molecular replacement parts become compromised. Many owners exist in a mentally cluttered state. Complaints of brain 'fog' early on in these patients typify the presentation. Later, they go on to develop hypoglycemic events. In the extreme cases, fainting and seizure disorders can result. Many of these patients have in common fuel delivery problems within their brain. Brain cells are more vulnerable to fuel delivery interruptions than other body cells. Two central reasons cause increased brain vulnerability to fuel interruption. First, the brain can only burn sugar for fuel. Therefore, the brain becomes vulnerable to injury when the blood sugar falls. Second, the brain has a high rate of fuel usage (high metabolic rate). If fuel supplies become interrupted brain cell's function quickly impairs.

The difference in brain tissue compared to most other body tissues concerns its independence from insulin and IGF-1. Thus unlike most other body cells the brain can take up sugar without either IGF-1 or insulin message content. It will probably turn out that the brain fuel uptake depends on insulin-like growth factor type two (IGF-2) that the choroid plexus and meninges manufacture and secrete at high levels. Prolactin is the most logical hormone to tell these areas to release IGF-2 because it releases during the stress response. At this time, this is only a suspicion because the textbooks contain sparse information. However, the unanswered question is: why would a healthy body's meninges and choroid plexuses make more IGF-2 than the liver's production of IGF-1?

Many owners suffer from various vague forms of mental dysfunction. Sometimes these conditions occur only because their physician fails to consider issues of fuel delivery to the brain. Fuel delivery problems to the brain largely result from imbalanced hormones.

The problem for most owners that suffer from low blood sugars involves a failure in their body's ability to mount an effective counter hormone response to insulin. The counter response hormones become necessary to counter insulin's desire to direct the liver to suck every last sugar molecule out of their blood stream. As discussed earlier, hormones operate on a system of balance. Balanced blood sugars only occur when the proper balance between insulin and the four counter response hormones exist. The counter balance hormones to insulin are glucagon, growth hormone, epinephrine and cortisol. By far the most important counter regulatory hormone to insulin, in the unhealthy body, is cortisol (chapter 7).

Healing these owners usually requires restoring hormonal balance. When was the last time a western trained physician was seen counseling about hormonal balance being central to healing these symptoms? Again, this is not meant as a criticism of the many fine physicians desiring to help their patients but rather as an observation of yet another evisceration of what the holism of science has revealed. Instead, in the place of healing, western physicians are trained to prescribe frequent feedings of carbohydrate, which predictably results in a fatter patient.

A return to hormone balance resolves brain fuel delivery problems. This approach contrasts with constantly loading the 'antique weight scale' with insulin and then constantly re-supplying the body with more sugar before insulin sucks the blood sugar down again. Instead healing the brain fuel delivery problem requires a more effective counter weight. Owners whose bodies for one reason or another, become enfeebled in their ability to secrete the ever increasing 'counter weight' of cortisol to the 'weight' of increasing insulin required by high carbohydrate diets, get low blood sugars.

Physicians who recognize the fundamental body theme of hormonal balance in the healthful state can counsel their patients to restrict carbohydrates. A restriction of carbohydrates lowers the need for insulin. Lowered insulin leads to a lessened need for the counter hormones, like cortisol. Exercise also has a profound stabilizing effect on one's blood sugars (see muscle chapter, explained in *Glandular Failure-caused Obesity*).

The above two lifestyle changes make mechanistic sense if one becomes cognizant of balance. In other words, less counter weight (diminished adrenal function and/or growth hormone secretion) means that one needs to decrease the need for making the weight (insulin) amount secreted into the blood stream. Attention to this basic understanding allows the 'antique weight scale of hormonal balance' to return to optimum. When this occurs, the symptoms of 'brain fog', anxiety secondary to roller coastering blood sugars, seizure disorders from low blood sugar, and weight gain from the commonly prescribed hypoglycemic diet, begin to resolve.

Part Three
Physical Health of the Brain and Nerves

4. The Blood Vessels within the Brain

The first vulnerability of the brain vessels results from the volume of blood flowing within the brain. The brain contains 25% of total volume of blood in the basal state. The brain blood vessel lining cells have a higher rate of exposure to rust producers (oxidizing agents) than in other parts of the body. Owners who have elevated levels of oxidizing agents (rust producers) and/or low levels of anti-oxidants become vulnerable to cranial blood vessel injury.

The second vulnerability of the brain's blood vessels arises because these vessels course through a closed box (the skull). Blood which leaks from a brain vessel has nowhere to go without squishing delicate nerves and ripping them from their precise connections. Processes that weaken the blood vessels do more damage to the brain than similar insults elsewhere in the body.

Last, nerve cells prove the most vulnerable of all body cell types to an interruption in oxygen and nutrient supply. Because of their high metabolic rate, neurons start to die, one minute after an interruption in blood flow occurs. Even the high energy consuming heart cell can be oxygen and nutrient starved for up to 4 hours before it dies (myocardial infarction). A partial explanation involves the fact that its high-energy requirements derive from neurons powering up their force fields (cell charge). Sufficient cell charge propagates their action potentials and keeps out injurious ions like calcium (see below). The brain creates a higher electrical charge than other parts of the body. The high electrical charge in the brain, powers the nerves transmissions between one another (the action potential). The neurons become vulnerable when the energy for current generation becomes compromised (see below for mechanism).

5. The Hormones Giveth and the Hormones Taketh Away One's Mind

The right types of informational substances (hormones) direct the process for how owner's preserves their nerve cells physical integrity. Only when the proper mixtures of informational substances courses through the brain blood vessels, will the nerve cells be directed to rejuvenate and repair. Adequate repair and rejuvenation activities mean the nerve cells receive the proper directions to spend their cell energy wisely. Some of these hormone mixtures direct appropriate absorption of minerals, vitamins, molecular building parts and fuel. Still other brain hormones promote adequate cellular infrastructure investment and rejuvenation activities. Cellular infrastructure investment activities include: new cell machines (enzymes); new cell factories (organelles); toxin and waste removal, etc. Nerve cell rejuvenation activities regard repair activities. Examples of repair activities are: new outside the nerve cell support framework replacing damaged molecules, rotten fats replacement, DNA repair and stabilization, etc.

The steroids like hormones (including thyroid hormone and Vitamin A) are the only hormones within the body that can go within any body chamber. Once these most powerful hormones penetrate one's mind, they instruct the nerve cell DNA programs. Which DNA programs activate or repress centrally determines how that nerve cell spends its energy.

Limits exist for all other hormone types (levels 2 through 4 discussed in the appendix) as to where in the body they can penetrate. Many other body hormones cannot penetrate the blood brain barrier. However, all the steroids, thyroid, and Vitamin A can penetrate into the central nervous system. Once inside the quality of their type and amount determines the appropriateness of the many different nerve cell's DNA programs. The DNA program contains the genes. Which genes turn off or on at any given time centrally determines how a cell spends its available energy. For this reason, lousy steroid amounts or types in the brain result in poor genetic program activation. Poor genetic program activation leads to the wrong types and amounts of protein synthesis. Like all other cells, brain cells need the right types and amounts of specific proteins or functional compromise occurs.

Processes that increase the "steroid pressure" and tone will give owners a longevity advantage (chapter 7). Processes that decrease the "steroid pressure" and tone within the brain will allow deterioration to occur more quickly.

Owners who have optimally functioning gonads and adrenals will have the ability to direct the wise use of nerve cell energy within their minds. Optimally functioning gonads and adrenals can do this because they capably create optimal "steroid pressure" and tone. In addition, the brain can make some of its own steroids. This means that even when the gonads and adrenals begin to fail in some owners, their brain has a back up system of it's own for the manufacture of steroids. The brain, therefore, has a degree of protection not afforded to other body systems when the adrenals and gonads fail. However, all three areas of steroid production (the adrenals, gonads, and brain) become potentially compromised when the body perceives stress. Stress redirects the nervous system energy into survival activities and away from repair and rejuvenation activities within one's brain.

Modern life's complexities are stressful: time deadlines, financial worries, job security worries, relationship worries, keeping up with the Jones etc. Stress damages certain brain tissues involved in learning and memory. Stressful living increases the lifetime exposure of these brain tissues to cortisol (one of the body's main stress hormones). Cortisol is a major player as an informational substance involved in redirecting cell energy into survival pathways and away from cellular maintenance activities. The body's cells can't discern if the stress is real or imagined.

Real or imagined stress causes cortisol levels to increase. Cortisol is one of the important informational substances that make up message content delivered to cells during stress. Excessive exposure of these brain structures to cortisol has been implicated as a major mechanism of cell death in the brain. The cortisol message channels energy into survival pathways. When energy directs into survival pathways a postponement in rejuvenation activities occurs. If stressful events occur occasionally, or are otherwise mitigated by adequate periods of behavioral and environmental restorative activities, the degenerative process slows down. However, if stress becomes chronic, the daily cortisol message continuously defers the rejuvenation activities. Adequate ongoing regeneration prove necessary to keep the brain in peak performance.

Chronically high cortisol production rates direct nerve cell energy away from rejuvenation activities and towards survival pathways. The lack of rejuvenation activities leads to an increase in brain wear and tear changes. This results from the chronic message of survival being delivered to one's nerve cells. During the stress response, the learning and memory centers in the brain are not a teleological part of the emergency cell team. The emergency cell team comprises the cells in the body, which preferentially obtain ample energy during the survival response.

Examples of these areas within the brain are the cerebellum and vision centers. Some examples of other body cells, which are part of the emergency cell team are: muscle, heart, and lungs. The emergency response cell team cells receive increased metabolic energy to mount the body's perceived survival challenge. However, they are asked by cortisol message content to put on hold critical cellular maintenance activities. The difference is that the emergency response cells of the body receive ample fuel delivered during the perceived emergency.

Thus, cortisol causes deferred maintenance throughout the body and the shunting of fuel away from the memory and learning centers, contributing to brain aging.

The effects of chronic stress on the brain exacerbate when the stressors prove unpredictable in nature and/or timing and intensity. The additional promoters of chronic stress changes involve a feeling of hopelessness and when the personality of the owner is emotionally reactive. Finally, the brain will age more quickly when there is less than optimal social support. In the end, all three of the above exacerbations of the stress response accelerate the brain-aging rate by increasing cortisol levels (Salpolsky 1992).

The destructive effects to one's brain from the chronic elevation of cortisol can be somewhat mitigated when a counter balance from the androgens arrives. Balance between the catabolic effects (body wasting effects) of cortisol (and the other stress hormones) with regular secretions of the counterbalancing anabolic hormones (the rejuvenating and strength giving hormones) has restorative potential. The anabolic class of hormones (the androgen steroids) plays a central and powerful role in the brain restorative process.

Remember, because cortisol contains catabolic message content, it uses up body structures for fuel generation. In addition, remember all steroids have the powerful ability to instruct one's cells DNA program. These hormone instructions concern, which genes turn off and which genes turn on. Therefore, the quality, timing and amount of each steroid-type interacting with a given brain cell forms a central determinant of how wisely that cell spends its energy.

All steroids are synthesized from cholesterol stores in the adrenal, gonads, and to a limited extent, the brain. Each steroid provides unique message content in how it directs body energy usage. Some of the steroids increase buildup activities within a given cell type and these are called anabolic. Some of them encourage burning different body structures for fuel to maximize survival during emergencies and these are called catabolic. Finally, there are the steroids concerned with maintaining the minerals within the body at an optimum level for structure and maintaining the cellular force field (aldosterone and Vitamin D). Like other body tissues, the brain, needs a balance between all three types of steroid message content.

Within the brain, the anabolic steroids are DHEA, progesterone, androstenedione, testosterone, and dihydrotestosterone. Different body tissues respond preferentially to the different anabolic steroids. Blood vessel health seems particularly responsive to DHEA and possibly progesterone. Brain myelin producing Schwann cells need a steady message from progesterone to optimize their nerve cell protective effects. GABA producing neurons in the spinal cord need adequate progesterone or anxiety and irritability occurs. DHEA is concentrated within the brain at five to six times the blood level when the brain remains healthy. Although each body tissue has a specific anabolic steroid, which it preferentially responds to, the take home point is that the brain needs the androgen class of steroids occurring in their optimal amounts before a return or maintenance of the healthful state becomes possible.

The anabolic steroids direct nerve cell energy into cellular infrastructure investment activities. Examples of this can be summarized in a broad way: toxin removal (taking out the cellular garbage), enzyme replacement (new cellular machines), rejuvenation of the cell membrane, and the manufacture of new organelles (cellular factories unique to each cell type). For longevity considerations the trick is to have enough anabolic tone influence (optimal amounts of DHEA, testosterone, progesterone, etc.) to counterbalance the possible deleterious effects of chronic stress elicited cortisol release. As mentioned earlier, certain brain structures with their increased metabolic rate are particularly vulnerable to increased cortisol message without adequate counterbalancing of the anabolic steroids.

Achieving adequate anabolic steroid levels within one's mind becomes possible only if several things occur regularly within the owner's body. First, there needs to be adequate functional capabilities in the gonads and/or adrenal glands. One or both of these paired glands needs to be sufficiently capable of producing the factory order of increased anabolic steroid production. If the bank vault becomes empty (ill or near dead adrenals and/or gonads), a response to stimulants towards increasing anabolic steroid production becomes impossible. Unfortunately, many owners exist who, through toxin exposure, surgical procedures, lifestyle, or poor genetic constitution of these glands, possess some degree of gonad or adrenal failure, which needs to be addressed before improved anabolic steroid output becomes possible.

Second, an adequate regular stimulus needs to occur to produce optimal anabolic steroids. Healthy sports competitions, regular aerobic exercise, warm nutritive relationships that are emotionally supportive, as well as positive emotions (happiness, joy, forgiveness, singing, and love) all directly stimulate more optimal anabolic steroid amounts. Of course, amorous romantic sexual attractions promote bank withdrawals in the capable gonad.

Finally, it should be stressed that the steroid hormones all derive from cholesterol, or more rarely, from plant derived sources containing high progesterone content. Natural progesterone can serve as a precursor for most other steroid biosynthesis (Lee, 1993). Progesterone easily converts, once inside the adrenal or gonad tissues, to many of the other types of steroids, including estrogen, if the body's intelligence sees fit.

This turns out to be a practical consideration because as bodies age, there becomes a decreased ability to manufacture steroids from the cholesterol precursor route. The failing rate-limiting step seems to be in the freeing up of cholesterol within the cell so it can be delivered to the mitochondria (the site of the first chemical reactions in the synthesis of the steroid hormones). Deficiencies of pantothenic acid and Vitamin A seem to greatly diminish the ability of these tissues to manufacture steroids.

Beyond the repair and maintenance of the neurons, destructive forces always lurk, which under certain circumstances, gain access to one's mind. One example of such a destructive process concerns those molecular substances, which tend to promote rust within one's mind. Thankfully, the properly nourished owner has adequate molecules to counter these rust promoters.

6. The Rust Promoters Versus the Rust Retardants

The next determinant of brain function regards the level of rust promoters versus rust retardants. Scientists call rust promoters oxidants. They call rust retardants anti-oxidants. A duplicity of saying the same thing exist by discussing a given elements electro-negativity. Electro-negativity denotes in chemical jargon the ability of a specific element to grab electrons (oxidize or rust) other elements or molecules. In order to avoid becoming the victim of what is not being said, one needs to remain mindful of these interchangeable terms that mean the same thing.

The top three rust producing atomic elements, out of more than one hundred, are: fluorine, oxygen, and chorine. The ability of an element to produce rust regards their power of electro-negativity. The fourth in line is sulfur but the body uses it to react with the first three on the list. Sulfur containing molecules like thiol, found in garlic, glutathione, MSM, and cysteine, all serve to neutralize the first three most powerful oxidants when they occur in the wrong places.

The higher the electro-negativity number of a certain element determines the ability of that element to rust or oxidize other molecules. This electro negativity scale gradates the rust promoting abilities relative to an interaction with all the other elements and molecular combinations possible. The most powerful electron hog (rust promoter) is fluorine followed by oxygen then chlorine and finally sulfur.

When any of these oxidizing elements penetrate into the brain, they had better be happy (stable) or the cellular consequence of rust formation results. Because human bodies contain greater than 60% water, some protection exists. Protection occurs when elements like chlorine bathe in sufficient water and become largely free of a tendency to bind to body structures. Sufficient water creates a way for chlorine to associate loosely (dissolve) with oppositely charged elements within body fluids (sodium, potassium, magnesium and calcium).

This quality seems largely absent for oxygen and fluorine in their ionic forms. Much attention regarding less potent oxidizing agents occurs within the media. It helps to be less gullible when one stays mindful of the big four electron hogs on the planet. These are the radicals of: fluorine, oxygen, chlorine, and sulfur. Most of the time, the oxygen and fluorine ion comprise the main rust promoters to be concerned with in one's mind. A prime example of the reactivity of fluoride occurs with its propensity to react with tooth and bone tissue. While it makes these tissues harder, what these media specialist leave out is the fact that fluorine makes these same tissues more brittle, as well. Brittleness measures one aspect of oxidation within body tissue. Here lies the concern of elements like fluorine and oxygen in the unpaired state within one's mind.

Oxidizing agents can damage one's mind by two different mechanisms. First, and more common with oxygen but less common with fluorine, concerns its unstable radical form. The oxygen radical denotes the state of unpaired oxygen before it steals an electron (s) from a weaker atom (less electronegative).

Oxygen cleavage explosions occur within the mitochondria of numerous body cells. Because tremendous amounts of oxygen cleave in half each day in an owner's life, a small amount of oxygen radical occurs as a by-product. Oxygen radical damage occurs whenever the split part of the two atoms, O2, gets outside of the 'armor' of the mitochondria chemical reaction chamber. Owners who lack sufficient ability to deal with oxygen radical leakage get diseases that result from oxygen radicals injuring body cells.

One prototypical disease associated with this defect, in the unpaired oxygen mop up team, is Lou Garrig disease (amyotrophic lateral sclerosis). Amyotrophic lateral sclerosis kills the motor nerves within the spinal cord because either an increased production rate or decreased ability to neutralize oxygen radical formation exists.

The second way that oxidizing agents (rust promoters) injure nerve cells occurs after one of these radicals hogs an electron. For example, the second mechanism occurs after the electron hog like oxygen and fluorine, have already stolen an electron from somewhere else. Scientists denote this state by acknowledging a negative charge to these elements. Scientists call oxygen that occurs in this state, oxide. They call fluorine that occurs in this state, fluoride.

Even after their radical form has hogged an additional electron, they still tend to bind to a positively charged body structures. When these hogs bind in this manner, they alter the recipient molecule's properties and shape. The fluoride and oxygen ion can do this. One needs oxygen for life and therefore curtailment here proves only possible by limiting intake of the salts of oxygen and in attempting to breath air that contains less oxidizing properties (commonly called clean air). Fluorine is the same as fluoride except the latter designates that it has already hogged an electron of its own. Already mentioned was the popular example of fluoride binding the tooth enamel and bone readily.

However, left unsaid, concerns the fact that beyond these tissues becoming harder, these tissues also develop more brittleness. Brittleness serves as another example of the rusting process (aging process). Fluoride and oxide within one's mind logically extend into the less than desirable category.

The example of fenfluramine needs to be recalled (see earlier discussion in the chapter) because it contains fluoride. The fluoride contained within fenfluramine has the potential to release fluoride within one's mind. The brain's number one protection from outside toxicities involves a highly functioning blood brain barrier. Pharmaceutical agents that penetrate beyond this barrier can cause great harm if they contain injurious atoms. The fluoride content of fenfluramine provides such an example.

A journal of the American Medical Association article disclosed direct evidence that fenfluramine (one of the components of the popular fen-phen diet) damages neurons cultured in Petri dishes. About the same time of that discovery, it was also discovered that fenfluramine was injuring heart valves (see earlier discussion). Three fluorine atoms occur on each fenfluramine molecule!

Other widely used prescription drugs as well, deliver fluoride to the brain. Prozac has the same amount of fluorine as fenfluramine. The other popular and related antidepressant, Paxil, has one fluorine atom per molecule. In addition, if one inquires into the chemical structure of these previously mentioned SSRI that doctors commonly prescribe to treat depression, they all contain an aromatic ring (a technical point for doctors). Fenfluramine has this same aromatic ring structure where the fluorides are attached in the same position as Prozac. These facts point to the possibility that the popular SSRI relate more to the recalled, fenfluramine than the medical literature reveals. Awareness of this possibility makes it worthwhile to consider more completely how one heals nutritionally from depression (discussed later).

Part Four

Physical Needs in the Brain and Nerves

The Politics of Scientific Information

The take home point here is not to vilify the profit-driven scientific community that operates in America today. The main point is to alert the reader to yet another consequence that the popularized science comprises only a small fraction of what science has revealed. Gullibility in this regard has health consequences that the above only serves as several examples of many. This will begin to change for the better as more people begin to realize that they have been the recipients of clever advertising campaigns. The PDR (Physicians' Desk Reference) actually proves less complete than it should in regard to what science has revealed. It contains wording that accentuates the up side of what the complex sells and simultaneously minimizes the risks involved. Anyone who doubts this trend can read for him or herself about any new drug that still has a patent advantage. The reason that it is important to read about patented drugs that regard this trend involves one method for increasing new drugs sales: Slam on the patent expired varieties.

In addition, these advertising campaigns contain designs that steer thinking in a beneficial way. The benefits of this approach lead to larger profits for their most lucrative products. When one understands the down side, there will begin to be a demand, at the consumer level, for a more complete discussion regarding the options for a given ailment.

One further point about the PDR concerns the realization that it has largely become an effective marketing strategy towards patients and physicians. These descriptions of the different drugs are sometimes without a picture of a drug's chemical structures. The lack of a chemical structure becomes very disabling, when one wants to understand the basics on the safety within.

One needs to stay mindful about the way drugs are classified. Drug classification can lead physician's thinking into erroneous avenues of understanding. The fenfluramine example being grouped outside the serotonin reuptake inhibitors (Prozac, Paxil, and Zoloft), when they share many suspicious overlapping structural and activity-related characteristics, again illustrates this point.

A long-held suspicion exists about under-reported side effect profiles. This suspicion becomes more justified when one becomes cognizant of the often-harried physician's work day. How much time do most doctors really have to read the fine print of these subtle PDR pieces of work? When the under reporting becomes outlandish, physicians eventually get suspicious and then they print warnings. More commonly, a chronic under representation exists for the potential to harm a given group of owners who take different medications. If owners were again taught some of the basics about the body processes, devoid of the complex's abstractions, they would better be able to alert their physicians about the first signs of trouble.

Mercury as a rust promoter needs to be discussed while on the subject of scientific incompleteness and inconsistency. Scientists have known for many years that mercury is a nerve toxin. Less appreciated even within the medical community concerns the duplicity of ways that pharmaceutical companies include mercury within vaccines by identifying mercury as a side name that few physicians and patients can recognize. This nasty little fact has finally come to light thanks to many doggedly stubborn owners who kept up the campaign against the mercury contained within these vaccines, but hidden under the ingredient name, thimerosal. Several decades prior, the previous code name for mercury was Merthiolate. Before that it was Mercurochrome. A new code name is probably forthcoming because of increased awareness.

This revelation has forced the manufacturers of many childhood vaccines to agree to reduce the mercury content within these injections to 5% of the previous amount. They now say that much less mercury proves necessary for them to stabilize the vaccine ingredients. This means that for years, countless children have been injected with a known and unnecessary neurotoxin. Coincidentally, as the amount of mercury received in immunizations increased, the rate of autism rose as well. The complex vigorously denies this association. Time will tell the truth as the health revolution practitioners continue to uncover what really happened to these children. The common flu vaccine still contains mercury (25 micrograms). In addition, some types of testosterone injections contain mercury.

ADHD and autism appear to have strong links to mercury toxicity but other interrelated considerations exist (explained below). For further information see the work of Jeff Bradstreet M.D., a pediatrician by training, who has devoted his career to discovering the true causes and effective solutions for both autism and ADHD. He treats about 1500 children a year with these disorders. He became involved when his son developed autism following his childhood immunizations. He went looking for the truth. Another knowledgeable pediatrician is Allen Lewis M.D. currently at the Pfiefer clinic in Chicago.

Arguably, it would be advantageous for physicians to receive their primary scientific information from unbiased sources of scientific inquiry. This will probably only become possible when enough patients stand behind their doctors and begin to demand a little house cleaning from the grips of the

FDA and rampant corrupt funding of university research by silent pharmaceutical interests. Socialized medicine has many of the same problems inherent in the current system because of the lobbying protectionism of any 'complex' interest before passage would become possible. In other words, the new socialized system would tax the citizens to ensure continued 'complex' profits.

Healing paths will probably originate outside of the current system. Movements like 'Keep it Simple' describe such beginnings. Here, doctors agree to charge less but accept no insurance or government programs of any kind for out patient care. Patients pay in cash, but at reduced charges, because their doctor no longer has to generate huge sums of money to pay for all the paper work and time spent arguing with insurance programs. In systems like this, the doctor-patient relationship becomes, once again, a private exchange and its focus regards the number one priority of placing that patient on a healing path.

Contrast this to the frenzied demands on a general practitioner's time today. **Very little of this time allows for focus on who the patient is, from where he/she has come, what their fears and hopes are, where they are going (someplace good versus someplace bad).** In the end, when change comes to health care practice standards, it will come from the patient's demands. **Politicians remain scared to death of angry voters.** This fact explains why, despite the complex's best effort otherwise, there has been a gradual acceptance of alternative modalities. Patients have legitimized chiropractic care, acupuncture, naturopathy, and massage therapy to their insurance companies. All the while, the various complex entities have been trying every dirty trick to attempt to marginalize these alternative therapies (see Methods for Dumbing Doctors Down section).

As mentioned earlier, John Lee MD summarizes the situation very well in the introduction of his book, ***Some Things Your Doctor May Not Tell You About Menopause***. He comments on how, over the last several years, there have been repeated attempts to marginalize the importance of his progesterone findings. However, he communicated that the complex underestimated the power of the international women's network that regards what works. In the end, accurate scientific information will become available only when consumers vote out those politicians that continue to receive 'honorariums' from the complex.

7. Taking Out the Brain Trash

The unique power supply to the brain presents unique challenges to keep the brain free of toxins. The main vulnerability within the brain lies in its obligatory requirement to burn only sugar for its fuel source. Sugar combusts within the nervous system at a high rate in oxygen's presence. Unlike most other body organs, the brain can only burn sugar in its power plants. Failure of the power plant energy supply when blood sugar supplies fall off, has toxic consequences to brain tissue. In addition, injury to delicate nerve cell contents occurs from the oxygen radical. Oxygen radicals create brain trash whenever inadequate backup systems occur. One back up system involves the oxygen radical mop-up enzyme machines. Oxygen radical enzyme mop-up machines clean up the occasional unpaired oxygen radical that escape outside the 'armored' mitochondria.

The nerve cell prevents the creation of oxidized cell components in two ways. **First**, the brain needs an effective set of enzyme machines hanging around to process the oxygen radical (reactive oxygen species) situation when it occurs. The enzymes within the nerves, which neutralize reactive oxygen species, are called super oxide dismutase and catalase. Oxygen radical formation occurs because of the shear volume of oxygen being processed for life-giving combustion reactions within nerve cell mitochondria. As stated previously, when this set of enzymatic machines becomes deficient, diseases like Lou Garrig result. These types of diseases kill nerve cells when oxygen radicals escape outside of the protection afforded within the mitochondria. When reactive oxygen species leak outside of the mitochondria, they damage the first structure that they contact. The damage from rust production processes eventually exceeds the best repair processes of the nerve cells.

A similar process occurs in the retinas of premature infants that require high oxygen content to remain alive. The high oxygen content that saves them also, in many cases, overwhelms the oxygen detoxifying systems and visual impairment results from death of the nerves behind the retina. Scientists call this retrolental fibroplasia.

The **second** form of brain defense with regard to oxidizing agents is more generalized. This system of anti-oxidants neutralizes many different rust promoters within the brain. Glutathione, lipoic acid, Vitamin C, vitamin E, garlic, and onions all provide common examples of substances that perform this important task. They each work by stabilizing many different rust promoters when they react with them. Some of these anti-oxidants are rechargeable and others are only able to work one time. Nutritional deficiency of these important protective molecules causes the nerves to rust more rapidly. The brain becomes one of the most potentially toxic areas in the body because the brain has 25% of the body's blood at rest. This is especially true with regard to the blood vessel lining cells' exposure to oxidant insults as the blood flows by traveling through the brain.

An additional consideration now occurs in regard to the overall effect of the rust promoters. This consideration concerns the nerve cell options once it suffers molecular component damage from an oxidant. When nerve cell molecular components become injured, a repair process needs to occur. Fat constitutes the largest proportion of a single molecular component within the brain and hence, remains the most likely brain component to suffer damage. An adequate cellular direction to invest in fat rebuilding activities logically follows. In addition, to appropriate informational substances, which direct the repair of damaged intracellular contents, the nerve cells need a highly functioning land-fill site (lipofuscin deposits) or incinerator (peroxisomes). The incinerator burns the damaged fats. The lipofuscin deposits within the nerve cells as storage sites for damaged fat molecules. Lastly, concerns the requirement that adequate molecular replacement parts remain available to remanufacture the damaged structures. In the case of damaged fat replacement, the owner needs to have appropriate dietary fat supplies or have a highly functioning methyl donor system to make these specialized nerve fats from scratch.

Lastly, before leaving the toxin discussion the owner needs to remain mindful of ingested substances that have the ability to cross the blood brain barrier and move on into one's mind. Once inside, the brain, fluoride-containing substances can breakdown into elements like fluorine (fluoride within the body). Too many elements like fluorine place a particular strain on keeping adequate anti-oxidants around. The less antioxidant around increases the need for repair or replacement of brain molecular parts.

Part Five
Physical Health of the Brain and Nerves

8. The nerve cell's cellular force field

The concept of the cellular force field was first discussed in the blood pressure chapter (more discussion now follows). Because nerve cells require optimal voltage to function reliably, more than in any other body cell, a brief summary is in order. Recall the analogy of the car battery. Car batteries operate on a similar principle, as do nerve cells. When the difference between certain mineral's concentrations maximize across a membrane these types of batteries charge up. The differences of mineral concentration in nerve cells, as well, become maximized, it fully charges. The greater the difference, between the two minerals (across a membrane), the more energy a battery will possess to perform electrical work. The nerve cell proves similar in that its membrane lining the cell maintains a concentration gradient between different minerals (electrolytes), which allows it to perform the work of living.

Powerful hormones need to occur, in adequate amounts, which direct the nerve cells' DNA programs. Proper DNA direction allows the nerve cell to make the enzyme machines, direct repair to cell structures, and direct the manufacture of force field generators (membrane mineral pumps) within the membrane. The force field generators (Na/K ATPase, otherwise known as a membrane pump) are necessary for an effectively performing force field. The strength of a nerve cell's force field directly relates to the amount of force field generators, the minerals respective availabilities, and the energy supply delegated to them.

One example of the importance of the nerve cell force field occurs with its ability to prevent calcium ion's inappropriate penetration. The nerve cell membrane only prevents the inappropriate penetration of calcium ion when it possesses sufficient strength of charge. Sufficient charge becomes possible only when adequate sugar makes its way into the nerve power plants. The power plants need sugar fuel, specific vitamins (see chapter 16) and adequate oxygen to combust, and eventually trap some of this energy. The energy-trapped charges up the membrane by pumping certain ions (minerals or electrolytes mean also the same thing) against their concentration gradient. This process constantly drains off the energy created in the mitochondria and redirects it into the energy contained in the membrane. Anything, which disrupts this process, allows the energy contained in the nerve membrane to run down. When the energy in the nerve membrane runs down harmful ions penetrate inside the nerve cell inappropriately (Salpolsky 1992).

Inappropriate calcium entry into nerve cells should not be confused with appropriately channeled entrance of calcium in order to perform cellular work. The difference with the latter concerns when calcium enters appropriately it remains tightly regulated and is quickly pumped outside again. This movement of the calcium mineral about a membrane is similar to how a battery discharges and recharges. In contrast, inappropriate calcium entry into nerve cells is similar to when a battery post becomes oxidized. Battery oxidation results when the minerals inappropriately leak outside the battery and react with the post. Visualize the buildup that accumulates on these aging battery posts. So it is with the inside of owner's nerve cells that for one reason or another become unable to keep calcium channeled within its appropriate pathways. When calcium penetrates outside of carefully gated channels, cellular gunk begins to occur. The cellular gunk occurs because inappropriate calcium reacts with delicate inside the cell structures. The calcium reaction damages these nerve cell structures.

This process describes the main mechanism for nerve cell death when either oxygen or sugar delivery become compromised. In each of these cases, the energy content of the nerve membrane falls off and calcium rushes inside the nerve cell. Nerve cell death begins to occur in as little as one minute (usually four minutes and in cold water drowning it can be a lot longer). In other words, calcium always lurks outside the cell wanting to get inside. The electrical charge keeps calcium out as long as the cellular force field remains strong. When nerve cell energetics become compromised, as in decreased oxygen, and/or decreased blood sugar, the force field's strength falls off dramatically. The energy contained within the nerve cell membrane rapidly depletes when the ability to recharge interrupts. A fall in membrane charge only takes a few minutes and when it occurs, massive amounts of calcium influx into the cell. Calcium can only flood into a nerve cell, by the inappropriate channels, when the force field has become compromised. When the force field compromises, calcium chemically reacts in harmful ways with intracellular contents.

Processes that increase a cell's ability to generate a maximal force field convey a longevity and performance advantage to the nerve cell. Processes that compromise the ability of nerve cells to generate an optimal force field, lead to cell injury (old age). Nerve cells become particularly vulnerable if their force field diminishes for a short time.

The two main hormones within the body that determine how powerful a nerve cell's force field becomes are aldosterone and thyroid hormone. Thus, a continued maximal nerve function only becomes possible when these hormones remain present in sufficient amounts (chapters 7 and 12). Over looking the central directive role, which these two hormones play often, allows owner's nervous systems to slip into the diminished energetic state mentioned above. The diminished energy state of one's nerve cells is best understood through the example of the common mineral imbalance of middle age. One important mineral imbalance, particularly important to nerve health, involves potassium.

Potassium Deficiency Will Diminish the Cell Force Field and Hurt Nerves at Eight Different Levels

Potassium is the main mineral within the nerve cells. Nerve cells, which possess adequate potassium, are afforded energy and protection. Unfortunately, the important role potassium plays within one's nervous system, remains mostly overlooked in the clinical setting. The failure to counsel owners on strategies, which will improve their nervous system's content of potassium, leads to many nerve health consequences (see below). Fortunately, once one remedies a potassium deficiency the owner begins to heal.

The potassium-depleted nerve cells exist in an irritable and weak state. Many owners are misled by their annual lab test results, which clearly states that they have a normal blood potassium level. This blood stream measurement constitutes the 2% tank of the body potassium. This fact occurs because only 2% of total body potassium occurs within the blood serum. The other 98% sequesters inside the body cells. The confusion arises when patients fail to appreciate that the 98% tank will greatly diminish before one ever sees a decrease in their 2% tank within the blood stream. The consequence of this misunderstanding results in a lot of owners with nerve cell potassium depletion but normal blood potassium test results.

The ability of a nerve cell to charge its force field directly proportions to the availability of potassium inside the cell. Potassium deficiency often results from poorly informed diet choices. The consequences of poorly informed diet choices usually delay its manifestation of the chronic disease expression until the onset of middle age.

The most common reason for potassium deficiency with the onset of middle age results from the American diet. Very little medical emphasis occurs in regards to the importance of the proper consumption of balanced mineral intake. Balanced mineral intake will promote the maximal nerve cell charges. Conversely, the chronic imbalance of mineral intake leads to around middle age to the tendency for mineral imbalanced related diseases. The reasons for this have been discussed in previous sections but a review, as they pertain to nerve health, follows.

Real food diets (natural food that has not been processed) tend to be high in magnesium and potassium. These foods are almost always low in sodium, as well (see mineral table). They tend to be intermediate in their calcium content. When an owner consumes real food, the minerals remain rather easy to obtain in the optimally needed ratios. In general, 4000mg of potassium, 1000mg of sodium, 500mg of calcium, and 300mg of magnesium a day will suffice. Owners that live in hot climates will need more sodium. Owners that live in colder climates may need less sodium In addition; owners that sweat while either working or exercising may need more sodium. These mineral intakes only apply for those with normal kidney and adrenal function. Owners, who chronically have been fed the reversed mineral ratios of the processed food diet, have nerves that become fatigued and irritable around middle age.

Nerve problems occur around middle age in America because processed food has had much of its potassium and magnesium removed. A compounding of the problem occurs through the addition of large amounts of sodium that lengthens the shelf life of the processed food. Shelf life lengthens because bacteria have even a harder time with survival in altered minerals than owners do. When owners eat these altered mineral contents for years, the nerves become less able to hang on to or procure the necessary potassium.

The nerve cell potassium deficiency process greatly accelerates in those owners who experience chronic stress. This occurs because the stress hormone, cortisol, increases potassium loss and conserves sodium. This fact forms the second tier of a complex problem. It would be very difficult for this to occur if a given owner ate a real food diet because there would be sufficient potassium around to accommodate its increased excretion rate.

The third tier of the nerve cell potassium deficiency problem occurs when the kidneys become damaged from chronic potassium deficiency. It has long been known that low potassium intake leads to a risk for kidney damage (hypokalemic nephropathy). Paradoxically, very little is said to patients in the clinical setting about this fact. The blood pressure begins to rise when the kidneys start to become damaged in this way.

High blood pressure injures the brain cells, as well. If the doctor understands nutrition at this early stage he/she will begin to counsel his/her patients regarding the importance of a more balanced mineral intake contained within real foods only. However, when the physician misses this healing opportunity, the patient will go on to develop more kidney damage. Once the kidney becomes damaged, blood pressure will be less responsive to a better diet. At this stage, high blood pressure medication may be necessary on a permanent basis. One of the reasons high blood pressure medication becomes necessary involves brain protection.

The fourth tier of the nerve injury caused by the potassium deficiency problem concerns the associated insulin resistance. Insulin resistance predictably occurs in the processed food diet situation around middle age. Insulin cannot facilitate sugar uptake in most body cells without a one-for-one association between sugar and potassium. This means that for every sugar molecule taken into a cell, there needs to be corresponding potassium taken up. When potassium availability becomes deficient, the secondary system within the liver activates. The problem here exaggerates because the pancreas senses the delay in the blood sugar falling when potassium deficiency occurs. In these situations, the pancreas eventually secretes even more insulin for a given sugar load as more potassium becomes available from within the cells. **This process describes one of the reasons for still gaining fat even though an owner eats less carbohydrate**. A given owner will always secrete more insulin for a given amount of sugar when their total body potassium depletes. The delay of blood sugar normalization damages nerves.

A larger insulin message, arriving at the liver, which results from the potassium deficient state, contributes to the fifth tier of potassium-related illness that damages nerves. The liver only needs insulin's message for it to begin sucking sugar out of the blood stream. However, like other body cells, the liver needs sufficient potassium to store sugar as glycogen. For these reasons, potassium deficiency accelerates the amount of sugar changed into fat and cholesterol within the liver.

In contrast, other body tissues require potassium to suck up sugar out of the blood stream. When insulin secretion rates increase, as in the case of potassium deficiency, the enzyme HMG CoA reductase will abnormally activate. This enzyme machine begins the process of turning sugar into cholesterol. **Here lies yet another simple explanation for how cholesterol tends to increase around middle age, but tends to remain neglected by the medical community**. High levels of liver manufactured fat and cholesterol (LDL) tend to damage the blood supply that feeds the nerves of the body. The blood vessels in these areas plug up when the macrophages lining the arteries chronically stuff themselves on excessive LDL cholesterol.

The sixth tier of damage, which low potassium states cause to nerve cells, arises from the lessened tolerance for aldosterone within the body. Aldosterone proves a fundamental player for two important nerve processes. One, it tells the nerve DNA that it is important to invest in updated cell charge components within the cell membrane (membrane pumps). Second, it is this steroid, which determines the rate at which cholesterol converts to pregnenolone. Pregnenolone is the steroid precursor for all steroids manufactured in the body. For this simple reason, aldosterone levels become the rate-limiting step for steroid biosynthesis within the gonads and adrenals.

Nerve cell health depends on adequate "steroid tone" and pressure. Adequate "steroid tone" and pressure cannot occur without sufficient aldosterone levels, which tell the steroid-producing tissues of the body to begin the steroid manufacture process. The steroid-producing tissues of the body are: the gonads, the adrenals and the brain. **Unless adequate aldosterone message content reaches these areas, the rate of steroid synthesis declines**. A fall in steroid synthesis means that the "steroid pressure" and tone will fall as well (a more enlightened discussion on "steroid tone" and pressure occurs in chapter 7). Consequently, the nerve cells have diminished message content to rejuvenate.

The nerves of the body rely on adequate aldosterone levels to help keep the steroid production rate at youthful levels and the nerve cell charge sufficient. The processed food diet, only compounds the difficulty of the body's steroid-producing cells receiving adequate aldosterone message content. Aldosterone deficiency will occur for two reasons. First, it occurs in the treatment of high blood pressure states with ACE inhibitors (chapter 4). Most of the time, these drugs become necessary if one fails to catch the low potassium diet injury to kidneys early on. It also occurs when an owner continues to eat a processed food diet. Chronic subsistence on a low potassium diet will injure the kidneys. When the kidneys become injured, blood pressure will rise. Not until over fifty percent of the kidney dies off will the common kidney function blood test (creatinine) begin to rise into the abnormal range.

ACE inhibitors work, in part, by decreasing aldosterone and therefore, conserving potassium. As explained earlier, they also lower cortisol, by a circuitous route, and this further conserves potassium and increases the rate of sodium loss. The more sodium lost, the lower the blood pressure. Potassium has long been known to directly lower blood pressure. The other mechanisms of ACE inhibitors were reviewed in chapter 4. The important point, in this subsection, concerns the many owners that fail to understand how their processed food diet proves central to their nerve disease process at multiple levels. If these people change their diets early on, their nerves will benefit in multiple ways.

The second way that potassium affects aldosterone, and therefore, the nervous system steroid levels, regards the fact that in some owners, atrial natruretic peptide (ANP), secreted within the atria, activates early on. This powerful hormone, released from the heart of some owners, over rides the stimulus to release aldosterone when a high sodium diet prevails. In these situations, this hormone, keeps these owners blood pressure low at a price to their health. The first price to these owners health arises from less aldosterone and this leads to a consequent reduction of their other steroids production rates. Second, they will still tend to have the consequences, other than high blood pressure, from diminished total nervous system potassium.

The seventh tier of potassium deficiency and the resultant nerve dysfunction arises from the diminished force field that falling nerve potassium levels cause. When nerve cells exist with diminished force field generating abilities, they become irritable. Certain owners prove more susceptible to this side effect. Because different bodies handle total body potassium deficiency in their own prioritized way. Some do a better job at conserving potassium within the nervous system until late in the deficiency process. The important point to recognize is that some cases of anxiety or irritability (restless leg syndrome?) have their origins in potassium deficiency states.

The eighth tier of potassium deficiency produced nerve disease present as weakness and fatigue. This situation occurs because total body potassium content serves as a determinant for the amount of cell protein possible within body cells. Nerve cells need protein for their function and health even more than other body cells. Potassium within the cells of the body has been known for many years to stabilize proteins by its association. Without adequate potassium, body protein dismantles. Nerve cell health relies on the ability of potassium content to stabilize nerve cell proteins.

The eight ways, which a potassium deficiency injures one's nerves, serve as an introductory example for how dietary deficiencies or excesses alter nerve function. In the next subsection, multiple other nutritional deficiencies that cause clinical depression will be introduced. Clinical depression can be healed when the nutritional problem resolves.

Part Six:
Nutritional Deficiency Caused Depression

Imbalanced amounts of the different neurotransmitters often result in clinical depression. Mainstream medicine adherents tend to lump all these cases into the vernacular of a biochemical imbalance. While the biochemical imbalance, accurately describes the cause of their clinical problem, the solution often proves nutritional. Unfortunately, instead of applying even a little effort as to how a poor diet might contribute to depressive illness, most owners receive antidepressant prescriptions.

Many patented prescriptions have been created to address nutritional deficiencies in peripheral ways. These medications circuitously improve depressive symptoms by keeping the deficient neurotransmitter around for a longer time within the active little spaces between nerves, the synapse. However, proper nutrition will increase the amount of neurotransmitter available within the different nerve cells of the body, as well. In addition, proper nutrition replacement therapy avoids side effects.

The science behind the necessary nutritional molecular components for optimal neurotransmitter production has been understood for years. Unfortunately, instead of advising owners on ways to increase their own neurotransmitter production rates, prescription medications remain the treatment of choice.

Certain nutritional factors need to exist before sufficient neurotransmitters can be manufactured. Optimal neurotransmitters amounts prevent depression. When a certain neurotransmitter's manufacture rate fails, predictable mental symptomatology follows. Paradoxically, rather than augment the deficiency through nutritional intervention, these owners receive counsel that they have a biochemical imbalance.

By labeling depression in ways that imply genetic determinism, the owner's ability to heal him/her self appears unlikely. The truth of this intellectual roadblock proves suspect but never the less perpetuates. A disincentive exists to share with doctors and patients the ability of directed nutritional reformation to overcome many inherited weaknesses within one's DNA. The appalling nutrition contained in the typical American diet accelerates the inherited weakness. In turn these inherited genetic weaknesses respond to symptom-control methods by peripheral pathways in the brain.

The symptom-control approach involves prescribing the various drugs that increase the length of time that the neurotransmitters occur within the little spaces between the nerves. These prescriptions do nothing to increase production of the deficient neurotransmitter. They only prolong how long the neurotransmitter gets to signal its message within the active little spaces, the synapse.

In marginally depleted owners, this approach has potential to help, but with a price. The price depends on the class of antidepressant agent given (see earlier discussion). Very few owners receive counseling concerning what needs to happen nutritionally, for normal neurotransmitter production rates to occur. Instead, they are told that they have a biochemical imbalance and this follows to imply that it is genetic in its causality.

Some owners prefer a trial of nutritional supplementation before they embark on symptom-control medicine. Nutritional supplementation covers the other side of the story of what science has long ago revealed about the cause of some depressive illnesses. The largely untold facts include the central nutritional molecular building parts and chemical reaction facilitators (vitamins). These molecular building parts and chemical reaction facilitators prove necessary within the brain for neurotransmitter biosynthesis to occur. If these factors arrive in reliable and constant supplies to the central nervous system the need for prescription medicine often disappears.

Many conventionally trained physicians receive little education about the important nutritional pathways that bring about optimal neurotransmitter levels. How convenient to leave some basic nutritional science out of the educations of the certified experts.

Earlier in this chapter, the most common neurotransmitters were reviewed and some of their manufacture requirements were discussed. The previous discussion contained the potential downside of several antidepressant classes. Here a brief summary follows on what nutritionally needs to pass into the brain in order for different neurotransmitters' biosynthesis to occur.

Serotonin (arousal states): Adequate tryptophan in the diet serves as its basic building block precursor. Sufficient stomach acid and digestive juices need to secrete once tryptophan occurs in a meal. Failure to separate tryptophan from a protein containing meal results in its deficiency.

Vitamins needed for its manufacture: tetrahydrobiopterin (made from folate) and pyridoxal phosphate (Vitamin B6).

Dopamine (pleasure and fine motor coordination): The amino acids tyrosine and phenylalanine can serve as its basic precursor building blocks. Again sufficient stomach acid and digestive juices need to secrete or deficiency occurs.

Vitamins needed for its biosynthesis: tetrahydrobiopterin (made from folate), pyridoxal phosphate (vitaminB6)

Norepinephrine (mental alertness): Dopamine is needed as its building block precursor. Sufficient stomach acid and digestive juices need to secrete or deficiency occurs.

Vitamin C is needed for its biosynthesis

Epinephrine (mental alertness): Norepinephrine serves as its building block. Stomach acid and/or digestive enzyme deficiencies lead to scarcity of this important neurotransmitter and hormone.

Sufficient SAMe allows its biosynthesis to occur. Because one SAMe donates its methyl for each epinephrine made, it becomes rapidly depleted without the methyl donor system adequately recharging it back into its active form.

Methyl Donors recharge system includes: Vitamin B12, Vitamin B6, folate, serine, and methionine. SAMe deficiency shows up as an elevated homocysteine level with laboratory testing of a blood sample. How many clinically depressed owners arise solely from a simple methyl donor deficiency nutrient?

Understand that tyrosine and phenylalanine lead to the sequential manufacture of dopamine, followed by norepinephrine, and lastly, epinephrine. Epinephrine deficiency is most likely because deficiencies anywhere along the assembly line will prevent its manufacture. Where the nutritional deficiency occurs becomes the point that a neurotransmitter's manufacture stops. In other words, epinephrine deficiency proves most vulnerable because it relies on the most vitamins for its manufacture.

Many depressive illnesses arise from deficient epinephrine neurotransmitter levels. One clue to the immense scope of the problem concerns the clinical observation that many dieters taking ephedra (epinephrine-like) note a marked improvement in their depressive symptoms. Many other benefits derive from epinephrine-like medication, such as: diminished insulin secretion, allergy relief, and mental alertness.

One needs to keep these benefits in mind and contrast them against the many patented and expensive drugs that would no longer be in demand if the public ever found out about these benefits. Re-including these facts into the ongoing mainstream media campaign against ephedra begins to provide the other side of the story for why the complex feels so strongly against ephedra. After all, there are several over the counter drugs that have proven to be much more dangerous. Where is the consumer protection from these patented drugs?

Histamine (consciousness and arousal): Histadine is the amino acid building block. Pyridoxal phosphate (Vitamin B6) is needed for its biosynthesis.

GABA (calm states): Glutamic acid is the building block amino acid precursor needed.

An important aside about GABA is that its production within the central nervous system depends on adequate progesterone levels. People that have diminished progesterone levels for too long tend to be anxious and irritable. This situation commonly occurs in peri-menopausal females up to two weeks before their periods (PMS).

The other irritability factor that always needs to be considered involves the amount of sodium relative to potassium intake. Potassium has a calming effect within the central nervous system (CNS). It probably has to do with an adequate force field (cell voltage).

Pyridoxal phosphate (Vitamin B6) is the vitamin needed for biosynthesis of GABA to occur.

The advice of a nutritionally competent physician will facilitate the correct replacement dosages and regimens. In addition, some attention needs to be directed at the integrity of the digestive tract. Improperly functioning digestive tracts will frustrate attempts to heal nutrition deficiency caused depression. In some of these cases, intravenous vitamin therapy may be warranted while the digestive problem resolves.

A caveat now occurs regarding supplementation to correct certain neurotransmitter deficiencies. The salt of glutamic acid is known as glutamate. It is popularly known as monosodium glutamate (MSG) and it often hides within ingredients such as vegetable flavorings, hydrolyzed protein and spices. Glutamate is the most powerful neurotransmitter for nerve excitation. Too much glutamate can excite a nerve cell to death. Nerve cell death results from over stimulation. Over stimulation of a nerve cell leads to a draining down of the nerve cell force field (cell voltage). When the nerve cell force field depletes, the massive in rushing of unwanted charged particles like calcium follows. Too much calcium within a cell binds to its enzymes and delicate structures and this causes cell injury.

Just eliminating this salt from one's diet can often enhance memory. This improvement occurs because nerve cells need to generate an adequate force field (cell voltage) to be able to work efficiently. Molecules like glutamate continually discharge the force field's energy. The memory nerve's force field depletes because the over stimulation of their membrane leads to the discharge of the concentration difference between important minerals. As the concentration difference between these important minerals about the nerve cell membrane decreases, the protection energy depletes (the force field has run down).

Acetylcholine (abstract thinking ability): The first building block precursors for its manufacture comes from consuming adequate choline in the diet, mostly from fish and eggs. The second building block precursor is acetate, which can be derived from all fuel sources (protein, fat and carbohydrates) but only when adequate vitamin levels are present (chapter 16). However, within the brain, it derives only from carbohydrate.

Low fat diet adherents make it hard on their methyl donor system. With appropriate types and amounts of fat intake, the methyl donor system donates a carbon at approximately one billion times a second. However, unless low fat diet adherents have even more methyl donors available than normal, their acetylcholine levels will tend to fall off. The acetylcholine levels will fall off because deficient fat intake leads to an increased need for the methyl donor system to synthesize choline from scratch. The more severe the fat deficiency becomes, the greater the burden on one's methyl donor system. The amount of methyl donor that one needs will sky rocket towards much higher levels per second.

An additional potential problem exists that regards the procurement of acetate within the brain for the manufacture of acetylcholine and other fat-building blocks within the brain. This problem arises from the fact that the brain only uses carbohydrate for its acetate creation (explained earlier). This limitation means that all five nutritional cofactors need to be present in order for the brain to convert glucose to acetate. Specifically the rate-limiting step in question involves the conversion of pyruvate to acetate. Scientists call the enzyme complex that performs this task, pyruvate dehydrogenase.

This enzyme needs five additional co-factors or acetate formation will not be possible. The five cofactors necessary are: Vitamins B1, B2, B3, pantothenic acid, and lipoic acid. Processed food often proves depleted in pantothenic acid and lipoic acid. The fact that it has been re-fortified with a little of the B vitamins proves unhelpful in these cases. This consequence results from the fact that like other chemical sequenced reactions in the body the depleted nutrient acts like a broken link in a chain. Everything stops at this point. What makes this situation even more alarming is that vitamin supplements often prove deficient in these two needed nutrients unless an owner specifically takes them individually.

Chapter 6: Attention Deficit Hyperactivity Disorder and Other Childhood Disordered Brain Function Pathologies

More than 9 million children take stimulant medications for inattention and hyperactivity. An additional 500 thousand suffer from autism. In between attention deficit hyperactivity disorder and autism are other brain dysfunction syndromes like: obsessive-compulsive disorder (OCD) and dyslexia. Jeff Bradstreet, MD. calls these the autism spectrum disorders. He points out that although they share overlapping common symptoms, which provide valuable clues for effectively treating them with holistic strategies, they also have their own unique features. The eventual outcome for a child with one of these disorders depends on whom the parents trust for their medical advice.

The human brain contains more fat weight than nerve weight. Brain fats are unique in their composition compared with other body structural fats. Because they are unique, their manufacture requires numerous minerals, cofactors and vitamins. An often-overlooked consequence of the brain's high fat composition concerns its rapid metabolic rate. A high metabolic rate means that these tissues are exposed to free radicals more often. Free radicals cause oxidation to the structural fats that make up the brain. Throughout life, replacement processes remedy this ongoing problem. The replacement of damaged brain fats can only occur smoothly when adequate molecular replacement parts exist. One acquires adequate replacement parts through proper absorption of the dietary fats that the brain needs or through nutritional supplementation.

Numerous government studies have documented that the majority of American children are nutritionally deficient at multiple levels. Some common examples are: Vitamin A, magnesium, essential fatty acids, zinc, Vitamin C, B Vitamins, and Vitamin E. All these nutrients that American children so profoundly lack also comprise some of the nutrients critically needed to manufacture new structural brain fats. Children experience additional vulnerability because these brains not only need to replace damaged fats but they also need to grow.

Somewhere between the child victim of a dysfunctional brain and the treatment offered by mainstream medicine, basic brain nutritional science remains ignored. Furthermore, the digestion impairments, toxic loads, metabolic and immune defects commonly found in these patients, are effectively downplayed or marginalized.

One pediatrician, Jeff Bradstreet, M.D. has devoted his practice to helping more than 1500 of these patients a year to improve their brain function through attention towards improved brain nutrition, immune function, liver detoxification and digestive tract healing. He reports success rates that leave prescription drugs, with all their side effects, in the undesirable and primitive category.

One of the consequences of living in a profit driven health care system concerns the vigorous attacks that arise towards people like Dr. Bradstreet because they effect drug sales. Healing has only one side effect: the impact on the complex's bottom line.

Mechanisms for Brain Malfunction in Children:
    Allergens, environmental toxins like mercury, persistent viral infections, maldigestion, intestinal inflammation, sulfation defects, inflammatory fats (the hydrogenated fats) that incorporate into the brain, altered mineral intake, and nutritional deficiencies.

Solutions to Consider (a brief overview)

    Specific molecular parts that replace and stabilize the malfunctioning brain components

    Special brain fats like; phosphatidal serine, phosphatidal choline (lecithin) and essential fatty acids. Avoid hydrogenated fats intake.

Specific molecular building components needed to make these specialized brain fats from, like, the methyl donor system (serine, methionine, folate, Vitamin B6 and Vitamin B12).

Specific minerals that the brain needs to power up its neurons and drive protective chemical reactions like; zinc, magnesium, selenium and potassium.

Digestive Enzymes that Deactivate Toxins, Help Assimilate Nutrients and Obliterate Allergens

Many of these brain dysfunction children continue to suffer because no one helps them improve their leaky gut and faulty digestive process. Orally supplementing with digestive enzymes helps with these three mechanisms of injury.

Improve the Detoxification Abilities of the Liver

Environmental toxin exposures, which are "safe" for adults, are poorly handled in infancy during a critical period of brain development.

Liver detoxification ability impairs with: nutritional deficiencies, increased GI tract toxin load, increased environmental toxin load, and genetic predisposition for a defect to metabolize certain toxins (sulfation defects).

These are more completely explained in the liver health appendix but the high prevalence of sulfation defects deserves brief mention. Decreased ability to sulfate biological molecules predisposes to leaky gut. Leaky guts allow toxins to seep towards the liver that are normally confined to the GI tract. Decreased sulfation ability also impairs the liver's ability to secrete toxin loads. Extra toxins in the blood stream penetrate into the brain and cause injury there. One study showed that 100% of autism spectrum disorder children suffered from abnormal liver detoxification pathways.

Supplementing with various forms of sulfur in these children therefore proves cornerstone. Examples of these supplements are: MSM, N-acetyl cysteine, garlic, onions and methionine.

The mainstream medical doctors are taught to treat ADHD with counseling and stimulant prescriptions. This approach ignores the basic nutritional science of what a healthy brain needs to maintain itself. It also ignores the common immune, metabolic and GI tract difficulties experienced by these children. In the end, the child's brain function will undoubtedly deteriorate until these holistic factors are addressed. The mainstream literature admits that drugs have not proved of value in the long term. They further agree about the side effects from their use including high blood pressure and growth stunting. Dr. Bradstreet, on the other hand, has proven the benefits of the above modalities but very few are listening. The health care revolution endeavors to change that.

SECTION 3: Skinny on Fat

Chapter 7: The Real Reason Americans get Fatter Each Year is a Secret

Obesity: Deactivating the Fat-making Machinery

Seven factors activate the fat-making machinery:

1. The glandular component
2. Reversed mineral ratios diet component (section 2)
3. Lack of exercise
4. Unmanaged stress (also discussed in chapters 13 and 14)
5. High carbohydrate diets (the "torture chamber" diet)
6. Vitamin And trace mineral deficiencies (nutritional deficiencies which propagate fat accumulation and impede its usage){see chapter 15}
7. The psychological compnent (see *Glandular Failure-caused Obesity and the writings of Dr. Herb Joiner-Bey*)

Overview of the problems associated with other popular diets

The Glandular component

Six glands control the amount of body fat:

1. Pituitary
2. Thyroid
3. Liver
4. Pancreas
5. Adrenals (adrenaline and steroid compartments)
6. Gonads (the ovaries or testicles)

The big problem in America is that most overweight owners have not had these glands' function checked in a scientifically sufficient manner. Obesity always contains a glandular component to its causality. Until one identifies the scope of the glandular component and it receives focus towards correction, the owner stays stuck within the "torture chamber" of worsening obesity.

Popular diets available today are incomplete for various reasons. The first problem concerns their incomplete attention to the fat-making hormones. Successful weight loss requires consideration of seven basic fat-maker related hormones - insulin, cortisol, androgens, estrogen, insulin-like growth factor type one (IGF-1), thyroid and epinephrine. In addition, indirect but important influences occur from the amount of growth hormone and prolactin secreted by the pituitary. One needs to consider these hormones first before starting any weight loss plan. Imbalances in the pituitary secretions cause disproportioned amounts in the basic seven hormones listed above. Obesity propagates as the result of inappropriately proportioned relationships between these basic seven hormones. Weight loss becomes prevented and fat production becomes promoted when these seven hormones imbalance.

Theoretically, there are even more fat-maker related hormones. The jury is still out on how they really relate to the overall fat-making machinery in the body. Rather than add these mysterious and inconclusive weight loss benefit hormones to the discussion, the tried and true hormones listed above will be the focus of this chapter. Meanwhile, the academicians can fight about these theoretical and peripheral hormones for gaining and losing fat.

Popular high protein diets fail to manipulate all seven basic hormones that contribute as determiners of obesity. A successful diet must affect the hormone-based urge to consume food. In addition, it must inhibit the fat-making hormones and encourage the fat burning hormones. The power of these hormone messages constitutes an important concept for weight loss and other health successes.

High protein/good fat and low carbohydrate diets improve the probability for weight loss by partially addressing hormone imbalance. Eating protein and good fats instead of carbohydrates **reduces insulin need**– the fat-maker. Using this principle also turns down the appetite center in the brain.

The Mineral Component

High protein diets often fail by creating a mineral imbalance between sodium and potassium. When mineral imbalances occur, weight loss curtails because the body requires increased insulin secretion for even a small amount of carbohydrate intake ((chapter 8). In this case, the failure rate becomes secondary to overlooking the importance of mineral balance.

The weakness in the high protein diet turns out to be the strength of some other diets. For example, the high fruit, vegetable, and unprocessed grain diets often have superior mineral balance content. These diets fail because of the other hormonal imbalances they perpetuate in the already obese owner.

(side bar - Correcting these diet defects will be explored throughout this section. The ideal diet combines the best of each diet and eliminates the part that sucks the owner back into the "torture chamber". Understanding how the seven different body hormones either help or hinder weight loss proves essential. Later, the mineral needs of the body will be explained. Implementing these interrelating factors allows overweight owners to start on healing paths.)

The Stress-Filled Lifestyle Component

Chronic mental stress provides another fat-maker messenger. Unlike physical stress, mental stress causes an increase of insulin within the body. Until the obese owner receives counseling on the ways to side step this hormonal havoc weight loss efforts will fail. How stress affects fat accumulation will be explained in the stress response discussion.

The Movement Component

Weight loss success cannot occur without an increase in body movement. Move or die. The body was designed to move around and resist the forces of gravity. Sedentary owners succumb to the shrinking forces that lead to old age: little muscles, little organs, weakened bones and loosened skin. The same lifestyle habits that lead to shrinkage in the above organ systems also contribute to an increase in body fat. Sedentary owners doom themselves to defeat until they assimilate an active lifestyle into the equation (chapter 8).

The Nutritional Deficiency Component

Another component of the successful dietary approach concerns the necessity of certain vitamins for the removal of body fat. The science is all there but it paradoxically collects dust. One of the reasons it remains largely ignored arises from the disjointed and circuitous manner that it presents within the medical textbooks. Until these nutritional facts are organized in a way that both doctors and patients can understand, fat will continue to accumulate from nutritional deficiencies (chapters 13-16).

Ironically, America is the land of the nutritional deficiency diseases: obesity, heart disease, high blood pressure and diabetes.

The final component for obesity's creation concerns the psychology of obesity's perpetuation. Stepping outside the ""torture chamber"" causes stress and anxiety. The comfort of the chamber, even though it tortures, is better than the unknown of feeling healthy and fully alive. This topic because of its bredth is beyond the scope of this manual and the reader is referred to the work of Dr. Herb Joiner-Bey.

Owners that understand the interconnectedness of these components are empowered to heal. Diets fail but insight heals. Healing often involves nothing more than a heightened awareness of how one became fat and how one loses fat. Awareness allows focus. Getting fat did not occur overnight. Likewise, shedding fat takes time. Most owners that follow the program outlined below will shed between fifty and one hundred pounds in the first year. In addition, they will gain back muscle, organ size, bone mass and skin health. In each success case, it all started with a brave first step into a new life of healing. Many other steps of awareness follow the first step. This chapter guides by creating awareness for an individual's solution to heal their weight problem.

The Glandular Component

Gland secretions play a powerful role in the creation of body fat and constitute the starting point for a successful weight loss plan.

Glands secrete information into the blood stream. The types and amounts of these various secretions determine how the body's 100 trillion cells spend their energy. Optimal secretions facilitate the right amount of 'raw blood fuel' (amino acids, fat, and sugar), cell nutrition, and cell function. Poor secretions facilitate manufacturing increased fat, decreased organ function, and accelerate the aging process.

The glands, listed above, secrete various hormones that affect the gaining and losing of fat. Hormones carry information to the body cells via the blood stream. The blood stream contains a 'sea' of information that changes, as the body needs change.

All hormones' message content (information) concerns how the cells direct their energy expenditure.

Obese owners have the problem in one way or another of too much body energy being directed into the storage of energy.

In addition, because obese owners have too much food energy directed into storage as fat, their cells are always hungry. These owner's cells will remain hungry until their hormone contained information changes into a message of fuel availability. Available body fat becomes fuel that combusts in the cell power plants.

The body stores energy mostly as fat. The ideally weighted person stores about 80,000 calories as body fat. The obese person stores many times this amount.

No matter what the body weight becomes, only 2,000 calories can be stored as sugar within the liver and muscle cells as glycogen. A cognizance of these relative amounts of storage abilities between these two fuel groups helps to elucidate the fundamental fat-making problem. Many pinheads pontificate the platitude about losing weight being a simple matter of restricting calories. Oh if it were only that simple. Hormones direct whether fuel stores or fuel burns up in the cell power plants. By definition pinheads do not remember their basic science.

Losing weight requires attention toward redirecting fuel energy away from storage as fat.

The hormones giveth and the hormones taketh away. Hormones direct how the body treats body fuel (sugars, proteins, and fat). The right hormones within, minute to minute, create a balance between storage and combustion of these fuels. Healthy owners always possess hormone balance. Unhealthy owners always suffer from hormone imbalance. Ironically, American health care often overlooks this basic fact for how one becomes fat.

Until the quality of the hormones within improve, weight loss efforts end in defeat.

Fortunately, out of the over 100 body hormones only 7 types centrally affect the making and losing of body fat. Two other hormones influence the central seven.

The glandular composite "hormone report card" is essential at the beginning of any weight loss effort.

The initial "hormone report card" includes:
1. **Fasting insulin and C-peptide levels**
2. **Fasting insulin-like growth factor type 1 (IGF-1) levels**
3. **Adrenal steroids (including aldosterone)**
4. **Androgen-type gonad steroids (from the ovaries or testes)**
5. **Thyroid hormones' levels (including reversed T3)**
6. **Estrogen status for both men and women**
7. **Epinephrine urinary output (metanephrine and normetanephrine) alternatively obtain a homocysteine level**
8. **Prolactin level**
9. **Growth hormone levels (surmised by looking at the amount of androgens and IGF-1 levels)**

Each of the first seven hormone types has a specific role in the overall message that directs the manufacturing of fat (energy storage). Prolactin has special fat-making properties through its effect on some of the first seven hormone types. Lastly, growth hormone directly influences the amount of IGF-1 released. In practice, it makes more clinical sense to measure IGF-1 levels instead of growth hormone levels.

Another fact about some of the obesity-causing hormones becomes important. Specifically, steroids and thyroid hormones are among the most powerful class of body hormones. I call these select few most powerful hormones, the level one-type hormones.

These most powerful body hormones, with the addition of Vitamin A, are the only body hormones that possess the ability to directly instruct the DNA (genetic programs) within the 100 trillion body cells. All other body hormones cannot directly instruct the DNA programs within cells, if at all. DNA programs (genes) activity determine whether or not body cells spend energy wisely or unwisely. Obesity results from the unwise use of available body energy. The hormone message content that the cells receive determines body energy usage. Message content (information) to all body cells conveys by the body hormones via the blood stream. The blood stream can be thought of as a sea of information that changes as the body's needs change. Bad information within the blood stream results from the wrong hormones secreting. Hormones direct how the body spends or saves energy. Too much energy storage message content results in excessive fat.

Many of the obesity-causing hormones are amongst the most powerful type because they uniquely direct the DNA programs into activity or silence. The activity or silence of the DNA programs within one's 100 trillion cells powerfully determines calorie expenditure. DNA program activity also determines repair versus disrepair within a cell. Parts of the reason owners gain fat results from their most powerful hormones, which instruct their DNA, being imbalanced.

Here lies the central explanation for why obesity associates with an accelerated aging rate. The hormone mismatches, which either allow or creates obesity, are among the most powerful body hormones.

(Side bar for physicians) Vitamin A and its Steroid like Properties

By its name, one immediately misunderstands Vitamin A (retinol). Unlike almost all other vitamins, Vitamin A contains message content by virtue of its molecular shape. In addition, Vitamin A has the ability to go anywhere within the body and deliver message content to the DNA program of a cell. In contrast, other vitamins work by facilitating chemical reactions within the cells. Vitamin A behaves more consistently as a hormone. By calling it a vitamin, this creates a tendency to hit an intellectual roadblock that needs to be crossed in order to appreciate the consequences of this molecule's deficiency or excess. A "real food" diet (chapter 8) would supply ample Vitamin A and little tendency to develop deficiency of this important substance.

Vitamin A must be obtained in the diet and can become toxic, at high levels, because at high levels it amplifies its instructional content of cellular DNA beyond healthful parameters. The only way to overdose on Vitamin A results from ingesting high dosage supplements (above 50,000 IU a day or about two carrots a day) for over three months. Some individuals can ingest much higher amounts without toxicity. After all, 50,000 IU's equals only 50mg. Too much Vitamin A causes thinning hair, dry and scaly skin, bone spur formation, and brittle bones.

Too little Vitamin A leads to diminished functional abilities of cells that coat the body (skin and cornea) and cells that line body cavities (the gastrointestinal tract and lungs). Conditions like ichthyosis vulgaris result from Vitamin A deficiency. Skin cancers are promoted by this deficiency as well. Yet, little encouragement comes from physicians for decreasing cancer risks by taking adequate Vitamin A. Adequate adrenal function depends on Vitamin A to instruct adrenal cell DNA activation programs. In the healthful state, the liver fills up with Vitamin A and releases it as needed.

Vitamin A denotes a complex of similar vitamins that promote cell maturity. Immature cells form a central property of

> cancer cells. AdequateVVitamin A complex intake provides a cornerstone for the prevention of cancer. Almost all cells contain DNA programs that respond to the message content of Vitamin A complex. Some Vitamin A derivatives occur in plant seeds. These prevent cell division until their removal when the right conditions occur. For example the right conditions occur when the planting technique proves correct. Likewise, within the body, Vitamin A's message content involves keeping the cells from undergoing rampant cell division. This fact continues to be almost entirely ignored by mainstream cancer specialist in their attempts to stop cancer cell division (tumor growth).
>
> Lastly, the thyroid hormone properly activates the DNA programs within the body's 100 trillion cells only if sufficient Vitamin A message content occurs. Some clinically low thyroid function patients arise solely from Vitamin A deficiency. When this causes the clinical symptoms of low thyroid function the thyroid test routinely done at the doctor's office will come back normal!

When the most powerful body hormones are out of kilter, not only obesity, but other health problems become encouraged because body energy becomes misdirected.

For example, instead of rejuvenation hormone message content directed, at cell repair processes being heard by body cells excessive body energy channels into to fuel storage activities (fat manufacture).

This fact partly explains why obesity increases the risk of heart disease, diabetes, high blood pressure, and arthritis (middle age related disease). Each of these diseases has a large component of causality in the abnormal hormones associated with obesity. This is good news because it means that by correcting the obesity-causing hormones it will also impact the middle age related diseases.

The basic seven hormone types, when imbalanced, cause obesity (note: these are all glandular secretions)

Thyroid hormones
Insulin
Insulin-like growth factor type one (IGF-1)
Cortisol
Androgens
Estrogen
Epinephrine

The additional two pituitary secreted hormones, prolactin and growth hormone, influence the amounts of the basic seven.

1. **Thyroid hormones** (T3 and T4) **direct the DNA to increase the manufacture rate of cellular mineral pumps and furnace combustion chamber components.**
   The lack of thyroid message content within an owner's body diminishes the furnace flames within his/her one hundred trillion cells. The most reliable manifestation of low thyroid gland function is a low body temperature upon waking.

   A poorly functioning thyroid gland leads to a decrease in its message content to the numerous body cells. One component of the thyroid hormone message concerns its directions to invest in furnace component upgrades. Scientists call the furnace or power plant of the cell the mitochondrion. Poorly functioning mitochondrion are analogous to heating one's home with a furnace that contains worn out components and plugged air filters. For the same reasons that these homes remain cold, an owner with worn out mitochondrion components in his cells stays cold.

Most body cells prefer fat as their fuel source. All body cells need certain key vitamins to process raw body fuels (protein, carbohydrate, and fat) into a processed fuel called acetate. Acetate is the simplest fatty acid. No matter what the raw fuel (protein, sugar or fat) consists of, before it can burn up in the cell power plant, it needs refining into acetate. The different raw fuels need specific and numerous vitamins to process into the refined fuel, acetate. Many owners have weight gain simply because they lack the necessary vitamins to turn raw fuel into refined fuel (chapter 16).

The cell furnaces can only burn acetate within their combustion chambers. This last fact is analogous to the requirement for refined fuels within power generators of the physical world. For example, automobile engine design usually requires the refinement of raw oil into gasoline. In general the combustion chamber of each power generator is designed to work only with a certain fuel type.

Similarly, the numerous body cell furnaces can only combust one fuel type. Therefore, many thyroid problems are made worse by specific vitamin deficiencies that impede the processing of raw body fuels into acetate. A diminished delivery of the refined fuel, acetate, will exaggerate weight gain because it tends to contribute to hungry cells (chapter 16).

Thyroid hormones deliver an additional message to the body cells beyond its heat creating effect within the numerous cell furnaces. The additional message involves its ability to direct the creation of membrane pumps that trap some of this heat energy for useful work. Again, this is similar to a car engine creating heat but some of the energy is used to move the car down the road by engaging the drive train. Power plants also lose energy to heat but some of this energy is trapped in the form of electricity.

The body cells also operate on an electrical system. A cell's ability to charge its membrane proves critical to life. The energy needed to charge the cell membrane derives from the energy trapped within the mitochondrion combustion chamber in the form of adenosine triphosphate (ATP). The more ATP (energy currency of the cell) available determines one aspect of how high a cell can charge its membrane. Membrane pumps charge the cell membranes. Membrane pumps need the energy contained in ATP to pump up the electrical charge (increase the voltage) contained in the cell membrane. The constant supply of ATP needs to occur or the electrical charge contained in the membrane diminishes and the cell dies.

Thyroid message content provides the informational direction that tells specific DNA programs to activate. In turn, these activated and specific DNA programs direct the manufacture of more membrane-contained mineral pumps. The zillions of membrane pumps within the membranes of all cells of a body are made from proteins, which are coded for by the specific DNA programs (genes) mentioned above.

The more mineral pumps within the cell's membrane; an additional determinant of higher membrane electrical charge becomes satisfied. **The greater the 100 trillion body cell's cumulative electrical charge, the more calories burned to maintain it.** In fact, the cell membrane mineral pumps comprise the reason that most calories burn up within the body. Fewer mineral pumps lead to fewer calories burned. Fewer calories burned leads to a lower metabolic rate.

Body cells utilize the electrical charge within the membrane to perform the cellular work of living. The more work performed, the more calories combusted. This is analogous to the charge within the membranes of a car battery, which can be drawn upon to power the electrical gadgetry within the automobile. Similarly, the cell power plants recharge the cell membrane like the car's engine recharges the car battery.

All body cells protect themselves and perform work by utilizing the energy contained in their membranes. Fully charged cells are maximally alive. Fully charged cells burn more energy (fat). The more energy consumed, the more calories consumed. Remember, the body cells cannot fully charge without the proper proportions of mineral intake within the diet (the third determinant of cell membrane charge).

For now, it is important to summarize the two main messages that the thyroid hormone conveys to many different body cells. 1) Carries to the DNA the message to invest in furnace component upgrades. 2) Carries to the DNA the additional message to create more mineral pumps within the membrane, which charges the cell electrically. Only when both of these processes occur smoothly can a normal amount of calories burn.

Certain DNA programs need the additional presence of sufficient Vitamin A message content to activate what the thyroid hormone message started. In this way, Vitamin A and thyroid hormones work synergistically.

2. Insulin Carries the Fat-maker Message and IGF-1 Competes with the Fat-maker Message

Insulin is made and secreted by the pancreas

IGF-1 within the blood stream is made and secreted by the liver

There are only two hormones that allow the cell fuel tanks to fill up. It helps to think of these two hormones as **"fuel nozzle" hormones**. Just as in filling a car with fuel, a "fuel nozzle" is necessary, so it is with most body cell. A molecular 'nozzle' is necessary to fill the 'tanks' of the cells with the fuel circulating in the blood stream.

The two "fuel nozzle" hormones are insulin and insulin-like growth factor type 1 (IGF-1). Healthy people have at least 100 times more IGF-1 compared to insulin in their blood streams. Each of these two "fuel nozzle" hormones has a preference for the cell types it prefers to fill up. Because roughly 100 times more cells exist that prefer IGF-1, it makes sense that healthy people have at least 100 times this hormone as compared to insulin. Only when the body becomes unhealthy and IGF-1 levels consequently fall off, will the body attempt to raise insulin hormone production rates to keep the total amount of "fuel nozzle" hormones constant. Hungry cells result when "fuel nozzle" hormones become scarce.

However, the insulin hormone contains message content that the IGF-1 hormone does not share. Insulin contains the fat-maker message. Overweight people have a problem with too much fat-maker message. Until the fat-maker message decreases, they will continue to gain weight, year after year.

Body fat is not possible without enough insulin message content to maintain it. The other six hormone types of obesity, when unbalanced, facilitate the amplification of the insulin message. Healthy people have almost no insulin in the fasting state but have high amounts of IGF-1 instead.

Unhealthy and obese people have higher fasting insulin and/or C-peptide and lower IGF-1 levels. Therefore, at the start of any dietary program obtaining these values for a baseline is critical for a successful weight loss. Insulin's major message concerns fuel storage.

Consistent with this fact is the increase in insulin following meals. The majority of the insulin message directs the liver to store up to 400 grams of glycogen within the liver. When the liver already has enough glycogen stored, the insulin message directs the liver to convert the additional sugar into fat and cholesterol.

The opposite situation occurs between meals because blood fuel tends to drop off. In these situations, fuel needs to be released from the liver and not stored. New supplies of fuel need to be present in the blood stream to constantly provide nourishment to the body cells. Blood fuel content delivery, into the body cells, is not possible without adequate "fuel nozzle" hormones available to facilitate this process. In healthy people, when the body's cell fuel levels begin to fall off, the resupply of fuel occurs via the other "fuel nozzle" hormone called insulin-like growth factor type 1 (IGF-1).

IGF-1 occurs at levels greater than 100 times that of insulin in healthy people. This hormone's design helps the body cells outside the liver and fat cells to procure the fuel they need. IGF-1 levels, within the blood stream of healthy owners, are 100 times insulin levels even following meals because its half-life is four days. In contrast, insulin's half-life is about ten minutes. IGF-1 levels increase slightly between meals, while exercising, and in the fasting state. Two other hormone types and two lifestyle habits need to occur for adequate IGF-1 levels to be maintained beyond middle age.

The two hormones are: Growth hormone and androgen. Growth hormone releases from the pituitary gland when blood fuel levels fall off (decreased energy substrate is the confusing term used in medical texts). Growth hormone release tells the liver to release more IGF-1 and fuel (sugar and fat). Androgens, like testosterone and DHEA, tell the liver DNA programs to activate towards the manufacture of more IGF-1. Androgen causes IGF-1 creation and growth hormone causes IGF-1 release. Normal blood stream IGF-1 levels require both normal growth hormone release and androgen levels (testosterone or DHEA).

Sufficient androgens, like DHEA and testosterone, direct the liver to make adequate IGF-1. There are others but for now these two provide the basics.

Sufficient growth hormone secretion causes the liver to release the manufactured IGF-1 into the blood stream

> **The lifestyle habit concerns the fact that the blood fuel falls between meals (fasting) and when one exercises. Consequently, these two habits encourage the release of growth hormone. This knowledge explains why chronically underfeeding (fasting) both in animals and humans results in a lengthened life span. The underfed human will tend to secrete more growth hormone. Increased growth hormone arriving at the healthy liver chronically will help promote elevated IGF-1 levels. Elevated IGF-1 levels provide the nutritional advantage to the organs, bones and muscles of the body. Whereas, elevated insulin provides the nutritional advantage to the liver where more fat and cholesterol manufacture occurs.**

Adequate IGF-1 in the blood stream facilitates the body cells outside of the liver in their procuring nutrition. Adequate insulin, but not too much, facilitates the liver and fat cells in storing fuel following a meal. While exerecising, between meals, or fasting, healthy owners draw down the stored fuel within their liver and fat cells, preventing obesity.

Unhealthy owners exist with a decreased growth hormone secretion rate and hence a diminished IGF-1 level. Death is prevented between meals when their blood fuel falls because two other hormonal aberrations save them. First, the stress response hormones release and activate catabolic pathways. Catabolic means that body structure dismantles to free up more fuel. The body structure is composed of sugar, fat and proteins. Second concerns the exaggerated amounts of insulin needed to help the body cells procure nutrition because IGF-1 levels have fallen. Remember, there needs to be a constant amount of total "fuel nozzles" around to fill the cell fuel tanks. Insulin, in large amounts (insulin resistance) gets past the liver and into the general circulation where it acts much like IGF-1.

Unfortunately, when insulin secretes in large amounts the highest concentration still arrives at the liver, via the portal vein, where the fat and cholesterol-making machinery preferentially activate. The liver and fat cells have the highest pure insulin-type receptor concentration of any cell type in the body at about 200,000 per cell. High insulin and/or C-peptide in the fasting state provide a good laboratory marker for these types of obesity prone owners. Modern literature calls these people Syndrome X, Metabolic Syndrome or Insulin Resistance Syndrome (expanded discussion in chapters 9 and 14).

Interestingly, the fact that these individuals have at the root of their problem a falling IGF-1 level, remains almost universally ignored. In its place, peripheral approaches like cholesterol lowering drugs, drugs that whip the pancreas into even more insulin production, and high blood pressure medication are prescribed. All these accepted approaches do little to heal the underlying problem and have side effects to these owners' health. Until steps are taken to raise these owners

IGF-1 levels, both obesity and accelerated aging will continue to propagate.

Healthy owners achieve the ideal balances between insulin and IGF-1. In these situations, insulin increases following meals and the IGF-1 stays unchanged. Balance between these two hormones allows the liver to uptake a proper proportion of fuel compared to the amount that other body cells are allowed to procure with the assistance of IGF-1 following a meal. The fuel stored by the liver in a healthy person becomes readily available between meals, when exercise or a fast occurs. In all three of these situations, as blood fuel begins to fall, growth hormone releases, which directs the liver to release the stored fuel (sugar and fat) and more IGF-1, but not protein. The extra IGF-1 released further facilitates the hungry body cells' uptake of nutrition.

Unhealthy owners that exist with insulin resistance (increased insulin need because of their diminished IGF-1) possess hungry cells. Hungry cells occur when excessive insulin secretes from the pancreas, providing excessive message content that allows the recipient liver to hog increased nutrition. Increased nutrition sucks up into the liver whether these owners have just eaten or attempt to exercise or go on a fast (explained later). These owners exist within the "torture chamber" of the "hungry cell syndrome". These owner's cells remain hungry until someone explains to them how to decrease their insulin needs. Only after insulin needs fall, will the cells beyond the liver and fat receive the nutrition they desperately require for rejuvenation activities.

Remember that only growth hormone prevents the catabolism of body protein for fuel between meals. Here lies the chronic weakening mechanism when unhealthy people are between meals, fasting or exercising. As their blood fuel falls in these situations the wrong hormones make body protein available for their fuel needs because growth hormone release proves inadequate.

Unhealthy owners also have diminished IGF-1, as a consequence of diminished growth hormone release, following meals and between meals. In both situations, this sets up the need for abnormal secretion rates of insulin (commonly referred to as insulin resistance). Remember, insulin contains the fat-maker message. The higher the insulin secretion rate, the higher the fat-maker message within. Syndrome X owners are doomed until their need for insulin lowers. One of the ways insulin needs fall off is when IGF-1 levels return to normal. IGF-1 contains none of the fat and cholesterol-stimulating message content that insulin contains. Rather, IGF-1 message content concerns itself with the procurement of nutrition (fuel) by other body cell types, outside of the liver and fat cells.

> (Side bar for physicians) The Myth of Insulin Logic
>
> Mainstream medicine's propaganda dogma grooms physicians and patients to focus on insulin as the nutrition uptake hormone. Meanwhile, they ignore the scientific fact that IGF-1 occurs at levels greater than 100 times those of insulin in the healthy individual. The disconnection between this simple optimal ratio maintains itself by arbitrarily measuring insulin in micro units or micromoles and IGF-1 in nanograms, throughout the medical texts. More disconnection results from the fact that numerous different names describe IGF-1. For example, the older medical literature describes IGF-1 in the following additional three ways: Nonsuppressible insulin-like activity of the blood, sulfation factor, and somatomedin C. In order for a physician to appreciate the important role that IGF-1 plays in the cells in obtaining nutrition he/she, would need to be aware of and have time to look up all four of these alternative descriptors for the same hormone. Reconnecting all four different names with the facts associated with them and a common measurement method, allows the important role of IGF-1 to emerge.
>
> Simple logic shows that there is not enough insulin to go around to all body cells. One liver or fat cell contains 200,000 insulin receptors. The 100 times more IGF-1 compared to insulin makes up the volume discrepancy needed to deliver fuel uptake

> message content to the other body cells. Remember, whatever the insulin secretion rate, the liver, because of its portal vein connection to the pancreas, will always receive the highest concentration of insulin message content.

It was briefly mentioned above that unhealthy owners have other hormone increases, which facilitate resupplies of blood fuel between meals. **However, there is a price paid from this aberration to the body structure in the form of lost muscle and organ mass. This largely ignored medical fact explains another consequence of the unhealthy body's lack of sufficient stimulus for growth hormone release.** Only when adequate growth hormone release occurs will there be a sufficient counter message to prevent protein destruction for fuel needs. Muscles depend on sufficient protein. Growth hormone's presence prevents the combusting of protein when blood fuel levels fall. Instead, growth hormone preferentially directs the liver and fat cells to dump sugar and fat into the blood stream while sparring protein. This fact partially explains why healthy owners have nice muscles while unhealthy owners do not.

The basic sequence of protein destruction, when unhealthy owners find themselves between meals and their blood fuel begins to fall, results from other hormones. The entire group consists of glucagon, cortisol and epinephrine. Like growth hormone they all facilitate the release of sugar and fat into the blood stream. Unlike growth hormone body protein dismantling (gluconeogenesis) becomes fair game when growth hormone levels prove insufficient. Here again, another vicious process destroys the physiques of countless middle-aged owners. **The importance of protecting their body protein content needs to be explained to them.** One of the central determiners of body protein content relies on adequate growth hormone levels for the above stated reason.

The other consequence of a falling growth hormone secretion concerns the fact that less IGF-1 releases into the blood stream from the liver. Less IGF-1 release means that the optimal 100:1 ratio between IGF-1 and insulin diminishes. When IGF-1 falls, insulin levels must rise to facilitate a way for the other body cells to procure nutrition. Remember that the "fuel nozzle" total hormone levels, between insulin and IGF-1, needs to stay constant or the body cells become hungry. Therefor,e a fall in IGF-1 necessitates a corresponding rise in insulin to keep the total "fuel nozzle" hormones' level the same.

Picture the anatomy of this imbalance: Portal vein connection between the pancreas and the liver. Secondary to this physiological secretion pathway, the liver will always receive the highest insulin message content for a given secretion rate from the pancreas secreting into the protal vein, which leads directly into the liver.

Remember, the insulin message concerns itself with storing food energy in times of plenty (following a meal). Therefore, the higher the insulin, the more that body fuel tilts towards storage sites (liver and fat cells).

In healthy owners, some insulin is necessary to allow enough fuel storage following meals in order to provide fuel in the between meal state (fasting and exercising). However, the 100 fold greater amounts of IGF-1 present in healthy owners following meals tips the blood fuel towards the body cells outside the liver and fat. This optimal ratio facilitates the sufficient nutrition of the cells throughout the body. Hungry cells occur when insufficient amounts of either insulin or IGF-1 occur. In addition, when insulin must increase to compensate for a falling IGF-1, the fat-making machinery abnormally activates.

The additional troubles within obese owners, such as other hormone abnormalities, chronic mental stress within a sedentary lifestyle setting, nutritional deficiencies, dietary indiscretions and/or mineral deficiencies all diminishes IGF-1 levels (discussions follow later in this chapter and section). The fall in IGF-1 levels means that the peripheral cells possess a decreased ability to uptake nutrition following meals because of the anatomical secretion pathway of insulin from the pancreas straight into the liver first. This anatomical fact results in the liver always receiving the highest concentration of insulin's message content. Abnormally high insulin levels with low IGF-1 levels means cells outside the liver have a decreased ability to obtain nutrition and fuel. Instead the liver, in these cases, obtains the lion's share of body energy and directs it into the storage pathways (fat).

This means that because insulin levels increase their livers make more fat and cholesterol for the same amount of caloric intake. Healing obesity involves facilitating a rise in IGF-1 levels. Weight can then be lost as insulin needs fall off.

Insulin has a half-life of 10 minutes. IGF-1 has a half-life of four days. Because healthy people have adequate IGF-1 levels while fasting or between meals they have no need for insulin during these times.

> **(Physicians side bar) Here lies another valuable clue: why would a body elevate insulin levels in the fasting state?** By definition an elevation of fasting insulin levels is either called Syndrome X or Metabolic Syndrome. The fact that IGF-1 levels diminish in this syndrome is almost completely ignored. Instead, usually a peripheral approach results in prescribing blood pressure medication, cholesterol lowering medication, and insulin increasing medication, which treats only the symptoms of this disease process.
>
> Insulin increases brought on by some diabetes drugs only worsen the obesity problem. The pancreas design was not intended to produce massive amounts of insulin to shore up falling IGF-1 levels. The pancreas is little and the liver is large. IGF-1 at amounts one hundred times insulin is easily produced and secreted by the large liver. The pancreas however has to work itself to death when IGF-1 levels fall even a little bit. The little pancreas was not designed to increase insulin production many fold in order to shore up a falling IGF-1 level. These owners eventually can exhaust their pancreas (beta cell burn out) and this leads to one form of diabetes (chapter 13).

As was previously mentioned, two hormones determine the amount of IGF-1 available and released (there are others but for now the all important first two are discussed). First, the amounts of androgen steroids like testosterone and DHEA secreted. Second, concerns growth hormone secretion rates.

Basically, growth hormone secretes when the brain senses that the blood fuel level has fallen (a decrease in energy substrate is the term used within the medical texts).

Blood fuel levels tend to fall with 2 situations
1. Fasting (between meals)
2. Exercise

The trouble with a sedentary lifestyle and obesity concerns two things:
1. Other associated hormone abnormalities prevent the fall in blood fuel
2. Exercise does not happen

Because of these two processes growth hormone secretion rates drop off. Elevated blood sugars caused by these other hormonal aberrations powerfully inhibit growth hormone release. Stress filled and sedentary lifestyles elevate the blood sugar, as well, and this inhibits growth hormone release for the same reasons (chapter 9). This leads to a decreased secretion rate of IGF-1. The fall in IGF-1 increases the need for more insulin. More insulin message content increases the production rate of changing sugar into fat and cholesterol. These are packaged into LDL cholesterol and move towards the storage depots in the abdomen and macrophages that line the arteries.

Scientific fact: High insulin levels turn on the cholesterol and fat-making machinery. Normal insulin secretion rates lead to a normal cholesterol and fat-manufacture rate. This simple relationship is largely forgotten within the hysteria to sell more cholesterol lowering prescription medication. Cholesterol lowering medication has side effects. Some authorities liken these side effects to the acceleration of the aging process.

Accelerated Aging shows up in the body kingdom periphery first and there is a scientific explanation but it's a secret

(explained like layers of an onion throughout the remainder of this text).

3. Androgen steroids: made in the adrenals and gonads (ovaries and testicles). Their message content always concerns rejuvenation and repair of body cells.

Two major androgen types, one secretes from the gonads and the other from the adrenals.
1. **DHEA secretes mostly from the adrenals**
2. **Testosterone secretes mostly from the gonads**

Remember that steroid hormones are among the most powerful hormone class. Only the most powerful body hormones directly instruct the 100 trillion cell DNA programs. Depending on the steroid type, certain DNA programs (genes) activate or shut down. What the message involves for a given steroid type results from its precise shape. Gene silencing, while a specific steroid binds to it, results in a cessation of protein synthesis for which that gene codes. Gene activation, while a specific steroid binds to it, results in protein synthesis unique to the gene activated.

Proteins constitute the metabolically active component of body tissue. In other words, proteins when active burn up calories. Examples of metabolically active protein types are: enzymes, mineral pumps and cell receptors.

This subsection begins the discussion of the first two types of steroid message content: anabolic versus catabolic. The androgen message (anabolic) concerns itself with rejuvenation (cell repair and build up) activities. The catabolic steroids deliver the opposite message. Catabolic message concerns itself with consuming body structure for the creation of energy. Body structure is made up of fat, carbohydrate and protein. High levels of catabolism make all three raw fuel sources fair game.

One facet of high levels of catabolic steroid's message concerns energy channeling for a perceived survival threat whether real or imagined. The stress response activates this system. **Body structure dismantles itself when the stress response activates in order to maximize available energy.** Stress steroids (the catabolic type) are only made in the adrenal glands. Both the adrenal and gonads manufacture the androgen steroids.

Healthy owners have a balance between survival message content and rejuvenation message content. Unhealthy owners are out of balance between these two opposing messages.

This subsection concerns the androgen message and how it curtails obesity. In the next subsection, the survival message (catabolism) elicited by stress will be reviewed in regards to its perpetrating obesity.

A few words on why only real hormone shapes carry accurate information

Hormones carry information via their precise shape. Steroid hormones are relatively small and simple in the world of other much larger hormones. The smaller the hormone, the more the message will change with even a slight change in shape.

In order to obtain a patent advantage, drug companies must change the shape of the natural body hormone. Natural body hormones deliver precise messages. Unnatural hormones, such as those being patented by drug companies, create profit but because their shape has been altered their message content changes, as well. One prominent example concerns horse estrogen collected from pregnant horse mare's urine. There is some human type estrogen within this mixture of horse estrogens given to millions of women. The pharmaceutical companies cannot get a patent advantage without selling the whole mixture or altering the shape of the hormone and thus creating a deviant product.

However, the mixture also contains unnatural-shaped estrogens that are not found in the human body. The altered shaped estrogens deliver abnormal message content. The message content differs because the shape differs. The unnaturally shaped horse estrogens deliver an altered message to the ingesting owners trillions of cellular DNA programs.

Uzzi Reis M.D. Ob/Gyn author of the book, *Natural Hormone Balance for Women* says it very well. "Are you a horse? Do you eat hay? Then why take horse estrogen?"

Estrogen's role in creating body fat will be discussed more completely in a following subsection. For now realize that estrogen promotes anabolism for fat cells in the body by a circuitous route. The higher estrogen becomes relative to androgen, the larger a women's breast and hips.

Summary recap: For now, it is only important to begin to appreciate that the different types of steroids need to occur in the proper amounts and timing or the message content reaching the DNA becomes altered. Unnatural hormones carry inaccurate message content to the trillions of body cells. Unnatural hormones carry faulty information because their shapes deviate from the natural hormone's shapes. When a steroid hormone's shape is changed to get a patent, the message content changes. Cells that receive altered directions on how to spend their energy manifest as side effects and eventually disease.

One of the side effects when the androgen message diminishes concerns the fact that the afflicted owner's body gets older. Bodies get older when their cells receive diminished instructions to repair and rejuvenate. Androgen-type steroids carry the rejuvenation message content to the body cells. Remember, the androgen message concerns rejuvenation instructions within the trillions of cell DNA programs. It is the lack of rejuvenation message content that accelerates the aging process. Some components of the aging process are the loss of muscle and bone but also the gaining of body fat.

The androgen message contained in testosterone and DHEA shed fat in one important way. Androgens direct the liver DNA programs (genes) to synthesize IGF-1. High IGF-1 blood levels mean that one requires less insulin for their cells to procure their nutritional needs.

Less insulin needed means that the fat-maker message diminishes. Many women notice weight gain after their ovaries are removed. Some of this tendency can be explained by the loss of androgen message content. Healthy ovaries and adrenals make androgens. Increased androgen message content arriving at the liver decreases insulin need because it tells the liver DNA to manufacture more IGF-1.

Weak adrenals incompletely compensate for the removed ovaries. Menopause also brings on diminished ovarian function. Health after menopause depends on healthy adrenals, which produce significant androgens. Many postmenopausal diseases have a component of causality in poorly functioning adrenals. Examples are: osteoporosis, obesity, and chronic fatigue.

A well run 24-hour urine test can check the thyroid hormones, adrenal steroids, and gonad steroids. Over a period, in a typical day, the peaks and valleys of hormone release will average out. In contrast, the standard mainstream approach entails a blood drawn sample for measuring one or two of these important hormones. The instant of the blood draw only measures that instant in time as to where the body directs its energy. Whether the values obtained prove the high or low for the day are not discernible with this approach.

For example, if the act of drawing blood causes stress, the rise in stress hormones, like cortisol, causes the displacement of the bound thyroid hormone fraction and thus artificially increases the true average of this hormone in one's blood stream. Forgetting this fact, doctors often falsely reassure low thyroid functioning patients that their thyroid tested normal when it is not. Taking the time to measure thyroid hormone production over a 24-hour period averages out these peaks and valleys.

The volatility of the blood stream levels makes sense when one realizes that the hormones direct how the body spends its energy. The many different activities and situations of life demand different message content to direct body energy appropriately. The resting state predominantly provides a time when body energy directs into rejuvenation activities. The right hormones need to occur to oversee this process. Likewise, exercise demands different body hormones to direct the freeing up of energy that allows this activity to continue. A blood sample taken in either of these situations would show entirely different results.

Remember that thyroid hormone, all steroid hormones and Vitamin A are among the most powerful body hormones because only these directly instruct the trillions of cell's DNA programs. Only these most powerful hormones directly determine a cell's genetic program activity. The genetic program activity determines which proteins are made. The amounts and types of proteins made by a cell determine its productive capacity, overall integrity, and repair rate. All the many other body hormones cannot directly instruct the DNA programs, if at all.

Keeping these facts in mind it is more logical that the overall mixture of hormones within constitutes an important determinant of health. The overall mixture of hormones within determines the informational direction of how the body spends its energy. Some bodies spend energy wisely and there occurs a continuum all the way down to those bodies that spend energy foolishly.

Healthy bodies have proper proportions of these important hormones directing their cells in the wise use of available energy. The opposite situation exists, in that unhealthy bodies spend their energy unwisely because their hormones are wrong. The wrong hormones result from nutritional habits,

lifestyle habits, patented forms of unnaturally shaped hormones and glandular failure.

All hormone message content concerns how the body directs its energy expenditure. Healing an unhealthy body cannot occur until better informational direction occurs, via the hormones, on how their body spends its energy. Remember, obesity has a component of too much message content directing body energy into storage. Hungry body cells result when too much energy channels into storage (fat).

"Steroid tone" provides a construct that helps quantify the quality of the mixture of blood stream information carried by these important types of body hormones. The steroids are among the most powerful body hormones because they each carry specific message content, inherent in their unique shapes, directly to the DNA. Each specific type's message individually direct the trillions of cell DNA programs (genes). Too much or too little of a particular steroid leads to either excess or deficiency for that message respectively.

Healthy people always have the proper amounts of these most important hormones. This occurrence results in the proper amount of repair to rest ratios within the body cells. Middle age begins to occur when the quality of the information delivered to the cells by these most powerful hormones begins to deteriorate. One of the consequences of middle age with a large component of causality in the deteriorating message content concerns obesity.

Almost all the body cells have a complete genetic program. The genetic program activity determines cell repair rates, rejuvenation rates, functional ability and the overall integrity of the cell. Paradoxically, mainstream medicine often overlooks the central importance, for continued youthfulness,

of bodies possessing correct message content directing their cells.

"Steroid tone" is measured by a well-run 24-hour urine test. It provides a "hormone report card" for these most important body hormones. The more optimal the amounts of the different steroids proportional to one another, the higher the "steroid tone" becomes. Adequate rejuvenation and repair activity occurring requires a sufficient amount of "steroid tone". A high "steroid tone" signifies that there are proper proportions of message content among the various steroids.

In other words, the catabolic message content balances with the anabolic message content. Unhealthy owners will have poor hormone message content. Their health will continue to deteriorate until improvement to the quality of the message that directs their cells occurs.

"Steroid pressure" provides another useful construct that helps to visualize the behavior of steroids once released from their glands of origin. Only the most powerful hormones (steroids, Vitamin A, and thyroid) can access all body tissue or chamber. There are essentially no barriers to their penetration. The amount of their presence within the body periphery (the joints, bones and skin) is determined mostly by their initial amount of release from their gland of origin.

Like smoke in a room, which moves from a high concentration to a lower concentration periphery, steroids similarly diffuse towards the periphery of the body kingdom.

A poor steroid generation rate at the source (the adrenals and gonads), diminishes the pressure head. It is the periphery tissues that suffer first. A falling "steroid pressure" manifests as wrinkled skin, painful joints and osteoporosis.

The periphery of the body kingdom is the most vulnerable because the presence of rejuvenation message content falls off here most severely because these tissues are furthest from the source of this information.

"Steroid tone" quantifies the quality of the steroid message content reaching the body cells. Different types of steroids have unique and precise shapes. It is the unique shape that conveys the message. Change the shape and the message content changes.

"Steroid pressure" quantifies the amount of a specific steroid reaching the body cells. For example an adequate androgen message directs sufficient rejuvenation activities. In contrast, inadequate androgen message content leads the body's cells to fall into disrepair.

The signs of disrepair show up first in the periphery:
>The skin
>The joints
>The bones

4. Cortisol: Stress Hormones and Weight Gain

The stress hormones, cortisol and epinephrine, are both made and secreted by the adrenal glands. This section concerns the cortisol component of the stress response. High levels of cortisol, as seen in the stress response, consume body structure to maximize energy; a catabolic effect.

The first facet of the stress response and weight gain

Sadly, the association between the chronic activation of the stress response and its tendency to promote obesity is often not mentioned within the mainstream medical approach. Even though the fact is when owners are sedentary and they continually experience mental stress, whether real or imagined, more insulin needs to be released. The more insulin released, the greater the message content to create fat. How can this be?

The body cannot discern the difference between mental and physical stress. Therefore, the physiological changes in both instances are the same. The physiology of the stress response largely involves outdated energy channeling when mental stress occurs. Even though mental stress does not need increased blood fuel (sugar, fat and amino acids) to survive it, the body responds by dumping fuel into the blood stream as if a physical challenge was forthcoming. In prehistoric times, the extra fuel proved advantageous because the fuel allowed increased strength within the muscles to respond to the physical danger.

Modern stress is largely mental in nature. Consequently, the extra fuel released has nowhere to go. The body eventually figures out that it has been fooled into dumping massive amounts of sugar into the blood stream and insulin secretes into the blood stream to rectify the situation. The increased insulin directs the activation of the fat-maker message, which causes problems in the setting of chronic mental stress.

This fact explains why the old adage about "walking it off" has merit. Exercise causes the extra fuel within the blood stream to be sucked into the muscles and combusted for the creation of energy. Exercise also increases androgen production, growth hormone output, and IGF-1 secretion rates. All these hormones combat the need for insulin (as previously discussed).

The stress response and the second facet of weight gain

The major hormone of the stress response is cortisol. Remember that cortisol is from the steroid class called catabolic. The message content of catabolic hormone concerns the consuming of body structure for fuel release into the blood stream. Unhealthy owners have other hormone increases as well. This facilitate fuel delivery with a price paid by consuming body structure between meals and when stressed. The price is paid to the body structure in the form of lost muscle and organ mass. This largely ignored medical fact is explained again by the fact that unhealthy bodies lack a sufficient stimulus or ability for growth hormone's release. Only when adequate growth hormone secretes, from the pituitary, will there be a sufficient counter message to prevent protein destruction for fuel needs. Muscles and organs functional components derive from protein. Growth hormone's presence impedes the combustion of protein when blood fuel levels fall. Instead, growth hormone preferentially directs the liver and fat cells to dump sugar and fat into the blood stream while sparing protein. This fact partially explains why healthy owners have nice muscles while unhealthy owners do not.

The basic sequence of unhealthy owner's body protein's destruction when they are stressed, between meals, or exercising and their blood fuel begins to fall, depends on other hormones. The entire group consists of glucagon, cortisol and epinephrine. Like growth hormone, they all facilitate the release of sugar and fat into the blood stream. Unlike growth hormone, body protein dismantling becomes fair game when growth hormone levels prove insufficient.

Here again, another vicious process continues to destroy the physiques of countless middle-aged owners until they understand the importance of protecting their body's protein content.

A deeper insight into the abnormal stress response occurring in the unhealthy owner

As if the body structure consumption facilitated by cortisol when growth hormone levels diminish wasn't bad enough, there is an additional obesity perpetuator and muscle loss facilitator to consider. Middle aged and obese owners have an increasing tendency for their adrenal glands to make more cortisol and less DHEA.

Healthy owners secrete two times the DHEA compared to cortisol during the stress response. This fact prevents the catabolic message contained in cortisol from becoming too aggressive. In this way, some of the body cells give up structure during the stress response while others continue repairing and rejuvenating.

Around middle age, a steep fall off in this optimal ratio between the adrenally released but opposing steroids occurs. Cortisol tends to greatly increase relative to DHEA.

Remember, DHEA is the major androgen steroid that instructs the liver to make IGF-1. IGF-1 facilitates muscle nutrition and impedes fat accumulation. A fall off of IGF-1 will necessitate an increased release of insulin. Insulin contains the fat-maker message.

This last fact, taken together with the need for increased insulin whenever mental stress occurs, without a compensatory "walk off the stress experience", explains how the fat-maker message becomes amplified. A falling DHEA secretion rate from the adrenal gland accompanies middle age. A chronic stress response amplifies this problem because more cortisol secretes relative to the DHEA released.

Until these owners improve their DHEA levels, manage their stress, and increase their growth hormone promoting activities, these owners' muscles and organs will shrink while their fat increases.

5. Adrenaline deficiency as a cause for obesity

Adrenaline carries out the receptor activation initiated by both cortisol and thyroid message content. Adrenaline (epinephrine) activates the receptors that these two more powerful hormones directed to be manufactured. Only when sufficient receptors exist, can its target cells hear the adrenaline message. When adrenaline releases under these normal circumstances, metabolism increases. When metabolism increases, fuel consumption increases. In addition, sufficient adrenaline proves as a powerful inhibitor for insulin release. Because the popular weight loss nutriceutical, ephedra, is molecularly similar to adrenaline, its demand remains strong.

Some owners suffer from various forms of adrenal insufficiency. It remains of little use to manufacture sufficient thyroid hormone and cortisol when the body experiences inadequate adrenal function from the lack of adrenaline. The manufacture of thyroid hormone takes place in the thyroid gland. The manufacture of cortisol takes place in the adrenal cortex. When the cortex fails, the diminished ability to make one or more adrenal steroids becomes the problem. Adrenaline manufacture needs to follow up on what both the thyroid and cortisol message started in the creation of adrenal receptors.

Overtaxed adrenal glands can often masquerade as a thyroid problem. These owners walk like a thyroid problem and talk like a thyroid problem, but they are not a thyroid problem. Patients feel lousy and intuitively sense something is wrong. These owners' standard fatigue work-ups come back normal at their doctor's office. A superficial inquiry leads to superficial platitudes and the statement that nothing is wrong. Some of these owners end up on antidepressants. How can this be? Further intrigue occurs when one includes the many depressed and overweight owners who note a marked lifting of their depressive like symptoms while taking ephedra (probably the real reason it gets bashed as dangerous while the more dangerous drugs, like aspirin, continues to sell over the counter).

A common example is revealed when one understands where adrenaline (epinephrine) derives from. Twenty different amino acids occur that, when arranged uniquely in sequence, types, and amount, become the various proteins. The body manufactures most of these de novo (from scratch). Eight essential amino acids must be obtained in the diet. The egg provides the only food source containing all eight. All other protein sources prove deficient in one or more amino acid. Adrenaline derives from the essential amino acid, phenylalanine.

The above discussion explains the importance of attaining adequate phenylalanine in the diet but a subtle and often-overlooked reason exists for adrenaline deficiency.

Protein disassembly requires adequate stomach acid and digestive juices to maintain essential amino acid supply lines. Owners who lack sufficient stomach acid and/or digestive juices tend to become deficient in essential amino acids necessary for the reactions of life. Deficient adrenaline manufacture describes one of the problems that can ensue due to ineffective disassembly of protein.

Another cause of adrenaline deficiency concerns the failure to obtain the necessary molecular building blocks for its manufacture. Most adrenaline derives from phenylalanine or the closely related amino acid, tyrosine. Physicians understand this much. Vitamins and cofactors, which prove necessary to make either one of these amino acids into adrenaline, often go unnoticed. Deficiency of any one of these halts this critical hormone's biosynthesis.

The nutrients necessary for the manufacture of adrenaline are: tetrahydrobiopterin (folate derived), Vitamin C, Vitamin B6, Vitamin B12, folate, serine, methionine, and SAMe (S-adenosyl methionine). The most common deficiency arises from a deficiency of SAMe, which evidences clinically as an increase of blood homocysteine levels. SAMe is part of the important methyl donor system and was explained in chapter 4.

A deficiency in one or more vitamins and cofactors results in health problems. These additional health problems develop because the adrenal secretes partially manufactured adrenaline (dopamine or noradrenaline) into the blood stream. When this occurs, deficiencies of one or more vitamins exist. Dopamine and noradrenaline (norepinephrine) have different shapes and consequently, each delivers a different message. A different message results when altered molecules bind to the adrenaline-like receptors.

When elevated amounts of noradrenaline enter the blood stream instead of adrenaline, a drastic increased tendency toward high blood pressure occurs. A single, simple vitamin deficiency can physiologically be the cause of elevated blood pressure. Some of these hypertensive owners may prefer taking vitamins. In this case, vitamins instead of blood pressure medicine lead to healing without the predictable side effects (chapter 4).

> **(Side bar) When was the last time a mainstream medical doctor inquired about these possibilities before prescribing medication? Please note, it is not the intent of this discussion to cast disparaging remarks on the many caring and kind physicians in practice today. It has been quite a shock to this author, while researching this work, the numerous holes in physicians (and this author's) educational exposure addressing healing versus symptom-control.**

> Usually the physician is not the one to blame, but rather, the way that simple concepts continually and knowingly continue to be withheld. The motive is money.

6. Insulin-like Growth Factor Type 1 (IGF-1)
The Sixth Hormone to Consider for Healing Obesity

Insulin-like growth factor type-1 has been discussed earlier in relationship to how it lowers the total body insulin requirements. It was also discussed earlier how it keeps the fat-making machinery, within the liver, quiescent. Before leaving the glandular component of obesities' propagation, a few summary statements need to be made about the important role IGF-1 plays in the body cell's nutrition status.

Rememer, insulin-like growth factor type-1 [IGF-1] occurs at levels greater than 100 times insulin levels when an owner remains healthy. IGF-1 acts like insulin outside of the liver and fat cells. The more IGF-1 in the circulation, the more the body cells outside of the liver and fat can uptake fuel and nutrients without excessive insulin. Growth hormone release promotes the healthy liver to release IGF-1 into the circulation. Androgens, like testosterone and DHEA, tell the liver DNA programs to activate and increase IGF-1 synthesis rates. In this way, when an owner remains healthy, the ample IGF-1 circulates within the blood stream, keeps his/her cells filled with nutrition.

As long as both a sufficient amount of liver manufacture and release of IGF-1 occur into an owner's blood stream daily, there will be less need for insulin release. Insulin release in healthy owners falls to very near zero between meals. However, unhealthy owners will tend to need massive increases in their insulin levels between meals because IGF-1 levels have fallen.

When IGF-1 levels fall, the cells beyond the liver and fat cells need increased amounts of insulin so that these cells can receive nutrition. The trouble with insulin level increases, to make up for the nutritional message ("fuel nozzle") deficit within the other body cells, regards its additional fat-maker role. Unlike IGF-1, insulin delivers a powerful message within the liver and fat cells to uptake excessive sugar and make it into fat and cholesterol. Additionally, because the pancreas secretes insulin straight into the protal vein, which leads directly into the liver, it receives the highest insulin message content before insulin spills out into the general circulation (beyond the liver).

Healthy owners gain weight less readily because their cells, like muscle and heart, receive nutrition with the help of IGF-1. Conversely, unhealthy owners have diminished IGF-1 levels so they will need excess insulin in order for their cells to uptake nutrition (cells need a "fuel nozzle"" to uptake nutrition). High insulin levels make an owner fat because the extra insulin delivers message content within the liver first. Only extreme amounts of insulin spill beyond the liver and out into the general circulation. This fact results from each liver cell containing around 200,000 pure insulin-type receptors.

Healthy insulin levels cause the liver to store just the right amount of fat and sugar within the liver and fat cells following meals. Between meals (fasting or exercising) healthy owners release stored fuel and IGF-1 together under the direction of increased growth hormone. In this way the healthy owner has sufficient blood fuel and ""fuel nozzle"" hormones to feed his/her cells from one meal to the next.

The Follow the Fuel and You Will Understand Diabetes chapter explains more of the particulars on how important a high IGF-1 level is in regard to body health. Here it is only important to understand how when IGF-1 falls, the insulin needs rise. Insulin needs increase because when one "fuel nozzle" hormones' level decreases, the other needs to increase. Insulin on the rise means fat making will also be on the rise. Conversely, IGF-1 levels, at healthy levels, facilitate muscle and organ development and nutrition and greatly diminishes the amount of insulin needed.

7. **High Estrogen** Levels Can Promote Obesity

Estrogen: a steroid hormone made in the adrenals and ovaries. The testes also manufacture a small amount. The estrogen message has a component in instructing cells to divide. High estrogen levels also initiate a circuitous message to increase body fat when its levels become too high compared to androgens (testosterone and DHEA).

When estrogen rises beyond normal levels a varying tendency occurs to promote two of the hormonal factors that create obesity. The ability of estrogen to raise insulin and lower androgens, in certain females, describes these two factors.

Three main clinical situations promote estrogen-induced weight gain. Not all female owners will express these tendencies equally. This variability may have a genetic basis. Not all women with increased estrogen states tend to gain weight equally. High estrogen states tend to promote weight gain in many female owners. This fact will be the focus of this subsection.

The first clinical example for estrogen-induced weight gain results from birth control pills. They predictably increase insulin in the body. The first mechanism for this situation arises from an abnormal hormone tandem that high estrogen levels cause.

The first part of the hormone tandem involves the fact that high estrogen increases the amount of growth hormone released from the pituitary gland. The increased estrogen states that result from birth control pills usage provide an example of this. Growth hormone will initially raise the blood sugar level. It is the second hormone in this tandem, that estrogen simultaneously inhibits, which alters the normal pattern of events.

When estrogen levels remain optimal, the release of growth hormone directs the simultaneous release of insulin-like growth factor (IGF-1), the second hormone in the tandem, along with the liver-stored sugar and fat. IGF-1 has powerful insulin-like blood sugar-lowering message content. This message content lowers the blood sugar that the growth hormone released initially elevated. Here, extra insulin is not needed.

Normally, this tandem hormone effect provides an effective way for the cells to receive fuel from the blood stream, between meals or with exercise, without raising insulin levels. High estrogen states, although they initially stimulate growth hormone release, counteracts the normal tandem by inhibiting insulin-like growth factor release (IGF-1). **The normal hormone tandem interrupts because high estrogen causes the simultaneous inhibition of IGF-1 release.**

As stated previously, IGF-1 delivers insulin-like message content for the uptake of nutrition in the cells outside the liver and fat. Its presence lowers the amount of insulin needed by the body. The IGF-1 released assists insulin by taking sugar out of the blood stream and into the cells outside the liver and fat. When IGF-1 levels diminish, the growth hormone released directs increased sugar release into the blood stream. More insulin becomes necessary from the pancreas to make up the deficit of total "fuel nozzle" hormones. The more insulin secreted, the more message content exists to make body fat.

The second clinical situation of estrogen-caused obesity involves increased prolactin levels caused by the increased estrogen state of birth control use and/or stress filled lifestyles. Prolactin inhibits ovarian androgen hormone formation and release. This hormone-induced mechanism, associated with obesity, generally does not operate in pregnancy because this physiologic state possesses a growing placenta. In the pregnant state, the growing placenta, more than offsets the prolactin-induced inhibition of the ovaries by serving as a hormonal factory for steroid production. Birth control usage fools the body into thinking it is pregnant. Prolactin levels rise in response to either increased estrogen or cortisol. However, in either of the above cases, no placental hormone factory exists to make up the prolactin caused androgen deficiency.

In a real pregnancy, the placenta manufactures androgens even though the ovaries become relatively dormant by the fifth month of gestation. When a female owner takes birth control pills, the body thinks it is pregnant. During birth control pill usage, prolactin levels rise because estrogen levels approach pregnancy levels. However, with birth control pill usage, no placenta exists to manufacture the androgen lost when the ovaries become inhibited by excessive prolactin.

Potential obesity problems occur because, like pregnancy, the birth control pills increase prolactin levels. Unlike pregnancy, there is no placenta (hormone factory) to correct the inhibition of steroid production within the ovaries. The potential for problems compounds due to the fact that the birth control pill does not contain androgens. They only contain abnormally shaped estrogen and progestins (abnormally shaped progesterone substitutes). Androgen production can fall within these owners and their adrenals are left all alone for this task. Some female's adrenals fail at the challenge of increased androgen production and obesity ensues.

The third clinical situation of high estrogen-induced obesity is beyond the level of this discussion. For those who are curious, it involves the dramatic increase of sex hormone-binding globulin that high estrogen levels direct. Androgen that may be produced by the ovary or adrenals, in high estrogen states, becomes trapped on a carrier protein in the blood stream at 98% of the efficiency level.

Hormone Mimics

Hormone mimics: environmentally present chemical compounds that resemble body hormones enough that they deliver message content when inside body tissue. Message content from these mimics are excessive, deficient, altered and/or prolonged. These properties alter the recipient owner's normal physiology.

Hormone mimics diminish the health of adrenals and gonads. Pervasive and insidious effects of hormonal mimics surface in the worldwide phenomenon of falling sperm counts in men. Androgen levels primarily determine a man's sperm count. Hormone mimics surface from environmental and nutritional sources. Around the world, chemicals like DDT and Agent Orange have been implicated in the estrogen mimic effect.

These mimics compete with men's androgen tone causing sperm counts to drop progressively each decade.

The numerous common chemicals that exert a biochemical message effect along various degrees of estrogen mimicry sounds fantastical. When one considers that all estrogen mimics share a similar molecular shape with their estrogen counterpart, it becomes conceptually consistent. The common shape, in the 'key' of estrogen is technically called the aromatic ring. Trouble starts because these diverse chemicals all contain the estrogen 'key' shape and once inside the body, they lead to an unnaturally high estrogen-message content.

In many ways, estrogen and estrogen mimics counter the effects of androgens like testosterone. The most frightening aspect of turning up the estrogen message in both men and women concerns their powerful cell division message that certain estrogen-types and estrogen mimics deliver. This can cause abnormal growths in the prostate tissues of some men - a prime cause of benign prostatic hypertrophy (BPH). In women, estrogen dominance (relative to progesterone) leads to an increased tendency towards developing fibrocystic breast disease, uterine fibroids, breast cancer, PMS, and others.

Saran wrap, plastic food containers, and the liners inside canned foods all contain estrogen mimics. As a general guide, the higher the fat content, the greater the tendency for hormone mimics to migrate into the food. Prime environmental hormone disrupters are DDT, PCB's, and dioxin that are widely dispersed throughout the environment.

DDT (a suspected carcinogenic in mammals) is an environmentally persistent insecticide that causes fragile and broken eggshells in wild birds. Estrogen-like substances stimulate cell growth in estrogen sensitive tissue.

Though banned in the late 1970's, PCB's used in transformers and other electrical components, still persist throughout the environment. Another common source of continued exposure is from foreign grown produce and fruits, which still contain the outlawed insecticides. The list of detrimental effects include severe birth defects in people and animals, cancer in animals, as well as a link to intellectual deficits in children. These mimics clearly tend to stimulate cell division inappropriately.

Dioxins have been shown to cause cancer in both animals and humans and have acted like estrogen in animal studies. In 1979, the Environmental Protection Agency (EPA) banned some herbicides because they were contaminated with dioxins, but there are still numerous additional sources including paper bleaching facilities, polyvinyl chloride factories and trash incinerators. The EPA and various industries modified their practices with some success, but it has proved difficult to eliminate them all. If consumers began a boycott of plastic and bleached paper products, the level of these disrupters would fall.

Plasticizer compounds may leech from landfills into the environment, but do not seem to linger in human bodies. Two types of plasticizers suspected to cause problems are phthalates and adipates. In lab animals, phthalates cause liver cancer and testicular damage. Adipates, in animal studies, link to shortened life spans and decreased fertility. Bisphenol A, a building block of plastic manufacture used in dental sealants and in food can liners, causes enlarged prostates in animals.

Several low cost strategies avoid ingesting estrogen mimics. Reduce consumption of suspect compounds by avoiding plastic containers and wrappers. Consider using alternatives to pesticides and insecticides on both lawn and pets. Wash fruits and vegetables thoroughly or buy organic foods. Limit consumption of suspect fatty foods where these compounds accumulate in the food chain. Watch for local fish pollution possibilities. When reheating food, don't use plastic as heat accelerates transfer of the hormone mimics into the food.

A Few Introductory Remarks about the Normal Female's Monthly Cycle

The healthy female's ovaries make appropriate amounts of androgens. In addition, the healthful state typifies by proper levels of estrogens, which cycle with proper levels of progesterone. Each month a new cycle begins and her cells receive the right amount of message content, which directs them to invest in rejuvenation activities. Rejuvenation activities keep the body young.

Around menopause, the ovaries begin to fail and give up their steroid production role to the middle aged adrenal. Many years prior to this, steroid production begins to diminish within the ovaries. When clinicians miss this or treat with aberrant shaped hormones, a female owner accelerates on the path to an old body.

Nutritional deficiencies play a major role in ovarian disease. Common factors include a chronic preference for the consumption of a 'processed food' diet versus a 'real food' diet (see earlier discussion). Ovarian steroid production provides an example of how nutrition affects ovarian health. One central facet of ovarian function determines the rate at which cholesterol converts to pregnenolone.

The amount of aldosterone present determines the conversion rate of cholesterol to pregnenolone. This fact about the steroid manufacture rate remains true for the adrenals, testicles, and ovaries. In the ovary, testicle, and adrenal DNA programs, adequate aldosterone needs to direct production of the enzyme, **cholesterol desmolase**. This enzyme makes steroid production from cholesterol possible. Cholesterol desmolase the initial enzyme for steroid manufacture, is also known as **side chain cleavage enzyme**.

A high potassium diet ('real food') stimulates aldosterone release from the adrenal glands. Processed food diets prove deficient in potassium and pave the road for dysfunctional ovaries. This fact provides an example of steroid interdependence in order for ovary health to become possible. Along with aldosterone, the healthy ovary needs vitamins C, Vitamins A, and B complex for adequate steroid production capabilities. The mineral zinc allows androgen steroid synthesis to occur at adequate levels.

Drastic mineral content differences exist between these two types of diets (see mineral table). Real food contains natural minerals in the proportions required for health. Processed foods contain drastically altered mineral content. Processing natural foods depletes the minerals magnesium and potassium. Shelf life of food extends by adding unhealthy amounts of sodium, calcium, hydrogenated fats, and sugar. Increased shelf life leads to more profits for the food industry. Processed food no longer contains the proper ratio of the four minerals - magnesium, calcium, potassium, and sodium. Ovaries need the correct mineral ratio more than other body tissues to maintain the aldosterone message content (chapter 12). Aldosterone message content determines the synthesis rates for all steroids within the adrenals and ovaries. Natural food diets facilitate an increased aldosterone level.

Owners who eat dead food diets (processed foods) become potassium and magnesium depleted at the onset of middle age. A deficiency of potassium creates the need for an increase in insulin to process the same amount of sugar (chapter 8). The greater the insulin level, the greater the fat-maker message becomes. In addition, potassium and magnesium deficiencies lead to high blood pressure, irregular heart rate, diminished adrenal and ovary steroid production, diminished red blood cell flexibility, and decreased cell voltages (a weakened cell force field). The 'why' and the 'how' of these facts are discussed in the appropriate sections throughout this manual. Proper mineral intake equals the healthful state.

Chapter 8: The "Torture Chamber" Diet:
(Lots of carbohydrates when one is already fat)

Lack of attention to the consequences from abnormal hormone levels occurs with the complex-endorsed diet. Abnormal hormones create abnormal urges in its adherent's feeding behavior. Abnormal hormones exaggerate feeding obsessions. The "torture chamber" effect describes the feeding obsessions that result from this official diet (The American Dietetic Association provides one example). As long as the American public believes in the diet, endorsed by the complex, there will be continued economic need from the complications of obesity. Examples of these complications are: high blood pressure, diabetes, and heart disease. The complex endorsed diet easily exposes itself when some basic missing facts return to the analysis.

> **A narrow band of truth occurs in the complex-endorsed diet but it concerns only one type of physique. The physique for which the complex-endorsed diet works occurs in an athlete who already exists at his/her ideal weight and/or peak performance. Peak-performing athletes attain optimal weight and have achieved optimal physical fitness. Through training, genetics, and/or age, they have the right balance of hormones.**

Owners at ideal weight and physical fitness levels have properly proportioned hormone-message content. This allows the proper appetite stimulation and exercise motivation to continue. They can handle increased carbohydrate intake that necessitates only a slight increase in insulin production because they have high IGF-1 levels. They tolerate slight increases in insulin because their lifestyles and/or genetics allow a sufficient amount of IGF-1 counter hormone. The counter hormone IGF-1, successfully counter weights the fat-building message of insulin. As middle age approaches, most owners are not endowed with superior amounts of androgen (chapter 7) and growth hormone, which are necessary for high IGF-1 production rates and release.

Little acknowledgment exists about basic scientific facts that discuss the relationship of dietary choices and hormone consequences to feeding behavior. Some notable exceptions are found in the Drs. Atkins', Schwarzbein and Sears' diets. Even less cognizance exists about the circular trap that feeding behavior dictates, which hormones secrete. This explains the vicious and circular trap overweight owners find themselves in, despite earnest attempts to diet (the "torture chamber").

When obese owners adhere to the complex endorsed diet's tenants, powerful hormones release. These stimulate a preoccupation with the next feeding and a decreased ability to shed fat. It is a travesty to withhold acknowledgment that the complex-endorsed diet creates a virtual "torture chamber" of emotional desires in the owner who expends effort to make positive health changes when his/her attempts to change are doomed. They destine themselves for defeat because of their unfavorable hormones. Weight loss efforts become hopeless until they obtain guidance about changing their hormones for the better.

Dr. Atkins was one of the first physicians to recognize the powerful role that hormones play in feeding behavior. He did this by reviewing what was known about the hormone, insulin, in basic medical physiology textbooks. He studied cultures that do not have high rates of obesity and obesity-related diseases. Dr. Atkins first began to apply what was known over thirty years ago about hormone levels and consequent feeding behavior. He correctly reasoned that insulin levels that are allowed to reach higher than optimum levels act as a powerful appetite stimulant. This creates an obsessive preoccupation for the next feeding event. He understood that insulin has a dramatic effect on the ability of the body to manufacture fat. He also understood how insulin prevents the body from accessing fat reserves.

Health benefits from lowering insulin levels are receiving renewed interest. Lowered insulin levels will decrease the stimulation in the appetite center of the brain and also increase the ability to use fat for energy. Obesity is on the increase in America and it can rarely be curtailed without an improvement in feeding behavior hormones.

It is important to extend the work of Dr.'s like Atkins, Bernstein, Sears, and Schwarzbein. Their important contributions allow consideration of the other obesity related hormones (chapter 7). Briefly, the other hormones, in addition to insulin, that need to be normalized before weight loss occurs are cortisol, androgens, estrogen, IGF-1, epinephrine, and thyroid. Attention to the rebalancing of these hormones provides an extension of these authorities work and a magnification of the weight loss possiblility.

The importance of real food versus processed food also needs to be added into the plan. Real foods provide the mineral nutrition necessary for maximum avoidance of the complications from obesity-related disease. The real food component of successful dieting explains why the opposite approach to dieting has some success. These diets, for which Dean Ornish and Nathaniel Pritikin, are most famous, do a better job of expressing the importance of real food in place of processed food. However, these diets fail their adherents because of the high insulin that results from the high carbohydrate content contained in these diets. In the end, both diet camps exist on the extremes. Each has some success, but each fails in maximizing success by ignoring either the hormones or the importance of real food.

Consuming real food (from the garden, off the tree, organic eggs, fresh fish, fresh chicken and meats that have not been canned or salted) helps avoid ingredients that are easily missed in the high

protein diet. High protein dieters need to take care not to consume high protein sources from processed food. Processed food is any food that comes in a box or a can. The requirements of putting food into a box or a can necessitates adding unbalanced minerals like sodium, which deviate from body design.

The diet that has the least success in the long haul is the ADA diet. The ADA diet takes the worst features from both diet extremes. It advises consumption of 50-60% of total daily calories from carbohydrate. Carbohydrate consumption in this proportion of total daily calories condemns the obese owners into the vicious ""torture chamber"" cycle. Weight gain consequences occur because of the obligatory rise in insulin levels. The "torture chamber" also involves a degree of other hormone imbalances.

A discussion of the additional hormones involved in obesity brings up a concept that Dr. Atkins calls **metabolic resistance**. Metabolic resistance describes those women for whom the low carbohydrate diet proves slow to effect weight loss. This author feels that the high protein diet approach fails to acknowledge that many of these women need the added benefit of androgen. Androgen deficiency explains some of the cause for this phenomenon quite well, as it is androgens that oppose fat gain. Fat gain opposition occurs because androgens provide message content to the liver to increase IGF-1 production. Increased IGF-1 production lowers insulin need (lowers insulin resistance).

Fat gain accentuates in some female owners because they have less androgen compared to men. The removal of the ovaries and the onset of menopause can exacerbate androgen deficiency. Consideration of the 24-hour urine test for steroid production will identify this type of metabolic resistance caused problem.

Once androgens improve, in as safe a way as possible, these female owners need to understand how to encourage increased growth hormone release. Exercise and fasting will stimulate the capable pituitary's release of growth hormone. The few women who prove unable to increase their growth hormone output by these methods may need growth hormone shots (chapter 15).

An additional cause of **metabolic resistance** concerns the increased production rate of the stress hormone, cortisol. High cortisol levels in the urine identify other owners who have trouble with weight loss despite strict adherence to a low carbohydrate diet. High stress will increase cortisol release. Increased cortisol in a setting of mental stress will elevate blood sugar inappropriately and it will only come down with exercise or increased insulin secretion. It is the increased insulin secretion brought on by stress occurring in a sedentary lifestyle that leads to obesity.

The intensity of the problem magnifies because weight gain prone owner's adrenal glands prove particularly adept at cortisol production when the stress response activates. These obese owners make more cortisol with the same amount of life stress compared to a non-obese owner. Increased cortisol causes an inappropriate increase in blood fuel that has nowhere to go in a sedentary owner until insulin releases. Only exercise and stress management will provide a way to stop this hormone cycle within the "torture chamber".

Thyroid hormone levels need to be carefully evaluated. The thyroid gland determines the rate at which calories burn in the cell power plants (see Thyroid subsection).

Estrogen levels, when high, as occurs in pregnancy and birth control pill usage, exacerbates the obesity problem in some female owners. Environmental estrogen problems can occur in men and women (see Hormone Mimics). High estrogen levels stimulate growth hormone release, but inhibit IGF-1 release. This aberration leads to insulin resistance because less IGF-1 becomes available to help insulin with fuel uptake by the cells. Consequently, increased insulin becomes necessary to bring the blood fuel level back to normal. The higher the insulin levels, the more liver fat-making machinery stimulated to make fat and cholesterol. More fat then becomes available for storage sites in the liver, arteries, and fat cells.

(Technical point for Physicians) Once again, the placenta rescues most pregnant women's from high estrogen states by increasing the secretion of human placental lactogen, which increases IGF-1 production within the placenta increases by 2-3 times normal blood levels. However, the high estrogen states of women on estrogen prescriptions do not have a placenta to correct the fall of IGF-1. High estrogen levels cause a fall of IGF-1 and these owners' livers make excess fat from the high insulin needed to correct the deficit. Note that it is the high cortisol levels of the pregnant state that are thought to cause insulin resistance (see cortisol discussion, in chapter 7, as to why this is so).

Epinephrine release occurs as an extension of the stress response. Like cortisol, it contains message content that instructs the liver to dump fuel into the blood stream. When mental stress occurs, there becomes little need for the extra fuel in the blood stream. Eventually, insulin needs to release to normalize blood sugar caused by mental stress's inappropriate elevation of the blood fuel. Increased insulin leads to an increased fat-making message in liver and fat cells.

A 'tug of war' exists between the hormones that help shed fat and the hormones that make fat. It is worthwhile to assess whether these interrelating hormones occur in excess, deficiency, or are present in the optimal amounts needed for a healthy body.

Thin people who eat as much as they want are not always fine specimens of raging androgen production. Deficiency in muscle mass usually provides a clue that increased androgen may not be the reason for perpetual thinness.

Emaciated skinniness in the presence of increased caloric intake can be due to poor digestive absorption of critical nutrients. Some of these owners contain weakened adrenals that prove unable to adequately secrete cortisol when they perceive stress (a subdued stress response). The clinical clue for these types, when they become unhealthy, concerns their tendency to suffer hypoglycemic events (chapter 13).

All of the Popular Diets Today Miss Vital Consideration for Weight Loss (each has part of the puzzle, but not the whole picture)

Two different extremes in diet philosophy have been introduced. Each presents a part of the puzzle that will help shed fat. Each also contains an impediment to weight loss. The best science in each diet's approach needs incorporation, while avoiding its downside.

High protein and fat with low carbohydrate diet plans are incomplete in their effectiveness because they do not contain the right mineral ratios. Their incompleteness sheds light on how some of the other diets have a weight loss effect. Some other diets have a weight loss effect because they inadvertently, partially address, mineral balance. The omission of mineral balance creates the hormone imbalances that lead to higher insulin need, which the high protein diet philosophy attempts to avoid. Mineral imbalance will occur any time processed food dominates in the diet.

On the up side, the high protein diet leads to lower insulin need. In contrast, the upside of the fresh and raw food diets occurs because it contains properly proportioned minerals that will better help with hormone balance. On the downside, these diets contain higher carbohydrate so the insulin need increases. **Higher insulin levels prove counter-productive to any diet effort.** Mineral intake balance also proves important to decrease this obesity promoting hormone's level.

The Body's Mineral Design Conservation Features are Obsolete in Face of the Processed Food Diet

The human body was designed for a natural mineral ratios intake. This consists of a minimum of three times the potassium as compared to sodium and there should be sufficient magnesium to counter calcium. **The sodium and potassium intake ratio more than reverses when one adheres to a processed food diet.** Magnesium intake is commonly deficient as well.

In prehistoric times a survival advantage occurred for anyone who could retain sodium. Natural food is relatively deficient in sodium content compared to potassium. When one eats natural food the potassium to sodium mineral ratio is greater than three to one.

Processed food has a drastically altered mineral content. Processed food diets have greatly diminished potassium and magnesium content. At the same time a processed food diet has a greatly increased amounts of sodium added to preserve the shelf life of the product. This combination causes a chronic imbalance between potassium and sodium (see mineral table).

The same owner types that once, in prehistoric times, had a survival advantage, now have a disadvantage if a processed diet is chronically consumed. These owners retain sodium inappropriately and have reversed mineral content included in the processed food diet (see mineral table). Around middle age owners on a processed food diet develop a whole range of health consequences. This leads to six potassium deficiency-related health consequences. **These owners who predispose to health consequences from the high sodium and low potassium diet, were the genetically superior human design machines of prehistoric times.** In modern times, as long as they adhere to a processed food diet, they remain on a rapid road to self-destruction.

Six Different Ways Obesity Propagates Secondary to the Mineral Imbalance Occurring Around Middle Age

1. Insulin resistance
2. Increased fat and cholesterol synthesis in the liver
3. Loss of protein content
4. Decreased steroid biosynthesis to keep blood pressure normal
5. Slower metabolic rate
6. Stress exacerbates the mineral imbalance and weight gain

All six of these factors need to be circumvented if one desires an effective weight loss rate. If one optimizes all seven hormones (chapter 7) that lead to obesity and corrects their mineral imbalance, their diet plan becomes more complete because they now apply the best from the different diets available. Concurrently, they also omit obsolete components of these other diets in light of new scientific understanding. These become important if one really wants to know what makes them fat. When owners know what makes them fat, they can make progress in their weight loss effort.

Chronic Mineral Imbalanced Diets Cause One Type of Insulin Resistance

The chronic consumption of a mineral imbalanced diet will lead to the need for increased insulin secretion (insulin resistance). Increased insulin becomes necessary because insulin needs sufficient potassium to get sugar into the cells. One potassium ion helps carry one sugar molecule out of the blood stream and into a cell.

The chronic ingestion of reversed ratios between potassium and sodium leads to a decreased availability of potassium for insulin-directed sugar removal out of the blood stream. The delay of the blood-lowering effect of diminished potassium eventually causes the pancreas to secrete more insulin.

The delay of potassium availability occurs after many years of consuming reversed mineral ratios. The blood stream amount of potassium contains only 2% of body potassium. The other 98% of potassium resides inside the cells. The potassium in the cells donates itself to keep the smaller potassium pool constant in the blood stream. Owners that eat processed foods will inevitably deplete their total potassium.

The potassium in the blood stream can be thought of as the 2% 'tank' of potassium content. It is the very last tank to deplete. The standard test at the doctor's office measures the serum component in the blood stream only. The blood stream value will only change when the larger tank severely depletes. The larger tank, containing 98% of potassium, resides inside the numerous cells. Cells, including red blood cells, will sacrifice their potassium content in order to keep the blood levels in the normal range.

Here lies the deception occurring in America today. Physicians wrongly reassure their patients about the potassium levels in their blood stream while they have not inquired about the status of the larger tank. Failure to consider the consequences that ensue when the body becomes chronically deprived of the correct ratios between potassium and sodium intake, leads to chronic degenerative diseases. Insulin resistance-related disease signifies only one of several consequences of diminished potassium compared to sodium content.

Examples of chronic degenerative diseases that have a component of causality as a consequence of imbalanced potassium to sodium intake are: adult onset diabetes, high blood pressure, high cholesterol, obesity, fatigue, and anxiety syndromes.

Insulin resistance can eventually progress into adult onset diabetes (chapter 13). The accompanying signs of obesity and an abnormal cholesterol profile often associate with adult onset diabetes. The mineral balance between potassium and sodium dramatically affects all three of these processes. Misery propagates when this important relationship remains ignored

One type of insulin resistance originates from a chronic imbalance between potassium and sodium intake. As the mineral imbalance increases, more insulin secretes to normalize sugar intake because most cells require potassium to bring sugar aboard. Each sugar transported, into most cell types, requires one potassium ion. The trouble arises from the fact that the cells donate their potassium to the blood stream when potassium occurs in scarce supply. The needed potassium donation occurs at the expense and sacrifice of the potassium content of other cells.

The pancreas senses that the blood sugar remains elevated and more insulin eventually releases when blood sugar-lowering delays. Insulin resistance describes the increased amount of insulin needed to do the same job for a specific sugar load. When an owner's pancreas exhausts its ability to produce additional insulin, adult onset diabetes results and blood sugar begins to rise. Many people's pancreases prove able to keep making more and more insulin and therefore these owners do not get diabetes. However, the high insulin levels make both of these types of owners obese and also to have abnormal cholesterol levels. The only difference between the two types of owners is that in one, the pancreas reaches exhaustion and blood sugar rises.

In both types, the high insulin levels promote the blood vessels getting clogged with fatty accumulations. The ability of insulin to lower the blood sugar depends on potassium availability. Less potassium availability will delay the rate that the blood sugar lowers to normal. The pancreas senses this delay and more insulin eventually secretes as the body cells sacrifice their potassium content, which insulin needs to work.

In these situations, the peripheral cells receive less nutrition. Most cells need adequate potassium to bring sugar aboard. In contrast, the liver uptakes a higher amount of sugar and processes it into more fat and cholesterol than is healthy because potassium is not needed by the liver when it converts sugar into fat. In order for the liver to store sugar as glycogen, there needs to be a fixed amount of potassium available. Again, the potassium deficiency changes the balance from the way that healthy livers store energy.

Blood vessels grow fat and people grow fat when the fat-maker message rises. Insulin always delivers the fat-maker message. Without insulin, there can be no fat. With high insulin there will be more body fat. The potassium deficiency of middle age explains one cause of insulin resistance.

Increased Cholesterol and Fat Synthesis in the Liver

An increased message content in the liver to make more cholesterol and fat occurs when insulin resistance develops. Cholesterol and fat are made from the sugar that does not enter other cells because of diminished potassium content. Diminished potassium content impedes the ability of the peripheral cells, like muscle cells, to uptake carbohydrate nutrition. The increased blood sugar becomes more liver accessible. The liver does not need potassium to suck sugar out of the blood stream and make fat and cholesterol. All the liver needs is adequate message content from insulin and it begins sucking out the blood sugar. The liver needs adequate potassium, like other cells, to store sugar as glycogen. Glycogen storage requires fixed amounts of potassium to sugar. Without adequate potassium, the liver is only able to make cholesterol and fat. Next, the increase in availability of sugar in the liver and the increased insulin message in the liver, accelerate the liver manufacture rate of cholesterol and fat particles, LDL cholesterol. Increased levels of LDL (triglycerides) cholesterol provide a hallmark of high insulin states. This mechanism explains the potassium deficient diet's contribution to this problem.

In the insulin resistant state, at the level of the liver, the low carbohydrate diet can fail to protect the owner because no one has counseled them about their potassium deficiency. **Potassium deficiency will lead to increased insulin production (insulin resistance) even on a low carbohydrate diet. If these owners restore total potassium content (it often** takes 3 to 6 months), their insulin needs will drop dramatically over time.

Many owners on low carbohydrate diets do not correct their potassium deficiency and this alone causes an increase in their insulin levels. The increased insulin levels direct the liver to produce greater amounts of LDL cholesterol from the little carbohydrate consumed. When LDL cholesterol levels increase, there becomes an increased risk for blood vessel disease and obesity. The increased insulin level directs both of these disease processes.

When an owner increases their potassium content, they will be able to tolerate more carbohydrates without abnormal increases in their insulin levels. **Obese owners are warned to initially curtail carbohydrates dramatically to decrease the appetite center activation that insulin directs. The more normal the weight becomes, the more carbohydrates from real food that can be consumed.**

The reason adequate potassium content in the body figures so importantly for controlling cholesterol concerns its ability to help normalize blood sugar with less insulin. Less insulin means less fat and cholesterol synthesis in the liver. The liver faithfully serves its owner and does as the message directs.

A 'tug of war' between glucagon and insulin occurs in the liver. The low carbohydrate diet, in the presence of adequate body potassium, will have more glucagon message content. More glucagon message content will, in physically active owners, curtail fat and cholesterol synthesis. This partially explains why owners on high protein and fat diets with low carbohydrate intake have decreased cholesterol levels.

The fact that one needs adequate potassium for their body to hold onto protein has been known by science for over fifty years. Decreased protein content results in shrinking muscles, organs, skin, and bones.

Mineral Imbalanced Diets Lead to the Loss of Body Protein

Owners that arrive at middle age with a history of consuming processed food diets will experience chronic protein depletion in their tissues. These bodies sacrifice cellular proteins in order to obtain sufficient potassium for the blood stream. This process takes many years to manifest. Even though their protein depletes at a slow rate, eventually, these middle-aged victims begin to look typical. Usually it manifests as an increased middle area from fat accumulation and smaller muscles in the limbs and chest areas. The protein depletion also shrinks the size of their organs.

The protein depletion process occurs because potassium in the cells stabilizes the protein content. When a cell loses potassium, the protein content will decrease. Little muscles, little organs, and shriveled skin, result from mineral imbalanced diets because processed food contains an altered mineral content.

Less body protein translates to decreased cell function in the effected cells and less need for cell energy. Less energy equates to fewer calories needed before weight gain occurs. Less energy also means less ability to participate in what life has to offer. The cycle of obesity breaks when a middle-aged owner begins to understand how to regain mineral balance. The first step of this process involves a commitment to real food diets that restore mineral intake in their proper proportions (see mineral table).

Mineral Deficient Owners Reduce their Steroid Production to Obtain Normal Blood Pressure

Year after year, the body, which chronically feeds on altered mineral ratios, faces a difficult choice around middle age. It can try to maintain steroid production, but in some its side effect causes the blood pressure to rise. Alternately, some bodies decrease steroid manufacture in order to normalize the blood pressure.

Owners that eat a real food diet can secrete optimal amounts of aldosterone without raising blood pressure because they consume the right ratios of minerals. Owners that eat processed foods consume mineral ratios that destroy body functions. These altered minerals eventually strain the ability of the kidneys to keep an appropriate mineral balance.

The altered mineral balance causes the middle age problem in both cases. Some bodies increase blood pressure to continue manufacturing adequate steroids that depends on adequate aldosterone production in the adrenal (see below). Other bodies diminish aldosterone production, but have a normal blood pressure. Although these owner's bodies have normal blood pressure, they will age more quickly because of their lowered steroid production rates. Lowered steroid production rates mean that there will be less rejuvenation message content. Less rejuvenation message content leads to the accumulation of wear and tear changes in these bodies. The more wear and tear changes accumulate, the older that body looks and feels.

Aldosterone gives the message to the adrenals and gonads to increase steroid production. Owners do not tolerate increased aldosterone levels with mineral imbalances between potassium and sodium. Potassium and sodium imbalanced owners conserve excess fluid when aldosterone elevates. Excess fluid leads to blood pressure elevation.

Mineral Imbalances Lead to a Slower Metabolism

The diminished protein content slows the metabolic rate. Protein content comprises the active metabolic fraction (the part that burns calories) of body tissue. Proteins, like enzymes and mineral pumps, consume energy and therefore, metabolize calories. Metabolism also slows with mineral imbalance because there is less electrical potential across mineral-depleted cell membranes. Mineral imbalance slows metabolism because it diminishes cellular charge. When the body rests, the majority of energy expends in recharging the trillions of cell membranes (the cellular force fields). These can only recharge adequately when the right mineral ratios oppose one another.

Each cell uses the cell membranes' charge energy to sustain life. Less membrane energy content occurs when the minerals alter from their optimal proportion. This is similar to what would happen to a car battery that had its mineral content altered. As the car battery membranes mineral concentration alters, so does its ability to perform useful work. Car batteries function better when the manufacture adds in the proper mineral proportions between the membranes. This fact proves as a prerequisite before maximal charge can occur. So it is with body cells, before they can charge, the right mineral proportions need to be available.

>**The food industry is not cognizant of this basic body design feature. Magnesium and potassium deplete in food from processing it. Next large amounts of sodium combine into processed food in order to retard spoilage. This formula of altered mineral ratios dumps into cells year after year (see mineral table). Around middle age, feeble cell batteries lead to weakness, fatigue, diminished calories burned, and weight gain (the "low voltage cell syndrome").**

Stress Exacerbates Mineral Imbalance

Stress will increase the need for insulin. Increased insulin leads to an increased fat-making message content. An additional way exists for chronic stress to make its recipient fat. It concerns the extra potassium loss that cortisol causes. Cortisol increases during the stress response. Increased cortisol causes increased sodium retention and increased potassium loss. This aldosterone-like effect of cortisol occurs because at high levels, cortisol will create message content similar to aldosterone in its sodium retentive effects. Sodium retention and potassium wasting are not a problem with normal levels of cortisol. At normal levels, cortisol is weak in its message content to retain sodium and excrete potassium.

Surgeons are well aware of this fact in post surgery states. The body cannot survive the stress of surgery unless there is a massive output of cortisol from the adrenal glands. The increased cortisol excretion rate depletes potassium. Surgeons routinely give intravenous potassium post-operatively because the owner's body will secrete increased cortisol in order to survive the stress of surgery. The increased potassium in the IV prevents a precipitous fall in body potassium. With mineral balance in mind, the real food diet that allows this is contrasted with the processed food diet.

Two Diets on Opposite Extremes in Mineral Content

Real food is high in potassium and magnesium, unprocessed, and low in sodium (see mineral table for specifics).

Fresh vegetables	Fresh fruit
Eggs	Fresh meat, chicken and fish
Low salt cheese	Brown sugar
Unprocessed rice	Unprocessed grains
Unprocessed nuts	Unprocessed beans (dry or fresh)
Potatoes	avocados

Processed food is high in sodium content, but low in both magnesium and potassium

Anything that comes in a box
Anything that comes in a can
Anything from a fast food restaurant
Anything that has more sodium content than potassium content
Some frozen foods have sodium added
Store bought bread, with a few exceptions
Condiments (catsup, soy sauce, salad dressing, steak sauce, and pickles)

A general goal is to obtain over four thousand milligrams of potassium, less than one thousand milligrams of sodium, over three hundred milligrams

of magnesium and about five hundred milligrams of calcium a day.

A word of caution becomes necessary for those owners that are already overweight. Overweight owners need further dietary restriction within the real foods that are high in carbohydrate content. Even though some foods are real foods, when an owner is already overweight, the high carbohydrate foods need to be further restricted. Carbohydrate curtailment allows insulin needs to drop.

A lowered insulin need forms the primary move for exiting the "torture chamber". Once one moves outside the "torture chamber", they can begin to lose weight. Weight loss accelerates when both the carbohydrate intake and the mineral imbalanced components are corrected.

As a normal weight approaches, there will be increased tolerance for more carbohydrate. Every owner's physiology differs and needs the counsel of a competent physician for sustained weight loss to occur.

A good place to start involves the almost complete elimination of carbohydrate contained real food and all processed foods. The high carbohydrate containing real foods are potatoes, rice, beans, grains, brown sugar, honey, and pasta. Following this initial approach will counter the IGF-1 deficit occurring in obesity by creating less insulin-produced side effects. Once the target weight, mineral balance, and hormone balance are achieved, some carbohydrates from real food sources can be allowed. Again, each owner's physiology is unique. The counsel of a competent physician is necessary.

As a general guide, keep carbohydrate consumption below 100 grams a day. Very few middle aged and Syndrome X types can consume more than this much carbohydrate a day without weight gain and exaggerated cholesterol and triglyceride increases.

Summary of the weight loss considerations:

1. Optimal hormone levels for insulin, cortisol, androgens, estrogen, thyroid, epinephrine, and IGF-1
2. An exercise program to counteract cortisol and increase growth hormone
3. Stress management
4. Real foods diet that provides a balanced mineral intake
5. Correct nutritional deficiencies (chapter 16)

Case History (application of weight loss principles)

Philip was a forty three year old professional that began to notice weight gain over the last several years. His weight gain occurred despite a vigorous work out schedule that was often one hour long for each session. Workouts included runs in the mountains, strenuous uphill climbs, and prolonged mountain bike rides. Despite his commitment to fitness training, he continued to notice a slow, but progressive 'fat tire' around his midsection. He attempted to follow the ADA diet and was always hungry. Food was constantly on his mind. He was in the "torture chamber". Hormones drove his excessive feeding behavior.

Eventually Philip came across some high protein diet books and figured it would not hurt to give this contrary advice a try. In these books, it was explained how to get insulin levels down and how this would greatly diminish the preoccupation with the next feeding event.

Through my counsel, Philip eventually went on to learn about several other hormones that effect feeding behavior and the tendency to gain weight. He also began to understand the hefty contribution of insulin to his high cholesterol level. To Philip's credit, he exercised regularly which increased his testosterone production and secretion from his gonads. Testosterone counteracts the desire of insulin to make fat by raising IGF-1 production. He came to understand that even with regular exercise, middle age leads to a tendency for decreased testosterone production.

Philip began to understand how increased carbohydrate consumption increases his insulin secretion that eventually tips the scale, in the setting of falling testosterone, for increased fat manufacture. The middle-aged body tolerates less carbohydrate because IGF-1 levels have fallen consequent to a fall in testosterone levels (note: DHEA is also important here).

Marked genetic variability occurs for how much insulin one needs to stimulate the liver into excessive production of LDL cholesterol. As a general rule, when LDL and/or triglyceride levels elevate, suspect high insulin as the culprit. Remember that both diminished thyroid function, specific nutritional deficiencies, and very rare genetic defects can cause the same abnormalities of increased blood fat of this type. Strict adherence to a low carbohydrate diet will dramatically lower LDL cholesterol in most people. The status of other hormones (thyroid, androgen, cortisol, IGF-1, estrogens, and adrenaline) importantly affects any weight loss effort. Finally, mineral balance and its influence on insulin levels need to be optimized if weight and cholesterol normalization is to be realized.

Individuals with high testosterone (athletes, young adult males, and body builders) can tolerate a higher carbohydrate intake. Likewise, an owner with mineral balance between sodium and potassium can handle more carbohydrate intake. In both cases, these owners need less insulin to move sugar into their cells. Less insulin correlates with a diminished fat manufacture rate.

It is the high testosterone and growth hormone, with consequent IGF-1 increases, combination occurring in youth that allows a decreased insulin requirement. The increased growth hormone levels increase IGF-1 release, which facilitates sugar uptake out of the blood stream without the fat manufacture message content contained in the insulin hormone.

Once fat begins to accumulate the body hormones must change in order to return to a trim physique. This summarizes what happened to Philip

before he realized this fundamental fact in the attainment of a more youthful physique again.

When an owner achieves his/her optimal weight, some increased (tailored to activity level) carbohydrate intake becomes allowed. Owners like Philip need to understand that by decreasing their insulin needs from cutting back on carbohydrates, they will decrease the stimulation of the appetite center in their brain.

As owners head into middle age, they destine themselves to failure if they adhere to the ADA diet. Failure usually manifests as a slow, but steady increase in abdominal obesity measured from one year to the next. **The "torture chamber" always wins until a hormonal harmony facilitates weight loss again.**

Knowledge provides power to take action in the destiny of one's physique. This happened in Philip's case as he applied basic hormone knowledge, his 'middle aged physique' began to rejuvenate to a closer version of his youth. He also noted a dramatic decrease of total cholesterol and LDL cholesterol (triglycerides). This means that Philip will have to watch carbohydrates more closely than others because a return to unfavorable cholesterol will always result if insulin levels again increase.

This dramatic improvement in Philip's LDL cholesterol and triglycerides occurred despite his eating four eggs with extra cheese every morning for breakfast. This effect explains the ability of the high protein and fat diet to raise glucagon while lowering insulin. The change in the hormone ratio will turn down the rate of liver synthesized cholesterol.

Philip had an added weight loss advantage by regularly engaging in aerobic exercise that burns calories but also stimulates the gonads to manufacture and release increased androgens. The ratio between glucagon and insulin will improve with regular exercise. Glucagon turns off cholesterol synthesis in the liver and increases this fuel in the blood stream. Without adequate exercise, the increased fuel release that the glucagon message directs will eventually require more insulin. Viewed in this way, it becomes clearer why regular exercise proves as one of the biochemical advantages for prolonged health.

Later in the workup process, I noted high stress operating in his life. Prolonged stress depletes adrenal glands and effects the adrenal secretion itself. Specifically, it increases cortisol release rates that direct energy away from cellular rejuvenation and into survival pathways. Prolonged stress causes the amounts of these opposing steroids to shift away from an optimal ratio between DHEA (an adrenal androgen with testosterone-like activity) and cortisol production. More cortisol and less DHEA production result from the chronic stress response. Increased cortisol is one of the hormones that direct the gonads to manufacture and release (by a circuitous pathway), less androgen. The increased amount of cortisol also directs the liver to dump sugar into the blood stream. Modern stress is usually mental in nature. This extra sugar cannot be used without physical activity. When this sedentary stress occurs, insulin releases to bring the blood sugar back down to normal.

When stress becomes the operational emotion, there needs to be consideration about the message content to raise blood sugar even when no carbohydrates are eaten. Now this discussion flips things on their head. As cortisol increases, the reoccurring body theme that the hormones need balance, comes into play. The only difference here concerns the fact that stress creates a situation where cortisol is the weight that needs the counter weight of insulin to put the breaks on the increase in blood sugar. This fact provides another mechanism for creating a "torture chamber" within, if prolonged stress occurs.

The fact that cortisol raises blood sugar makes sense teleologically, when one remembers the advantage of increased blood fuel in physical survival situations. Prehistorically, when a human ran from the jaws of some large animal, a rapid rise in blood sugar conferred a survival advantage by increasing the physical strength. Ample fuel in the blood stream facilitates muscle fuel delivery. The problem today occurs because many stresses are psychological (mental). The predominance of psychological stress means that no flight ever comes. The stress molecules circulate and direct valuable energy inappropriately. **One of the inappropriate consequences of mental stress concerns the increased blood sugar that it causes.**

The final point about Philip was the hardest part for him to realize. Mineral imbalance in middle age plays a substantial role in fat production. Little recognition occurs between the connection for mineral balance and fat reduction. This information remains missing from many diets offered today.

Philip eventually began to appreciate the many similarities between car batteries and his cells. He began to realize that he would not alter the intended mineral composition of a car battery any more than he would his trillions of cells. This relationship helped him to understand that unless he took in mineral ratios similar to body design, his many cell batteries would deplete. When minerals are consumed in the proper design ratios the cell batteries can charge. Only a body that has fully charged cell batteries can sufficiently liberate enough potassium into the blood stream to help sugar enter cells. Adequate potassium lowers insulin requirements dramatically. The mineral determinant is the fifth determinant of how much insulin a body needs to normalize its blood sugar. All five determinants were eventually improved in Philip's life.

In summary, the five basic determinants of insulin requirements are:
1. **Carbohydrate load**
2. **Mental stress load**
3. **Exercise level**
4. **IGF-1 levels (dependent on both growth hormone and androgen levels). Excessive estrogen can also decrease IGF-1 despite growth hormone and total androgen levels being normal or high.**
5. **Mineral ratios of intake within the diet.**

When these five basic determinants become optimal an owner will have a normal insulin level. Other factors exist (chapter 7), but these make up the central players of the fat manufacture rate potential in a body. They need to be reconciled first and the other factors can be worked on later.

Chapter 9: A Deeper Understanding of Syndrome X: a deadly form of obesity

As was mentioned earlier, Gerald Reaven MD, of Stanford University, coined the term, Syndrome X. This term describes those owners who have embarked on an accelerated path to old age. These owner types age because their blood vessels 'rust' and then go on to develop consequent blockages. Dr. Reaven believes that Syndrome X results from having high blood insulin. He explains the clinical signs of this syndrome as the result of the high insulin state. His opinion of the clinical signs of the high insulin state are: increased abdominal fat, high blood pressure, increased blood triglyceride level, elevated LDL cholesterol, increased skin tag growths on the neck and under the arms, increased blood clotting tendency and an accelerated rusting [oxidation] rate within the blood vessels.

The author of this book feels that the signs of high blood pressure, increased blood clotting tendency and increased rusting rate are better explained by three additional primary antecedent factors. The first concerns the chronically elevated production of cortisol caused by a stress filled lifestyle. The second involves the fact that these owners tend to consume a processed food diet. The third factor and perhaps more central to the underlying cause of this syndrome concern the fact that they have a diminished IGF-1 level.

Recognizing Syndrome X:

The first step involves an owner standing in front of the mirror and noticing whether or not his or her trunk contains their predominant area of obesity. High insulin levels deposit fat here preferentially.

The second step is to notice if his or her cholesterol and triglycerides are elevated. High insulin secretion rates drive the elevation of cholesterol and triglycerides in most owners.

Third step is to obtain a fasting insulin, C-peptide, and IGF-1 level. Many physicians are misled when the fasting insulin comes back normal. They fail to realize that insulin's half-life decreases with a diminished IGF-1. An elevated C-peptide catches these cases of occult Syndrome X. In addition, measurable insulin in the fasting state is abnormal (see below). Many labs have been lowering the lower limit for normal IGF-1. Some labs now say 80ng/ml is normal. As the population becomes fatter the normal IGF-1 skews predictably downward. All physically fit and young people have at least 250ng/ml serum levels. Many have much higher levels.

Fourth strep involves looking for skin tags, new moles, suspended by a narrow stalk, most pronounced on the neck and armpits. Insulin is felt to be a growth factor for these moles.

Fifth step involes noting whether or not, high blood pressure exists. High insulin levels leads to increased levels of blood pressure elevating hormones and decreased levels of blood pressure lowering hormones.

Sixth step concerns whether or not he or she appears older than his or her chronological age because Syndrome X patients tend to motivate by stress. Stress increases the fight or flight emergency response hormones and decreases the repair hormones (explained below).

> **Seventh step** involves ascertaining a given owner's emotional well being because of the increased stress response operating within the Syndrome X owner's life, the blood-clotting tendency elevates. Specifically, the stress response causes an elevation in the acute phase reactants (introduced below and more completelydiscussed in chapter 14). One of the acute phase reactants is called fibrinogen. Fibrinogen, when elevated, increases the tendency for blood vessels to clot from within (explained in the physicians side bar below).

Syndrome X is also known as Metabolic Syndrome and Insulin Resistance Syndrome. This syndrome has been largely attributed to increased insulin secretion rates. Elevated insulin levels describe only one of the hormone aberrations causing Syndrome X. This syndrome becomes more interesting when the other hormone abnormalities are included.

> One big hormone player remains strangely absent from the analysis of sufferers from this syndrome. Although IGF-1 occurs at levels many times those of insulin in the healthful state it remains almost devoid of discussion. Its old name, the nonsuppressible insulin-like activity of the blood stream, sheds more light on its importance. To this author, it seems rather odd that it has been dropped from even a cursory consideration. Especially when one realizes that a major cause for increased insulin need derives from a falling IGF-1 level.

Exaggerated insulin release rates, following mental stress, or following a carbohydrate meal, are only required when IGF-1 levels begin to fall. Healthy individuals have 100 times IGF-1 compared to insulin levels within their blood streams. Because IGF-1 has a half-life of four days, once it releases into the blood stream, it hangs around much longer than insulin's five to ten minute lifespan. When either or both androgen or growth hormone levels begin to fall, the liver releases less IGF-1. IGF-1, occurring at high levels, greatly reduces the amount of insulin released because it facilitates the body cells outside of the liver and fat in their procurement of nutrient uptake. As IGF-1 levels begin to fall off, secondary to sedentary lifestyles, chronic stress, frequent feedings, or the poor hormonal levels mentioned above, more insulin release becomes necessary (insulin resistance). More insulin becomes necessary because the peripheral cells outside the liver and fat have less IGF-1 to assist in nutrient uptake.

Insulin, however, contains message content that IGF-1 does not share. The insulin message directs the liver to manufacture increased amounts of sugar into both fat and cholesterol. IGF-1 message content does not direct this process. The progressive inverse changes in the amounts of a Syndrome X individual's insulin versus IGF-1 levels provides a more complete explanation for their primary hormonal defect.

When IGF-1 levels remain high, the body cells, outside of the liver and fat, procure an increased proportion of blood fuel. However, because of the anatomical location of the pancreas dumping insulin directly into the portal vein, the liver always receives the highest amount of insulin message content.

Exaggerating the effect concerns the fact that the liver and fat cells have the highest pure insulin-type receptor concentration of any cells in the body, occurring at 200,000 per cell. A falling IGF-1 level tips the advantage to the liver procuring more fuel for the manufacture of cholesterol and fat.

Recap Fact: the higher the insulin and the lower the glucagon level within the liver, the more active HMG CoA reductase. HMG CoA reductase is the enzyme, which makes cholesterol in the body. This detail explains how the high insulin states, like adult onset diabetes and Syndrome X, develop abnormal cholesterol profiles.

Once again, instead of the medical industrial complex revealing this simple scientific relationship, the more lucrative cholesterol-lowering drugs fill media advertising space. How one heals from Syndrome X involves an emphasis on the methods that will increase one's IGF-1. Improvement here leads to an improved cholesterol profile without side effects or toxicities.

The overall genesis of the typical Syndrome X individual results from his/her high insulin only after his/her

IGF-1 levels begin to fall. Once IGF-1 falls, either the stress response or increased carbohydrate consumption leads to an exaggerated release of insulin. Increased insulin release preferentially tells the liver to make sugar into fat and cholesterol. Insulin levels become even higher in those owners who chronically subsist on a processed food diet.

Processed food diets provide reversed mineral content that deviates from body design. Reversed mineral intake leads to insulin resistance around middle age. In addition, the vitamin deficiencies, which are inherent consequences of subsisting on a processed food diet, prevent adequate blood vessel repair and blood fuel removal processes (chapter 16).

Syndrome X owners exist on an accelerated track to an old body. Their fundamental defect concerns their elevated insulin levels. One cause for increased insulin need, results from falling IGF-1 levels. This syndrome worsens in a setting of increased stress, because it leads to lower IGF-1 levels. Increased stress will accelerate potassium loss, as well. Low potassium and low magnesium diets with elevated sodium intake will contribute further to the disease process.

In many ways, a high stress hormone output could help explain how Syndrome X patients age so quickly and have high blood pressure, as well. This is better illustrated by the fact that chronically elevated cortisol tells the body that an emergency situation chronically exists. When the body perceives an emergency (real or imagined) the body's energy redirects into survival pathways (catabolic instead of anabolic). In the Type A personality or Syndrome X owners, the survival pathway becomes the norm instead of rejuvenation activities.

When body energy chronically directs into survival pathways, wear and tear changes will become more likely. **Wear and tear changes within the body cells manifest clinically as an old appearing and feeling body.** Wear and tear changes become more likely, secondary to the lack of cellular repair activities. Cellular repair and rejuvenation activities cannot occur unless sufficient anabolic message content reaches the cells. This helps to explain why Syndrome X owners tend to age so quickly. Not only do they tend to have high insulin derived disease but also high cortisol derived disease, as well. Cortisol directs body energy into catabolic pathways. Too much catabolism within the blood vessels leads to wear and tear changes.

After all, in one way or another, the initial blood vessel lesion (rust) grabs hold when the blood vessel repair processes fail to keep up with the injury rate (excess iron or fluoride ions). The degree of anabolism determines the repair rate. Conversely, the amount of catabolism puts repair on hold and survival pathways activate instead.

The severity of the Syndrome X exacerbates from the consumption of processed foods.

> (Physician side bar) Dr. Reaven is right about insulin having some role in the blood pressure elevation of these owner types. One of the reasons that elevated insulin raises blood pressure concerns the fact that it powerfully stimulates the blood vessel lining cells' production of endothelin. When endothelin production increases, blood pressure rises. High insulin levels also diminish the ability of the blood vessel lining cells to produce nitric oxide. The diminished production of nitric oxide further reduces the body's ability to maintain an appropriate blood pressure level.

Large amounts of insulin within the blood stream require large amounts of cortisol to effectively counter insulin's behavior of moving every last sugar molecule out of the blood stream. Remember insulin levels need to rise abnormally only when IGF-1 levels fall. Almost always the fall in IGF-1 levels has a component of causality in a diminished growth hormone secretion. Bodies that cannot produce sufficient growth hormone need increased insulin and increased cortisol in order to maintain their blood sugars between meals (chapters 10 and 12).

> (Side bar for physicians) Syndrome X owners have long been known to have an increased prevalence of gout.

> Mainstream textbooks often fail to explain why this association occurs. If one adds back in the protein sparing effect of growth hormone, it begins to become clear. Additionally, concerns the fact that unhealthy owners need increased cortisol, glucagon, and epinephrine to keep their blood sugars elevated between meals because their growth hormone levels have fallen off. These two facts, taken together, elucidate why gout risks increase with Syndrome X.
>
> Syndrome X owners have an accelerated rate of gluconeogenesis. Gluconeogenesis creates increased nitrogen waste that normally releases as urea and only small amounts of uric acid. However, with the high carbohydrate production rates, caused by increased gluconeogenesis, the uric acid production rate goes up, as well. Some owners have a weakened, genetically determined, ability to convert excessive uric acid production into urea, and gout ensues.
>
> Rather than give these patients toxic prescriptions to treat their symptoms of gout, it seems worthwhile to spend a little effort on getting their growth hormone levels back up to par. This approach becomes even more critical when one adds in the knowledge of the association between body protein content maintenance and youth preservation. Without someone helping these Syndrome X owners to regain their protein content, they are destined to age at accelerated rates.

Cortisol counters the effect of insulin by increasing the blood sugar levels. Cortisol, however, directs body energy and molecular building parts into survival pathways and out of repair and rejuvenation pathways. Anti-oxidant synthesis and blood vessel repair defer with a chronically high cortisol level.

Modern life stress further exacerbates the increased need for insulin. When the owner also experiences chronically high levels of cortisol release, the body energy directs away from cellular rejuvenation activities. Syndrome X causes the inefficient use of molecular building parts for repair activity by the body. The correction of this dysfunctional process begins when the healthy and appropriate ratio of cortisol and insulin returns to normal within the blood stream. This can be substantially accomplished by nutritional rather than symptom-control treatment plans. Before a description of those strategies occurs, a syndrome closely related to Syndrome X will be described. This syndrome can be treated with very similar nutritional strategies used for the treatment of Syndrome X.

The Type A personality is a closely related condition typified by a hard driving (intense), hurried, over achieving and aggressive type of individual. These personality traits have long been associated with an increased propensity for acquiring heart disease. The trouble is that the mainstream education stops at a superficial level of explaining this association. A deeper hormonal explanation exists for why these types of individuals develop the inflammatory type of heart disease at an accelerated rate.

All body hormones contain message content inherent in their precise shape. All hormone message content concerns how the body becomes directed to spend its available energy. The stress response hormone's release is quite active within the Type A individual. The body cannot discern whether a stress is real or imagined. In addition, once the stress response initiates, body energy redirects into surviving a physical stress. This largely outdated hormonal response has health consequences in the modern world because most stress has become mental in nature. There are three big health consequences within the blood vessel that result from chronic mental stress (Type A personality). These mechanisms are included in the side bar for the reader's doctor to review because the second consequence is generally considered to be above the laymen's level of how to heal from obesity.

(Side bar for physicians) First, the survival message contained in the hormonal stress response directs body

energy away from rejuvenation activities and into mounting energy for increasing physical strength. Ongoing blood vessel rejuvenation activities are crucial if one is to avoid the consequence of disrepair damage and eventual inflammation. Survival mode that occurs occasionally is without consequences. However, some personalities are always in survival mode. The body cells are faithful servants to the message content that they receive.

The opposite extreme of message content occurs within the blood vessels of those owners who are happy and physically active. Regular physical exercise and effective stress management promote the increased release of the rejuvenation (androgens) hormone's message content. Within the blood vessel, the rejuvenation hormone's message content tells these individual's cells that it is important to invest in repair and regeneration activities. Ongoing repair activities are necessary to prevent the wear and tear changes within the blood vessels, which lead to inflammation.

The second way that the stress response leads to blood vessel inflammation, when it becomes chronic, involves the fact that certain inflammatory proteins release. C-reactive protein is only one of several of these types of proteins released within the stress response. Collectively, these proteins are known as the acute phase reactants. Other acute phase reactants include: fibrinogen, complement, interferon, haptoglobin, ferritin, and ceruloplasmin. The increase of these protein types in a setting of physical stress makes sense. The physical stress of combat or running from a large animal requires the increased activity of the immune system, blood clotting and remanufacture of new blood cell components. Each of the above acute phase reactants contributes to this overall scheme for surviving physical trauma. However, in the setting of chronic mental stress, when these acute phase reactants elevate, the increased tendency for blood vessel inflammation occurs.

The above cause and effect relationship of the acute phase reactants and chronic stress develops a more comprehensive picture. An elevated C-reactive protein is only a small part of the overall picture of blood vessel inflammation. Other specific acute phase reactants, like ferritin and fibrinogen, contribute directly to blood vessel inflammation.

Healing Type A personality individuals' blood vessels becomes possible when they understand the bigger connection of the scientific facts. Rather than being led down the well-worn path of the hopeless mantra about the cruel hand that genetics has dealt so take your cholesterol lowering prescription, healing becomes possible. Healing occurs when a Type A personality gains insight into the importance of increasing his/her positive emotions and physical activity level while decreasing his/her stressful behaviors.

The third facet for how the stress response causes blood vessel inflammation, which occurs chronically in the Type A personality, involves the obligatory increase in blood fuel. This third facet concerns the outdated survival response, which directs the massive dumping of fuel into the blood stream. Extra fuel within the blood stream confers a survival advantage for mounting the increased strength required with surviving physical stressors. However, mental stress causes the release of increased blood fuel, as well. This response occurs because the body cannot discern the difference between mental and physical stress. The body is smart enough to eventually figure out that the mental stress caused increases in blood fuel has nowhere to go. Increased amounts of insulin then secrete from the pancreas to direct the uptake of the unneeded fuel into the liver. This fact helps to unite the Type A personality to the Syndrome X owner for how each of their blood vessels become inflamed.

There exists one key difference between the classical Type A personality and the classical Syndrome X owner. The syndrome X owner's primary defect results from a fall off in their IGF-1, usually from either or both a fall in androgens, growth hormone secretion rates and/or liver injury. In other words, glandular failure originating in the pituitary, adrenal, liver or gonads brings about a diminished IGF-1.

> In contrast, the classical Type A personality suffers a drop off in his/her IGF-1 levels because chronic stress elevates his/her blood sugar, secondary to elevated cortisol. Remember that growth hormone cannot release until the blood sugar begins to fall. Here lies the fundamental pathology obstructing longevity in a Type A personality. Their IGF-1 falls off when their growth hormone fails to release because the stress response chronically elevates their blood sugars. This association makes it clearer why exercise becomes so important to restoring health to the Type A personality body. Exercise provides a mechanism to draw down the blood fuel levels and hence growth hormone release can occur. (see Blood Vessel Inflammation discussion in chapter 14)

Finally, in order to complete the current discussion of syndrome X (note:a more comprehensive discussion about inflammation follows in chapter 14), the importance of IGF-1 levels needs further emphasis. Healthy owners predictably have high normal IGF-1 levels. IGF-1 is synthesized within the liver in response to sufficient DHEA (simplified). Growth hormone secretion from the pituitary causes the IGF-1, stored within the liver, to be released. Healthy owners have at least 100 times the IGF-1 in their circulation as they do insulin. IGF-1 acts like insulin for the cells outside the liver and fat. High IGF-1 levels lower the amount of insulin needed within the body. IGF-1 levels provide a mechanism for fuel uptake by cells outside the liver and fat cells between meals. In contrast, insulin's design facilitates the liver and fat cells to remove fuel out of the blood stream following meals.

Troubles start around middle age in sedentary and stressed owners. These two lifestyle traits combine to diminish IGF-1 levels. A lower IGF-1 level means that insulin secretion must rise to abnormally high levels in order to attempt to offset the decrease in IGF-1 levels (thus keeping the total amount of "fuel nozzle" hormones constant).

This detail explains why Syndrome X types present with elevated fasting insulin and/or C-peptide levels. Healthy owners have essentially no insulin in the fasting state. Most mainstream labs allow some insulin in the fasting state before it is considered too high. However, this belief proves inconsistent with what role insulin serves when one remains healthy.

The body is smart and consistent. Insulin's design helps to store fuel in the liver following meals so there will be enough fuel released from the liver between meals to keep the blood fuel constant. However, a rise in IGF-1 facilitates the uptake of nutrition between meals, which growth hormone release directs, while sparing body proteins usage for fuel. Remember, growth hormone release also directs the liver to simultaneously release sugar and fat into the blood stream that was stored in the liver following the last meal under insulin's direction.

Following meals, the healthy body relies on sufficient insulin to store adequate fuel for the next between meals state. In the between meals state, sufficient growth hormone release tells the healthy liver to release the stored sugar, fat, and IGF-1. In this way, the healthy body's cells have access to sufficient blood fuel at all times while protecting their protein content from combustion for usage as fuel.

In contrast, unhealthy people do not release sufficient growth hormone. Instead, they release excessive cortisol, glucagon and epinephrine between meals in order to keep their blood fuel elevated. Body protein now becomes fair game for fuel usage and because IGF-1 levels are down, more insulin needs to be secreted between meals. Insulin secretion in the between meals state is abnormal. It only becomes necessary when IGF-1 levels have fallen.

(Recap side bar for physicians) Why would a healthy body instruct the liver to draw down the blood sugar further in the between meal state? Unhealthy bodies do this only because they lack "fuel nozzle" hormones (a fallen IGF-1 level) for their cells, as in muscle and organs. In order to keep alive they accept the complications of increasing insulin output enough to spill over into the general circulation and allow these cells their "fuel nozzle". The major complication results from the fact that whatever the insulin secretion rate, because of the pancreas-portal vein connection to the liver, the liver receives the highest concentration of its message content before the other body cells can get any insulin "fuel nozzles". This means a contradictory message occurs within the unhealthy body's liver during the fasting state.

The contradictory message within the unhealthy body results from the fact that insulin, within the liver, opposes the other body cells procurement of nutrition between meals (fasting state). Remember that the liver and fat cells have the highest pure insulin-type receptor concentration per cell at about 200,000. A high insulin release rate becomes necessary to get insulin beyond the liver and into the general circulation but this also excessively stimulates the cholesterol and fat-making machinery. This leads to the liver performing counter-productive tasks during the fasting state. Some liver cells, under the influence of insulin, begin sucking sugar out of the blood stream while the body is in the fasting state, and thus, worsens the falling blood sugar. Other liver cells, under the influence of the counter hormones, cortisol, glucagon and epinephrine, tell other liver cells to dismantle protein (gluconeogenesis) to make sugar and release it into the blood stream. The end result accelerates protein degradation and increases the manufacture rate of fat and cholesterol. These side effects occur just to keep the unhealthy body's blood sugar elevated between meals.

Remember that normally, between meals, the healthy liver responds to growth hormone's release by simultaneously releasing IGF-1, sugar, and fat into the blood stream. Growth hormone's release also protects body protein content between meals. Healthy bodies, avoid competing messages at the level of the liver between meals (fasting state), and conserve organ and muscle protein stores, as well.

SECTION 4: More Medical Myths That Promote Suffering

Chapter 10: Diminished Adrenal Reserve Caused Disease

The adrenal glands sit on top of each kidney. They are about the size and shape of an acorn. The 'seed' makes the epinephrine and is directly 'wired' into the sympathetic nervous system. This sympathetic nerve connection facilitates the release of epinephrine. Epinephrine conveys an overall body message of both alertness and increased metabolism. The 'cap' makes the adrenal steroid hormones (aldosterone, DHEA, progesterone, androstenedione, and cortisol) from cholesterol. Aldosterone proves as a key hormone in the regulation of salt and water balance and its amount also controls the rate of all other steroid's manufacture rates. DHEA and cortisol can be thought of as counter regulatory opposites.

As previously explained, when cortisol levels rise, the message that directs cellular energy into survival pathways increases. The primitive survival response is the same whether a stress proves real or imagined. It is also the same whether it proves physical or mental in nature. The fallout of this truism means that whatever the stress, massive fuel dumps into the blood stream. Physical stresses need extra fuel to survive them but mental stress does not. Cortisol provides blood fuel by dismantling body structure. The body composes itself from sugar, fat and protein. By definition, hormones that dismantle body structure for fuel needs are called catabolic.

This redirection of cellular energy occurs whenever cortisol levels rise beyond a very low threshold. In the healthy state, low levels of cortisol (below the threshold) provide anti-inflammatory, cellular rest, sodium, and fluid retention, and maintain blood vessel responsiveness to epinephrine's message.

DHEA and androstenedione are from the androgen class of hormones that direct body energy into cellular infrastructure investment activities that lead to cellular rejuvenation. Note that the androgen steroids provide the opposite message compared to the catabolic hormones. As an aside, insulin proves anabolic for fat and cholesterol accumulation. While true anabolic steroids tend to build up the protein component of the body tissue (muscles and organs functional components). Proteins comprise the metabolically active component of body tissue. In other words, they burn up calories. Examples of proteins that consume energy while they function are: enzymes, some hormone types, cell receptors and membrane pumps. The more of these one has, the more calories burned. The more calories burned, the faster the metabolic rate.

The role of progesterone within the adrenal also seems to counter the salt and water retaining effects of cortisol and aldosterone. In women, progesterone is manufactured in both the adrenals and ovaries.

Some women have weakened adrenals and when ovarian progesterone production slows, just before their menstruation, their progesterone levels fall too far. Just before their menstruation, these women experience first hand the fluid retaining effects that occur when progesterone levels suddenly plummet. They can also experience anxiety and mental irritability (PMS). These symptoms shed light on the calming effect of progesterone within the central nervous system. In fact, it has been known for many years that high doses of progesterone produce anesthesia from the increased GABA that results within the neurons of the brain and spinal cord. Progesterone rises considerably during pregnancy. Pregnant women also possess a calming beauty and note frequent urination. Both of these facts further support progesterone's powerful messages within the body.

A 'tug of war' exists between the adrenal androgens and cortisol message content. Modern life complexities often cause chronic stress that increases cortisol output relative to other adrenal androgens. Typical modern stress comes in the form of deadlines, job insecurities, complex multiple task responsibilities, and incessant noise, to name a few. If one adds the increased consumption of carbohydrate, which increases the need for more cortisol in many middle-aged owners, gland exhaustion becomes possible. Increased cortisol is needed to balance the effects of increased insulin within the blood stream of unhealthy owners (explained below). One gains insight into this modern day problem, when considering the counter-regulatory response necessary to keep extra insulin behaving within the blood stream.

Low blood sugar often provides the first clinical sign that the adrenal glands are beginning to fail in their output of cortisol (stress hormone). Increased cortisol becomes necessary in order to deal with the stress of modern life and the stress of having extra insulin. When the cortisol level becomes inadequate the first symptom is often 'brain fog'. 'Brain fog' provides a warning sign that something is wrong with hormonal balance. The loss of balance incrementally leads insidiously to an amplification of the mental problem.

Balanced hormonal responses create a cellular communication harmony that underlies the healthful state. As the adrenals lose their ability to respond to the demands for balance, 'brain fog' ensues.

As stated above, the main androgen types of steroid hormones within the adrenal glands are DHEA and androstenedione. While DHEA is only made within the adrenal gland, androstenedione is made by the ovary and adrenal gland. DHEA only will be discussed here, but the reader can also extend this as applicable to androstenedione. Different body tissues prefer to interact with different androgens.

DHEA proves particularly important in females as it displays the utility of peripheral conversion into the more powerful androgens, like testosterone, once inside the target cell (muscle, ligament, bone). Peripheral conversion spares females the masculine effects of dumping straight testosterone into their blood streams. DHEA (and androstenedione) are much weaker androgens than testosterone. DHEA, like other androgens, directs cellular energy into cellular infrastructure investment activities (an anabolic effect). Regular infrastructure investment proves necessary for continued health. Testosterone and DHEA differ in the strength of their message content to direct masculine traits. The female body initially secretes a weaker androgen like DHEA, and later peripherally converts it to testosterone within the cell. This approach leads to a diminished masculine message carried within the blood stream.

As the adrenal loses its ability to keep up with the demands for its hormonal products, DHEA manufacture can be the first to drop off. This imbalance is often missed clinically. At this level of dysfunction, there are only subtle clues. Females are more vulnerable to the ravages of diminished DHEA production as there is less androgen output from their ovaries, relative to the male testes. These patients tend to present with increased fatigue, some with increased fat, and the earliest signs of deteriorating musculoskeletal structures.

As stress continues, the adrenal glands cease to make adequate cortisol to counter balance insulin's blood sugar lowering message and this causes 'brain fog'. 'Brain fog' often indicates adrenal imbalance has continued long enough for moderate body cellular damage to occur. Cellular damage occurs secondary to the prolonged survival message that directs the body's energy away from rejuvenation activities.

At a cellular level, the lack of rejuvenation activities leads to old cellular components: old cell factories (organelles), old cellular machines (enzymes), and diminished cellular charge (the battery) – simply stated, old age.

The body has a backup system within the gonads for specific steroid type hormones (not cortisol or DHEA). The amount of DHEA produced within the healthy adrenal gland can be a thousand times more than the amount of testosterone produced within the ovary. The amount of androstenedione production within female ovaries, under the best of circumstances, approaches one-fifth the adrenal amount of DHEA normally produced. The ovary has little ability for the manufacture of DHEA. Internal havoc is probable when the adrenal becomes wounded. The wounded adrenal gland led to the description of **diminished adrenal reserve** over fifty years ago.

Diminished Adrenal Reserve Syndrome

In the 1950's, John W. Tintera MD pioneered the concept of adrenal exhaustion. He noted that adrenal exhaustion often results from prolonged stress and added this to the previously accepted causes. Some of the other causes were various infections, hemorrhage, and genetic defects for certain adrenal steroids manufacture and medication side effects. The focus here regards how stress leads the way to diminished adrenal function and how this will always manifest with a tendency for low blood sugar episodes.

In 1955, Dr.Tintera published a paper in the New York State Journal of Medicine that included over 200 cases of patients with sub-optimal adrenal function. He discovered that 100 percent of these patients had low blood sugar episodes along with their other complaints that occur with the diagnosis of adrenal insufficiency. He called this state of sub-optimal adrenal function, hypo-adrenal-corticism.

Years later, it was established that cortisol, secreted from the adrenal gland, proved as a powerful counter regulatory hormone to the blood sugar-lowering effects of insulin. As the adrenals in these patients began to fail in their ability to counter the message of insulin, these patients would present with low blood sugars. The low blood sugars resultrd from too much insulin and not enough cortisol to balance out the message content.

The body design includes a system of counter balanced hormones. When secreted, a given hormone always needs a counter-balancing response from an opposing hormone or group of hormones. The balancing hormones direct energy expenditure so energy never moves too far in one direction.

In these cases, insulin desires to remove every last sugar from the blood stream while cortisol moderates the effect of insulin. The balance between these two hormones avoids going too far in any one direction for energy expenditure. Disease results when this balancing system impairs. Dr. Tintera correctly deduced that when prolonged stress depletes the ability of the adrenal to respond as a counter balance to insulin, blood sugar regulation diminishes. Patients with impaired adrenals are unable to secrete sufficient cortisol so their blood sugars become unstable. These patients remain more vulnerable to the threat of hypoglycemia.

Over fifty years later, new hormonal understandings about the ideal blood sugar regulator between meals being growth hormone comes into play for the youthful body to continue (explaied in chapter 13). For now, it is only important to realize that growth hormone levels fall first in these patients. This exaggerates the need for insulin within the body (insulin resistance). In the between meals state, instead of growth hormone causing the continued secretion of blood fuel, cortisol needs to pick up the slack. **Dr. Herb Joiner-Bey** points out that increased cortisol secretion proves violent to body structure because it accelerates protein dismantling where growth hormone does not. In fact, growth hormone proves as the only hormone to protect body protein content between meals and while exercising. Healthy bodies have ample protein content within their muscles and organs. Unhealthy bodies do not.

Hormones always need opposition from counter-hormones to maintain balance. It helps to understand balance if one envisions an antique weight scale. In general, whenever there is a hormone secreted (weight), there needs to be an adequate counter-hormone response (counter - weight) or health cannot be maintained. Healthy owners have balanced 'weight scales'. Their bodies secrete the very best hormones in their optimal amounts. Their counter response hormones also secrete in the optimal amount and with appropriate timing.

Improved laboratory testing developed over the last 40 years has led to more accurate testing methods of patient's hormone profiles. Unfortunately, owners in America live in a profit driven health care system. The profit motive leads to the

$25,000 solution receiving press coverage while the $1,000 solution remains ignored. The basic knowledge of what science has revealed empowers an owner who suffers from diminished adrenal function. This approach opens up options that can lead to healing instead of symptom-control. In addition, this knowledge allows awareness of some inconsistencies perpetrated by the profit motive of the medical industrial complex.

Adrenal Health Determines Immune Systems Readiness and Appropriateness

Many owners in America wake up tired, catch colds and coughs frequently, and deal with stress poorly. Many have diffuse aches in their muscles and joints. The majority are depressed and have lost their zest for life. Most have allergies or asthma that worsen with prolonged stress and fatigue. In the more severe cases of diminished adrenal function, chronic degenerative diseases like rheumatoid arthritis, systemic lupus, ulcerative colitis, Crohn disease, and fibromyalgia syndrome surface. Many of these ailments appear to be from divergent sources. Often, each of these afflictions trace back to a poorly functioning adrenal system.

The science behind the dysfunctional adrenal gland system conflicts with the symptom-control medicine approach. The complex panders the symptom-control, medicinal philosophy. Many physicians have no idea that a deeper understanding of adrenal function can often lead to considerable improvement in the above disease processes. They have been groomed to think of the adrenals in a very superficial and piecemeal way.

Medical textbooks are curiously deficient in the discussion of interrelated consequences of a diminished adrenal reserve. Instead, their discussion focuses only on the most extreme examples of adrenal dysfunction. Examples of these extremes are Addison's disease (cortisol deficiency) and Cushing's disease (cortisol excess).

A peripheral discussion might surface regarding the role of the adrenal hormone, cortisol, for its role in the prevention of hypoglycemia. Cortisol proves as the major player in the prevention of hypoglycemia for many middle-aged owners. Most textbook discussions concern hormones within the adrenal gland, but fail to unite the fact that adrenal steroid hormones secrete together in a preformed ratio. A reoccurring tendency within the medical textbooks also exists to completely ignore the concept that some owners may have diminished adrenal function under conditions of stress. Unless stressed, these owners' level of dysfunction is not as severe as those of an Addisonian patient.

Doctors are taught to think about disease of the adrenal, in a piecemeal fashion. Cushing's disease exemplifies this. A hallmark of this disease involves losing muscle and gaining body fat. A consistent failure exists in emphasizing the reason body fat goes up and is not directly related to the markedly elevated cortisol levels.

Initially, cortisol promotes fat and sugar dumping into the blood stream. Increased body fat proves secondary to elevated blood sugar spikes. The elevated blood sugar results from the high cortisol message content which then directs the liver to release its stored sugar into the blood stream. The sugar dumping amplifies because cortisol also encourages the liver process called gluconeogenesis. Gluconeogenesis denotes the conversion of amino acids into sugar. This source of sugar also dumps into the blood stream. The body eventually realizes that the blood sugar has elevated inappropriately.

Elevated blood sugars suppress growth hormone secretion but promote excess insulin releases into the blood stream to counter this situation. The increase in insulin required to make the blood sugar normal, leads to the increased making of body fat. Remember, whatever the insulin secretion rate, the liver always receives the highest concentration of its message content (basic anatomy of the pancreas portal vein connection to the liver). The liver and fat cells also have the highest pure insulin-type receptor concentration at about 200,000 per cell.

High insulin states, within the liver, cause the blood sugar to preferentially suck up into it. The liver turns varying amounts of this sugar into LDL cholesterol (chapter 13).

Lost protein proves secondary to two other abnormal hormonal processes that occur with chronic stress (elevated cortisol) and elevated insulin levels. The first part results from the fact that elevated cortisol levels lead to increased prolactin release. Increases in prolactin levels inhibit the gonads' release of androgens that constitute a counter weight to the high level of insulin's ability to make patients fat. Remember that the androgens promote muscle and organ growth and repair. The inhibition of the gonads is often left out of the discussion.

Also left out of the discussion concerns the additional fact that a slight elevation in the blood sugar will inhibit growth hormone release. Diminished growth hormone release will lead to a diminished ability to hold onto body proteins (chapter 7) and diminished IGF-1 release. Remember, IGF-1 is insulin's helper and occurs at levels one hundred times those of insulin in healthy owners. As growth hormone secretion falls off, less IGF-1 secretes and this leads to excessive insulin need (insulin resistance). This last little detail ties in those Syndrome X (also known as Metabolic Syndrome or Insulin Resistance Syndrome) patients to a variant of Cushing's disease pathology (physician's sidebar chapter 14). This specific disease example points to the incongruous discussion between the various hormone abnormalities in the way physicians learn to think about adrenal disease.

The examples of Cushing's and Addison's Diseases provide extreme examples of adrenal dysfunction. Cushing's Disease produces extremely high cortisol production rates. Conversely, Addison's disease has an extreme deficiency of cortisol. The deficiencies are so significant that viability can only be maintained by taking cortisol supplements.

What about those owners whose adrenal abnormality lies somewhere between these two extremes of adrenal dysfunction in stressful situations? Both of these situations have health consequences. In the wounded adrenal

responder, additional life stress pushes them towards the need to lay down (much like early Addison's Disease). In the over reactive adrenal responder (Syndrome X types), the excess secretion of cortisol for surviving trivial life stress leads to a chronic mild elevation of the blood sugar. This tendency causes an increased insulin need and also a decreased ability to secrete growth hormone.

Mainstream medicine most often recognizes the extremes of adrenal dysfunction. The consequence of this concerns owners who suffer, but are not in immediate danger of death. This common medical practice is analogous to only considering thyroid dysfunction if it is on either extreme that puts the patient at risk of death.

Science could help owners with the above diseases improve their adrenal system's function. Curiously, this is not the case. Medical educations do a better job at alerting physicians to the subtleties of altered thyroid function and the diseases that follow. Before ways to heal from these diseases are discussed, there needs to be a discussion about two important facts. First, steroids have a powerful nature when compared to other body hormones. Second, different disease presentations result from the same common deficiency of cortisol and/or DHEA. Much is known about the first fact and an introductory discussion follows. Very little is understood about the second fact and this awaits further scientific investigation before a plausible explanation sufaces. Be aware of this current mystery.

The common property of steroids, Vitamin A and thyroid hormone must be emphasized. These hormones are the most powerful of all hormones in the body. These steroids include testosterone, estrogen, DHEA, androstenedione, cortisol, progesterone, and aldosterone. There are other steroids of less importance. The power of this group lies in the fact that only these hormone types carry their message directly to all the DNA programs throughout every cell in the body. No other hormones directly influence the DNA (genes) program.

These hormones interact with the genetic program. They directly determine which genes turn off and on. Gene activity determines which body proteins are manufactured. Healthy bodies have the exact amount of protein types needed. The only way to achieve the right amount of protein types requires possessing the right amounts of these powerful hormones that direct one's DNA. The quality, type, and amount of these powerful hormones determine how wisely the cells will spend their available energy. These hormones carry their message by virtue of their unique and precise shape. The steroids, Vitamin A, and thyroid, differ from other hormones by binding directly with many DNA receptors. They have access to every body chamber.

The unique property of these hormones allows them to be the determinants of which DNA programs activate or repress. Owners that have the proper quality, amounts, and timing of these hormones, receive a tremendous health advantage. The effectiveness of these hormones determines the quality and amounts of the lesser hormones manufactured (see appendix). Therefore, these hormones prove as the most critical of all the hormones in the body. Ways to heal begins with considering their quality within an owner.

The power of these hormones lies in their control of the genetic program. An excess or deficiency provides an abnormal message content to the DNA of the cells. When the wrong DNA programs activate or repress, the cell spends energy unwisely. Energy used foolishly on the wrong proteins, wrong repair to rest ratios, wrong immune activation level, wrong amount of cell product, etc. describes a disease process.

Though diseases have predictable results, identical excesses or deficiencies will initiate different diseases in different owners. This part remains only partially understood and the understood portion involves complex science that occurs beyond the scope of this manual.

Any of the six links in the adrenal system chain will cause disease when it becomes defective.

In today's world of harried physicians and managed care, the owner needs to be aware of the six levels, which the adrenal system can fail. Erroneously, most attention toward adrenal health inquiries limits the focus to one or two levels only. Consequently, many owners' diagnosis remains incorrect and/or they receive symptom-control treatments. Thus, owners miss out on ways to heal themselves. *The Body Heals* explores the six levels of the adrenal system and how any one of these being defective leads to the above-mentioned adrenal system related diseases

Uniting high stress and a defect within the adrenal system make any of these adrenal system diseases worse.

1.	Allergies	4.	Systemic lupus
2.	Asthma.	3.	Rheumatoid arth.
3.	Colitis	6.	Crohn disease

In this subsection, the reasoning will be introduced as to why mainstream medicine's fear of steroid replacement often fails to be substantiated. *The Body Heals* contains a more detailed explanation as to why many well-meaning physicians looking for a diminished adrenal system function fail to find it. They have not been trained to evaluate all six links in the adrenal system. **The chain links in the adrenal system includes:**

1. **Hypothalamus in the brain**
2. **Master control panel gland for hormone glands, the pituitary (which hangs on the underside of the brain)**
3. **Healthy adrenal gland function**
4. **Blood stream transport system**
5. **Complete, intact characteristics of the DNA receptor waiting for something to do within the target cell.**
6. **Result of DNA program activation is the manufacture of certain protein-composed receptors for the 'lesser' hormones.**

A defect at any of the six levels clinically behaves as if the adrenal system isn't functioning properly. Most physicians receive little instruction for evaluating the integrity of the entire system. The profit in treating symptoms of the above diseases overrides the incentive to educate physicians about the other side of the scientific story. Some lonely thinkers clunk along with some really good healing insights, while the complex supports effective ways of marginalizing these scientific discoveries.

One of the heroes in the lonely thinker/scientist category is William McKenzie Jefferies, MD. Dr. Jefferies, the author of *Safe Uses of Cortisol,* 96, brings over 45 years of clinical insight to the discussion of illness secondary to a malfunctioning adrenal system. His career in Endocrinology included professorships at both Case Western Medical School and more recently at Virginia Medical School. All of the above diseases he discusses and reviews in his book. This book is a must read for an owner with any of the listed diseases secondary to a poorly functioning adrenal system. One needs an education in order to step beyond symptom-control and into healing.

Many physicians have been effectively taught to fear cortisone treatments over the long haul. This training has been so well performed that many physicians are automatically negative in their response to hearing the word cortisone or steroid. This effect results from successfully confusing physicians and the public between the effects of cortisol within physiologic doses versus higher doses given to treat disease.

Further confusion results from not educating physicians in the basics of how the precise shape of the steroid delivers accurate message content. Only altered steroid shapes can get a patent advantage. However, altered steroid shapes deliver inaccurate message content to one's DNA programs. Inaccurate message content leads to side effects and toxicities.

Perhaps even more damaging to overall middle-aged health concerns the fact that the optimal adrenal secretion contains preformed ratios between the different steroids listed earlier. To only replace one, when several prove

deficient, creates even more message content disharmony. The above diseases arise from an adrenal deficiency. Each unique deficiency has different proportions of the various adrenal steroids that are not getting to the afflicted owners DNA programs.

Without a complete inquiry into all six links, these diseases continue to smolder until they erupt. Diseases that erupt require symptom-control and symptom-control has side effects.

The media campaigns have persuaded physicians and owners to fear even small doses of the natural body manufactured cortisol. This occurs despite the fact (evidence to be discussed shortly) that the diseases mentioned before have a deficiency of cortisol function in common. These diseases often directly result due to a failure to receive adequate adrenal steroids to the DNA program.

An extension of Dr. Jefferies' work addresses the emerging realization that healthy, activated adrenals, secrete a mixture of steroids in preformed ratios. This optimizes the message content of a healthy owner whenever the stress response activates. Only giving cortisol in all instances of the above diseases results in the potential for a lessened healing response. A lessened healing response ensues due to the exclusion of the other adrenal steroids, which the adrenal normally produces.

Keep in mind that other adrenal steroid imbalances may contribute significantly to a disease process. The 24-hour urine test for adrenal steroids often proves as the best method for detecting these defects in steroid production. However, many physicians are unable to interpret these tests. Until physicians receive education in this area, they will remain unable to prescribe the optimal replacement of real message content.

The clinician must consider, while measuring the cortisol level of those with the potential for diminished adrenal reserve, that borderline patients tend to have deceptively normal blood cortisol levels while low stress prevails. However, during stress their adrenals' production of cortisol diminishes relative to need in order to remain symptom free. In these cases of diminished adrenal reserve, blood testing or a 24-hour urine test for cortisol production can be deceptively normal. Some of these patients will require an ACTH (Cortrosyn) challenge test before their diminished reserve shows up on laboratory tests.

The ACTH challenge test measures the ability of the adrenals to increase cortisol production when stimulated. Since ACTH is the actual hormone that stimulates the adrenal to release cortisol, a challenge with this hormone should increase cortisol in the blood stream, within thirty minutes. A normal response is two times greater than the blood level before the adrenals are challenged with ACTH.

Many owners, with diseases related to adrenal deficiencies; fail to achieve this increase in cortisol production. Consequently, many of these diseases intensify when an owner experiences stress. Stress increases the need for cortisol within the cells. The cell DNA needs cortisol to survive various stresses of life. The above diseases come about when certain cell DNA programs receive defective amounts of the adrenal steroid message. If any of the six links of the adrenal system break, a deficiency results. A broken link causes a defect for all levels below it. All six links need to be intact or the above types of diseases begin to manifest.

Physiologically, the ability to handle stress depends on adequate increases in cortisol. Adequate increases in cortisol direct energy into survival pathways. As stated previously, surgeons see first hand the importance of cortisol production. Its sufficient presence determines the ability to survive the stress of surgery. Following the stress of surgery, a patient will die if their adrenals prove incapable of increased cortisol production. When cortisol release skyrockets into the body, potassium loss increases. Consequently, these two facts are routinely provided for post-operatively. Potassium and cortisol are administered in the post-operative period. This precaution prevents severe complications in case a post-surgical owner's adrenal glands are not up to the task.

One of the best ways to screen for defects in the first four links of the adrenal health chain is to obtain a **24-hour urine test**. The urine test misses the last two links in the adrenal health chain. Unfortunately, very few physicians can interpret the complex issues that arise from the results of this test. Also, the standard method for which the 24-hour urine test is calibrated is to give the patient instructions regarding a normal stress day. This raises the question about missing those patients that only become adrenal compromised during times of stress (when an increased need occurs for cortisol that they cannot provide).

Fortunately, there are valuable clues that will show a deficiency in the adrenal system (all six links in the 'chain'). These clues can occur within the blood stream whenever a white blood cell differential is performed. If the eosinophils, (a type of white blood cell), are elevated, the adrenal system may be deficient. Two other types of white blood cells, the neutrophils and the lymphocytes,, also provide clues by their numbers. If neutrophils decrease and lymphocytes increase (a right shift), another red flag of adrenal insufficiency should go up. When either clue occurs, the physician should thoroughly check the six levels of the patient's adrenal system. A cortisol deficiency will allow abnormalities of these white blood cell types. All of the diseases (listed at the beginning of this subsection), have a high likelihood of increased eosinophils within their clinical picture.

Another valuable clinical discovery indicates that patients with an adrenal system deficiency consistently wake up tired. This is especially true when their disease process activates. This contrasts to the low thyroid patient who tires in the afternoon.

Occult infections and hidden malignancies can present with some of the same clinical findings as adrenal deficiencies. As a precaution, rule these out before initiating a treatment plan for an adrenal problem.

Chapter 11: Hormone Replacement Therapy in America

The Modern Females Dilemma

A defective ovary system can lead to the same clinical picture as the adrenal system weakness (chapter 10). However, the origins of the diseases differ because of different defects in the 'chain links' of the ovary system of health. If the physician fails to evaluate all six links in the 'chain', the disease will be treated in the symptom-control paradigm. Female owners interested in healing need an education in how these glands work and what they need at all six levels within their ovarian system.

Healthy females have highly functional ovaries and highly functional adrenal glands. Around age thirty-five, many female owners begin to experience various levels of hormonal decline. The clinical clues are there, but the physician needs to know how to look for them.

Prescribing abnormally shaped replacement hormones causes problems. The shape determines the message content. Abnormal shapes do not contain the intended body message content that female owners require. Since the aberrant message content directs DNA programs in unnatural ways, these patented versions always have side effects. This chapter contains scientific revelations on this subject. Other pertinent information relates how natural female hormones keep middle age at bay. Both declining natural hormones within and unnatural ones, with their always-present altered shapes, lead to diminished outcomes.

Diminished outcomes predictably occur whenever the body cells natural message content disrupts.

Message content disrupts when hormone replacement consists of altered shaped hormones. Natural hormone's shapes are altered to gain a patent. Without a patent, less financial advantage ensues. Financial advantage has nothing to do with healing. How one heals, involves replacing the lost message content by nutritional, lifestyle, and real hormone replacement. This chapter discusses the problem of symptom-control; why real hormones are better; how nutrition affects the ovaries health; and the six links in the ovary chain of health.

Introduction to the Imbalanced Hormonal States of Female Owners

The general imbalance, in pre-menopausal female owners today, results from too much and the wrong types of estrogen-message content. Too much estrogen occurs relative to the availability of the counter-regulatory hormone, progesterone. For post-menopausal females, the imbalanced hormone situation can be more variable, but progesterone deficiency is always present (see below).

The important difference between natural progesterone and the fake progesterone substitutes (commonly called progestogens and progestins) remains widely misunderstood. Lack of this knowledge has led countless female owners to suffer from unnecessary and chronic diseases. Natural progesterone plays an important role in maintaining female health.

Estrogen and progesterone are some of the most powerful hormones. Their quality and amount directly interact with the cellular DNA program. Different types of estrogen substitutes compound the problems created by fake progesterone by creating additional poor message content. Health consequences occur when DNA programs receive poor directional information. The abnormal monthly cycle of a female describes the effects that occur when DNA receives poor message content.

Steroids, like estrogen and progesterone, are relatively simple molecules within the domain of the larger hormone molecules, like insulin. The smaller the hormone (message carrier), the more exact the shape that the hormone needs to have in order to preserve message content.

In the size class of the steroids, changing a single angle in one chemical bond between carbon and hydrogen changes the message content and/or strength.

It has been known for almost fifty years that changing the angle between one carbon and hydrogen in estradiol changes the potency of the message content by a factor of thirty. Chemists denote this change as beta to alpha angle rotation.

The most powerful estrogen-type in humans is Beta-estradiol. However, common estrogen replacement prescriptions contain, Alpha-estradiol, which is thirty times more powerful than the naturally occurring human form, Beta-estradiol. In addition to the alpha-type estrogen that horses make, they also make horse estrogen-message content. Horse specific estrogen-message content is contained in both equilin and equlinin. Many women are taking these powerful and altered message type estrogens in the prescriptions given to them for hormone replacement. These altered hormones are collected from the urine of pregnant horses or made synthetically from soy or yams. Either of these prescribed replacement hormones send the wrong message to the female owners' DNA.

The Monthly Cycle and Imbalance

Estrogen stimulates cell growth in estrogen sensitive tissues (breast, uterus, fat, and liver) for the first half of the female menstrual cycle. If left unopposed, the stimulant effects of estrogen lead to common ailments such as fibrocystic breast disease, uterine fibroids, breast cancer, uterine cancer, and unnatural growth of other estrogen responsive tissues.

In the second half of the menstrual cycle, in the healthy state, progesterone counter regulates much of the estrogen-message content. Progesterone directs influence over DNA programs in the same cells that estrogen influences. Progesterone deficiency is a common problem.

The first of four reasons for this deficiency concerns the multitude of pervasive 'estrogen mimics' within the environment. This increases the total estrogen message for many women when compared to their ability to manufacture progesterone.

Secondly, the progesterone part of hormone replacement therapy intensifies the problem by using unnatural progesterone substitutes (fake hormones). Unnatural progesterone substitutes can inhibit natural progesterone production, which is needed for the counter-regulation of estrogen and other youth-preserving processes.

Thirdly, progesterone deficiency relates to a nutritionally poor diet. Certain nutritional elements are necessary for adequate progesterone production. Each of these factors that contribute to estrogen dominance will be explained shortly.

The fourth factor relates how female hormones become unbalanced and eventually produce disease. This common situation results when female owners are prescribed the wrong types of estrogen (not to be confused with factor two above, which is caused by the prescribing of abnormally shaped progesterone substitutes).

Mainstream medicine adherents prescribe their female patients many different natural and unnatural estrogens as a mixture. When the estrogen-message content imbalances, the wrong cellular message occurs chronically.

Four Factors Leading to Estrogen Dominance Relative to Progesterone

1. **Estrogen mimics in the environment (chapter 7)**
2. **Unnatural progesterone in hormone replacement therapies decreases real progesterone levels.**
3. **Nutritional deficiencies exacerbate the progesterone and estrogen imbalance (discussed within the six links in the ovarian chain of health, link three).**

4. Hormone prescriptions commonly contain abnormal estrogen-message content

In order to understand how prescriptions commonly disrupt the natural message in a woman's body, the natural state needs to be defined. When treatment strategies facilitate a recreation of the natural state, healing becomes possible. Wisdom exists in the power of the female body to heal.

Three natural estrogens produced within the human body allow balanced health. Each natural human estrogen-type has an optimal percentage of the total estrogen-message content within the body. When balanced, a coherent cellular message manifests. A deviation from the optimal relative percentages leads to an imbalanced hormone message with cellular consequences. For example, estriol has weak cell division stimulation tendencies, but it provides the majority type of the natural form of human estrogen-message content initially released from the ovary.

Good reasons exist for why the weakest estrogen initially releases within the pelvic cavity in the highest concentration (see below). Estriol proves very powerful in the maintenance and health of the vulva and vaginal tissues. It doesn't need conversion to the more powerful estrogen-types.

This contrasts to Beta-estradiol and estrone, which contain powerful cell division message content directed at estrogen responsive tissues. This fact helps one begin to see the advantage of their minority position.

Unfortunately, the patented pharmaceutical estrogens are the powerful cell division message type. This situation is completely avoidable if the patient obtains a prescription filled by a **compounding pharmacist**. This method of prescribing hormones recreates natural estrogen-message content made with natural estrogen ratios via a patch, cream, capsule, sublingual drops, or vaginal gel and customizes these prescriptions. A natural ratio and type between these three is individualized and **determined by the 24-hour urine test results**. This leads to a natural cellular message in the estrogen responsive tissues. The restoration of the natural estrogen message constitutes the first step in healing from estrogen dominance.

Symptom-control medicine ignores the unique natural estrogen-message content found in the human owner. The typical prescriptions contain either abnormally shaped versions or nonhuman estrogens from horse urine concentrate. The earlier example of attempting to make even the slightest change to atural estrogen by changing the angle between one carbon and hydrogen in estradiol reveals the abberation of such practices.

In the natural condition, humans make small amounts of the much weaker beta-estradiol. This alone is a very powerful estrogen in the scheme of things. Imagine the potential consequences when the message content is multiplied by a factor of thirty. Yet, this occurs in millions of women who ingest or apply unnatural mixtures of estrogen or abnormally shaped hormones. This leads to estrogen imbalances, the number four factor. The fourth factor is the topic of this subsection. Physicians may be unaware of this chemical fact because they receive medical information through sources that are 'friendly' to the interests of drug companies (medical schools and journals).

If women are healthier with natural estrogen, why aren't more pharmaceutical companies manufacturing this? Natural prescriptions cannot be patented and hence, less profit potential arises. Remember, in order to obtain a patent, the natural estrogen or progesterone shape needs to be changed in some way. Small changes in molecules of this size prove impossible without changing the message content inherent in the precise shape.

Within the various birth control pill formulations, the shapes change even more radically compared to the natural shape of estrogen and progesterone. This example cites the estrogen molecule alterations from the natural human shapes, but what about the consequences of altering progesterone, the counter hormone to estrogen?

Abnormal Shaped Progesterone Substitutes as a Factor in Real Progesterone Deficiency for Its Message Content

Synthetic alteration of progesterone's natural shape profoundly affects a woman's health for two reasons (factor two above). First, only one type of progesterone exists in nature. The natural form proves necessary for the building block molecule for many other steroids creation.

Second, like other natural hormones, the exact inherent shape of progesterone carries an exact message that the cells need in the second half of a female's monthly cycle. It counters many of the effects started by estrogen in the first part of the menstrual cycle. The progesterone content, which rises in the second half of the female cycle, counters the cell division and fluid retaining effects of estrogen. Without adequate progesterone, females will tend toward estrogen dominance based disease such as fibrocystic breast disease, breast cancer, uterine cancer, premenstrual bloating, uterine fibroids, and migraine headaches. With the shape alteration of patented progesterone substitutes, the message content changes and these tasks cannot be preformed effectively. Hormonal balance occurs when the balance-counter-balance mechanisms function properly. This includes proper timing and an adequate amount of real progesterone and estrogen.

Progesterone serves as a building block molecule for other important steroids manufactured within the adrenals and ovaries. This molecular building block provides one source for testosterone, cortisol, and some estrogen. When owners have synthetic progesterone prescriptions in their body, the likelihood increases for creating an imbalance in the synthesis of other steroids.

The message content of molecules the size of steroids, like estrogen and progesterone, is inherent in their precise shape. When the shape changes minutely, so does the message delivered to the DNA. Healthy people have real hormones that carry accurate message content. Unhealthy people are the consequence of unnatural message content being delivered to their DNA.

Estrogen Dominance

Conspicuous clinical signs of estrogen dominance:

1. **Pre-menstrual breast pain**
2. **Poor sleep quality**
3. **Fluid retention more than twenty four hours before the onset of the menses**
4. **Increased tendency toward premenstrual tension (increased irritability and combativeness) up to fourteen days prior to the onset of menses**.

Remember, as estrogen dominant imbalance persists, an increased likelihood develops for diseases like: fibrocystic breast disease, uterine fibroids, breast cancer, shortened menstrual cycle, endometrial cancer, menstrual cycle migraines, osteoporosis, and weight gain. Mindfulness for what the female body communicates through symptoms and signs creates awareness about estrogen dominance.

Clinical signs deserve attention into the 'why' and the 'how' of estrogen dominance. A brief review of the six links in the 'chain' of the estrogen and progesterone system will follow in the ovary system. Within this discussion, there is an explanation for how estrogen dominance accelerates the changes of middle age. Attention to these six links will increase the odds of a female owner having the best hormones that are consistent with good health.

Six Links in the 'Chain' - Good Health of the Ovarian System

Six links in the health of the ovarian system include:

1. **Hypothalamus**
2. **Pituitary**
3. **Ovary**

4. Blood stream transport system
5. Nuclear receptor at the DNA level within the ovarian hormone responsive tissues
6. Receptors manufactured as a result of ovarian hormones activation of certain DNA programs causing direction for the manufacture of new receptors (other steroids and the 'lesser' hormones)

Different female owners suffer from different points of break down in the six links of the 'chain' within their ovarian system. Menopause results from a broken link at level three, the ovary. Some systemic illnesses affect level one, the hypothalamus. Some hormone abnormalities at the pituitary (link two) inhibit the ovary. The broken link must be correctly identified to restore hormonal balance.

Link One - Hypothalamus

The hypothalamus controls all the other links within the ovary system. Under activity of the first link creates under activity of all successive links of the chain. The amount of ovary stimulant information that the hypothalamus sends out is largely determined by the amount of estrogen it senses. Too much estrogen reaching this level weakens the link. When the hypothalamus turns down its informational direction of the ovarian system, other important hormone consequences ensue. As long as the female ovarian system remains in balance, turning down the volume can be appropriate. When certain estrogen prescriptions penetrate into the body, the hypothalamus gets fooled and doesn't direct the manufacture of other important hormones.

Sometimes various estrogens are prescribed without consideration for how this practice will decrease testosterone-like steroids. The ovary, while releasing progesterone and estrogen, also releases testosterone (an important androgen)-like steroids, as well. Rejuvenation requires the testosterone message. In this way, female owners who take too much estrogen can short-circuit a powerful androgen message. The androgen message decreases because artificially high estrogens, within certain female owners' bodies, have fooled link one, the hypothalamus.

In the example of estrogen replacement, androgen deficiency results because hormonal replacements usually do not contain androgens. The hypothalamus assumes when estrogen elevates, testosterone is elevated as well. **In chapter 12, in the subsection on '"steroid tone"' the central role testosterone like androgens play in rejuvenation will be further explained.**

Larger amounts of estrogen inhibit the amount of stimulatory information that the hypothalamus sends into the ovary chain of health. When the ovary remains healthy, it produces progesterone, estrogen, androstenedione, and testosterone. Estrogen replacement strategies usually do not contain the androgen lost when estrogen levels elevate artificially. Both androstenedione and testosterone constitute ovarian androgens. These pills fool the hypothalamus by the mechanism described above.

Link Two - Pituitary

The master gland, the pituitary, regulates the other hormone glands. It manufactures many competing hormonal messages for release. The hypothalamus acts as the main director of the messages released by the pituitary. The pituitary then releases specific hormones directing the ovary. Hormones contain message content. A gland's importance lies in which hormone messages it releases. The quality of the mixture that the master gland secretes tells the ovary how to expend energy. This becomes the dominant message. Adequate and rhythmic release of leuteinizing hormone (LH) and follicle stimulating hormone (FSH) released from the pituitary, nourish the ovary by giving specific direction to continue its natural cycle.

Adequate release of adrenal corticotropic hormone (ACTH) stimulates the ovary to increase steroid biosynthesis.

The associated release of aldosterone provides a circuitous, but important pathway, as well.

Conversely, within the master gland (the pituitary) exists another powerful hormone, prolactin. The ovary becomes inhibited when prolactin releases beyond low levels. Even though many physicians have been groomed into the 'knee jerk' summary that prolactin stimulates milk production, the evidence clearly implicates prolactin as a powerful inhibitor of ovarian function.

The confusion arises because they also know that during the pregnant state steroid production becomes very high and the prolactin level also elevates. One solves this false discrepancy about pregnancy and prolactin inhibition of the ovaries when the additional placenta hormone factory receives recognition. Even though prolactin inhibits the ovaries, in the pregnant state, the placenta cranks out huge amounts of steroids, which explains the increase.

Four common clinical states occur that exist without the benefit of a placenta but where prolactin, produced within the pituitary, induces ovary inhibition. In these four situations, a placenta remains absent. Only a placenta will make up the difference in the lost steroids produced by the ovary when prolactin levels rise.

The four states that stimulate the pituitary to release high levels of prolactin include: low thyroid function, birth control pill usage, chronic stress, and high serotonin. In these cases, the production of the ovarian component of body steroids greatly diminishes because these situations lead to increased prolactin. Steroids are so powerful, if any one of them diminishes, the DNA content of the body will go either dormant or hyper. Most people have a pretty good feeling that when the DNA misbehaves a danger to over all health exists. With an appropriate prolactin level, healing transpires.

Mechanisms for the increased pituitary release of prolactin:

1. **Birth control pill usage**
2. **High serotonin levels**

3. **Chronic stress**
4. **Low thyroid gland function**

Increased prolactin levels are caused by increased estrogen contained in birth control pills. Prolactin inhibits ovarian hormone formations and release. This fact provides another hormone-induced mechanism associated with obesity that does not operate with pregnancy. The pregnant state has the growing placenta, which generates the needed steroids. The placenta manufactures androgens even though the ovary becomes relatively dormant by the fifth month of pregnancy. When female owners take birth control pills, the body thinks it is pregnant and prolactin levels rise. Prolactin levels rise when estrogen levels approach pregnancy levels.

Potential obesity occurs because like pregnancy, the birth control pills increase prolactin levels. Unlike pregnancy there is no placental hormone factory to correct the inhibition of the ovaries in steroid production. Additional potential problems exist. Birth control pills do not contain androgens, only estrogen and progestins (abnormally shaped progesterone substitutes). Androgen production can fall, and some adrenals fail, in the challenge to increase androgen production and obesity ensues.

High serotonin levels can occur when SSRI-type anti-depressants are taken (chapter 5).

Chronic stress tends to raise prolactin levels. Prolactin levels elevate when increased cortisol release stimulates prolactin as part of the stress response.

Low thyroid gland function will stimulate the hypothalamus to release thyroid-releasing globulin (TRH). TRH proves a very powerful secretogogue for prolactin release from the pituitary.

Link Three - Ovary

A healthy female owner's ovaries make appropriate amounts of androgens. In addition, the healthful state typifies by proper levels of estrogens, which cycle with proper levels of progesterone. Each month, a new cycle begins and her cells receive the right amount of message content that directs them to invest in rejuvenation activities. Rejuvenation activities keep the body young.

Around menopaus,e the ovaries begin to fail and give up their steroid production role to the middle aged adrenal. Many years prior to this, steroid production begins to diminish within the ovaries. When clinicians miss this or treat with fake hormones, a female owner jumps on an accelerated path to an old body.

Nutritional deficiencies play a major role in ovarian disease. Common factors include a chronic tendency toward the consumption of a 'processed food' diet versus a 'real food' diet. Ovarian steroid production provides an example of how nutrition affects ovarian health. One central facet of ovarian function is determined by the rate at which cholesterol converts into pregnenolone. One hormone controls the rate of this process, aldosterone.

Aldosterone levels determine the rate of this important step necessary in the creation of all steroids. This fact about the steroid manufacture rate remains true for the adrenals, testicles and ovaries. The ovary, testicle, and adrenal DNA programs need adequate aldosterone message content to start production of cholesterol desmolase. This initial enzyme involved in steroid manufacture is also known as a side chain cleavage enzyme.

A high potassium diet ('real food') stimulates aldosterone release. Fresh meat, vegetables, and fruits provide high potassium. Processed food diets prove deficient in potassium and pave the road for dysfunctional ovaries. Remember, processed food constitutes any food that comes in a box, can, and bag or from a fast food restaurant. This fact provides an example of steroid interdependence for ovary health to be possible.

Along with aldosterone, the healthy ovary needs Vitamin C, plus the vitamins in A and B-complex, for adequate steroid production capabilities. The mineral zinc allows steroid synthesis to occur at effective rates. Adequate zinc also prevents the excessive conversion of testosterone into estrogen.

(Recap) The mineral type content between these two diets show drastic differences. 'Real food' contains natural minerals in the proportions required for health. Processed foods have drastically altered mineral content. The minerals, magnesium and potassium, deplete in processing natural foods. Unhealthy amounts of sodium, calcium, hydrogenated fats, and sugar are added to extend shelf life. This equals profits for the food industry. Processed food doesn't contain the proper ratio of the four minerals - magnesium, calcium, potassium, and sodium. Ovaries need the correct mineral ratio to maintain the aldosterone message content (chapter 12). Aldosterone message content determines the rate of all steroids synthesis within the adrenals and ovaries. Natural food diets facilitate an increased aldosterone level.

Owners who eat 'dead food' diets tend to become potassium and magnesium depleted at the onset of middle age. A deficiency of potassium creates the need for an increase in insulin to process the same amount of sugar (insulin resistance). The more insulin released the greater the fat-maker message within the body. In addition, potassium and magnesium deficiencies lead to high blood pressure; irregular heart rate; diminished adrenal and ovary steroid production; loss of body protein content and a simultaneous increase of fat production; diminished red blood cell flexibility and decreased cell voltages (a weakened cell force field). The 'why' and the 'how' of these facts are discussed in the appropriate sections throughout this manual (chapter 8). Proper mineral intake equates into a better ovary and adrenal gland function.

Link Four- Bondage Fraction versus the Free Level of Ovarian Hormones within the Blood Stream

Transport of ovarian steroids describes the fourth link in the ovarian system of health chain. Three different methods exist for the transport of ovarian steroids within the blood stream.

1. **Within the red blood cell membrane (major fraction)**
2. **Trapped on bondage proteins, western owners are often misled because of an incomplete inquiry into the level of ovarian hormones released and trapped within this compartment (see below).**
3. **Small amounts travel free by themselves within the blood stream.**

The ovarian steroids, estrogen, progesterone, testosterone, and androstenedione, are usually transported within the red blood cells. While in transport within the red blood cell, estrogen can be acted upon by enzymatic machines and transformed into more powerful types of estrogens. By this mechanism, the initial release of estrogen-types changes in the periphery. The initial types of the different estrogen's relative percentages, which are secreted from the ovaries, can be altered while in route to the distant target cell.

The liquid component of blood, plasma, also transports some ovarian hormones (testosterone, androstenedione, estrogens, and progesterone). The higher the thyroid hormone and estrogen level within the body, the higher the transporter 'bondage' protein levels. When they occur at high levels, these hormones instruct the liver to make excessive bondage proteins for all steroids within the blood stream.

Some physicians are misled into thinking a blood drawn laboratory test looks good, when in actuality, the bondage proteins, being abnormally high, captivate the steroids within the blood stream. Steroids need to bind to the DNA before they deliver their message content. Trapped messages circulating around and around within the blood stream prove worthless.

A higher bondage protein level means that a hormone measured within an owner's blood may be misleading if the transport (bondage) protein level proves either higher or lower than normal. The name of the transport protein for testosterone and estrogen is referred to as sex hormone binding globulin (SHBG).

The blood stream must contain this important protein for ovarian function. Deviations from normal levels do two things to steroid message content. First, it alters the rate at which the liver can inactivate steroids in the blood stream. The higher the levels, the less readily the liver inactivates them. Conversely, the higher the level, the less readily the body cells access their informational content. High levels slow the ability of steroids to gain entrance into their target cells' DNA programs.

Remember that the blood cells contain and free a fraction of the various steroids that have the ability to get into the 'target' cells. Only when the steroids make it into the target cells can they activate the various DNA programs. When the DNA programs receive message content, they direct the cell's energy expenditure. Conversely, 'bondage' protein (SHBG) levels determine the amount of steroid that fail to escape from the blood stream. Steroids, trapped onto bondage proteins, prove unable to deliver message content into cells until another hormone event changes their equilibrium. This last detail is beyond the scope of this book. These are the variables to consider concerning steroids when interpreting blood test results.

Looking at only steroid levels in the blood can be misleading. A modest improvement in accuracy can be achieved with the inclusion of an SHBG level. When this protein's level rises, large amounts of steroids circulate without a destination. A 24-hour urine test for steroid hormone excretion proves more accurate for these reasons.

The level of effectiveness of a steroid to bind and activate its DNA-associated receptor (link five) is a concern. Failure to consider the links that make up the ovary system chain has led many clinicians to falsely conclude that all is well.

Link Five - Integrity and Amount of Functional DNA Associated Nuclear Receptors Within the Target Cell

Once an ovarian steroid successfully travels within the blood stream and enters the target cell, it needs to activate its DNA-binding receptor. Without binding its receptor, it cannot activate or repress a cell's DNA program. When defects occur within the receptor link, the message content of a steroid fails to be heard. A simple example of level five-associated receptor formation regards the interdependence between progesterone and estrogen to manufacture each other's DNA associated receptors.

A dysfunction in the fifth link can mislead clinicians because patients often have normal blood and urine tests for different ovarian steroids. The prematurely aged female body will warn an astute physician that a level five problem operates.

Whenever hormonal dysfunction happens at this level, the preceding four levels operate effectively. However, diagnosis remains difficult. Even the best and most thorough tests available are not sophisticated enough to measure dysfunction in the message content that the DNA receives. Specific accuracy awaits further discovery.

Adequate zinc plays an important role in preventing improper steroid receptor interaction, once the steroids arrive at the DNA-associated receptor. The DNA-associated receptor contains zinc (zinc fingers). Zinc is to steroid-receptor activation what oxygen is to burning fuel within the mitochondria. Just as oxygen deficiency diminishes the power plant flame, zinc deficiencies prevent steroids from activating the different DNA-associated receptors. Many owners have zinc deficiencies. DNA-associated receptors refer to the types of receptors for all steroids, Vitamin A, and thyroid hormone. If the owner experiences a level five problem, they should ask their physician about their zinc status (hair analysis or red blood cell content).

A properly functioning fifth link forms a prerequisite for the sixth link to function. The sixth link concerns protein receptors that are manufactured or repressed, on additional DNA segments, when the DNA activates or represses by a specific ovarian steroid. These activated or repressed DNA segments result in the increase or decreased amounts of receptors for the 'lesser hormones' (see appendix). In contrast, the fifth level concerns hormone receptors manufacture levels determined for the most powerful hormones only.

Link Six - Receptor Manufacture, for the Lesser Hormones, Depends on the Success of Ovarian Steroids Activation of

certain DNA Programs (optional reading for the scientist type of reader)

The sixth link concerns the receptor formation amounts for the lesser hormones. These lesser hormone receptors only occur as a result of successful activation of the DNA associated nuclear receptor. The result of DNA activation by a specific steroid directs recipient cells to manufacture specific proteins. The instructions for the manufacture of specific proteins are contained within the genetic code - the DNA segment activated. Specific proteins directed to be synthesized lead to new receptors being made from these proteins. These specific receptors are manufactured for other steroids and other 'lesser' hormones. Hormones can't deliver message content without their specific receptors.

Most of the discussion at this level is beyond the scope of this book but a basic appreciation is warranted. At the sixth level interdependence of the different steroids, Vitamin A, and thyroid hormone, takes place. However, the final hormone receptors created at level six are constructed to receive the messages contained within the lesser hormones (see appendix).

An example of the lesser hormones' receptor being decreased by estrogen's influence on the DNA program, occurs within the liver. High estrogen states influence the liver DNA to suppress growth hormone receptors associated with IGF-1 release. When these receptors diminish, which triggers the release of IGF-1, growth hormone will tend to raise the blood sugar without compensation, by increasing IGF-1 levels. This increased estrogen-caused defect leads to the need for increased insulin release in order for the growth hormone-caused blood sugar rise to return to normal. The increased insulin then turns on the fat-making machinery within the liver. This is an example of a level six problem, which leads the female owner to get fatter until someone helps her to normalize her IGF-1 again.

To eliminate confusion of the ovarian system, visualize six links in a chain. If one of the links breaks, the ovarian system failure profile appears. Common examples of this dysfunction include: hot flashes, irritability for up to two weeks prior to the onset of menses, insomnia, forgetfulness, breast tenderness, cyclical migraine headaches, fibrocystic breast disease, uterine fibroids, some breast cancers, some uterine cancers and some cases of obesity. Also, the consequences of diminished androgen eventually present as joint aches, osteoporosis, premature wrinkles, and fatigue. These occur clinically regardless of which link fails. Even a well-run battery of ovarian steroid tests, including urine and blood samples can be deceptively normal. In these cases, listening carefully to the body and finding a doctor who will look thoroughly for clinical clues is critical.

The content of this section should alert the owner to the complexity of inquiry necessary to establish the level of ovarian function. Superficial inquiries have side effects and little to do with healing but form the standard of care for symptom-control medicine. With opportunities for healing in mind, the time has come to discuss how various hormones interact as informational substances.

Chapter 12: Information Carried in the Bloodstream

The amount of communication that occurs between different cells via the informational substances proves critical to health. These substances secrete at numerous sites within the body and exert distant cellular communication. Glands create specific informational substances. These are designed to connect with a certain group of receptors. The blood stream carries the information toward the target cell. The shape that results from this combination generates a specific message within the target cell. The blood contents functions as a stream of information molecules.

Informational substances are of two types, the delayed response and rapid response. The term delayed denotes the ability to effect the activity level of a cell's DNA program. Activated DNA programs make new cell proteins possible. One of the proteins made possible by DNA activation is the manufacture of certain receptors for the rapid response hormones. The rapid types depend on proper amounts of the delayed type of informational substances activating enough DNA programs so there will be receptors when these 'lesser' hormones release (the rapid response type).

The term 'rapid' denotes informational substance types that only effect existing receptors and cellular machinery's activity levels. These types of informational substances prove rapid in their message delivery since they have no ability to directly instruct the DNA programs. When DNA programs activate or silence, the protein levels are effected only after a delay within the target cell. Rapid response informational substance side steps this and stops short by having message effect on what already exists within a cell.

Adrenaline and insulin provide common examples of the rapid response type of informational substance. In general, rapid acting informational substances affect existing cellular machinery. Adrenaline and insulin only have effects on the activity level of preexisting cellular machines (enzymes).

In contrast, delayed informational substances determines the types of cellular machinery and receptors created. Cellular machinery types and amounts are created when the delayed informational substances instruct the DNA programs. Only when DNA programs receive instruction are cellular machines and new cellular structural components manufactured. These delayed types of informational substances act by binding directly to cellular DNA and turning off or on different genes. Examples of delayed informational substances are thyroid hormone, Vitamin A, and all steroid hormones.

In general, the rapid response informational substances, in general, derive from amino acid metabolites, amino acid combinations, or hormonal fat precursors. The final shape carries information and is created from these variously arranged molecular building blocks. Molecular building blocks, after processing into the manufactured hormone, carry information by virtue of their final shape. Several sites of manufacture exist for each of the different types of rapid response hormones. Once released, the closest target cell receives the highest message content and the farthest receives the least. In this way, the site of release sometimes controls the response.

Without proper activation by enough types and amounts of delayed response-type of informational substance to the DNA programs, the rapid response hormones develop a diminished ability to deliver their message content. Rapid response informational substances depend on the delayed informational substances for their receptor formation. Without a receptor, they remain unable to deliver their message content. The rapid response informational substances can only affect the activity level of existing cellular machinery and structural cell components. One of the structural cell components involves the receptor types it contains. In general, only the delayed informational substances determine the manufacture rate of cell repair, cell structures, and new cellular machinery.

Basic medical physiology texts are full of molecular and metabolic pathways that describe the individual rapid response type of informational substances. These descriptions detail the rapid response informational substances. It is more practical to simplify things down to the overall big picture. In this case, the big picture of the rapid response type of hormones means that they only effect existing cellular infrastructure and machinery. All rapid and delayed response hormones transport within the blood stream. The blood stream provides the mode of transport for the messages contained via hormonal-type informational substances. Within the nerves, these same substances are called neurotransmitters and the blood stream remains uninvolved.

Communication occurs among the cells via numerous informational substances that flow within the blood stream. Factors that improve the quality of the tone in this informational highway reflect themselves in improved owner health. Conversely, factors that decrease the quality of the informational tone within the bloodstream predictably decrease health.

Traditional scientific dogma states that the central nervous system is the center of communication. This dogma erodes in the face of new data. Contemporary biochemical studies reveal that information from numerous cells direct the central nervous system, as well. The classical notion of the central nervous system still has some truth in the control of its command of conscious thought processes, body movement, and tissue tone (as far as the nerve part of the central nervous system goes). Examples of nervous system movement include voluntary and involuntary types. Voluntary movements include ambulating, the mechanics of talking, and conscious urination. Involuntary movements directed by the classical nervous system are the heart's beating, most unconscious breathing, and digestion. Blood vessel tension, airway tension (bronchial tone), and intestinal tone, all evidence tissue tone orchestrated by the central nervous system.

Not all cells have a nervous system connection. All cells have an informational substance connection (see below). All cells depend on the quality of informational substances. Informational substances direct the cells in their energy expenditure. Whether or not cells receive quality information proves central to longevity.

Remember, quality informational substance content forms a prerequisite to health. Healthy owners have optimal types and amounts of informational content flowing through their bloodstreams. This occurs at appropriate times and intervals and allows maximal cellular efficiency and harmony. Conversely, unhealthy owners have reflective poor qualities of types and amounts of informational content within their blood streams.

Their informational tone is out of sync with the needs of their cells that need proper informational direction on how to expend available energy. The quality of the informational substances within the blood stream determines energy usage patterns.

Good health cannot occur if the informational substances circulating in the blood stream fail to be the types and amounts that promote maximum cellular efficiency and vigor. Stressed owners carry and secrete informational substances that communicate stress messages to every cell. Common negative emotional energies such as fear, anger, guilt, and sadness communicate to cells. Unhappy owners communicate 'unhappiness' messages to their cells via their informational substances. Chronically sad owners secrete informational substances that decrease the readiness of their immune system cells. This decreases their ability to defend against rogue cancer cells, foreign invasion from yeast, bacteria, or viruses and toxins.

Conversely, happiness, love, thankfulness, forgiveness, and hope, stimulate the immune system to increase its effectiveness and this communicates through informational substances, as well.

Scientists call informational substances, hormones. Some of these same substances are also called neurotransmitters when nerves secrete them. Numerous cell-types secrete hormones. Each hormone conveys a specific message. The message content depends on the shape of the hormone plus the cell receptor-type that it interacts with. An informational substance conveys varied content depending on the receptor it interacts with. The combinations of shapes between the hormone and receptor creates message content. Many different receptors exist that a hormone type can interact with. The resulting message depends on the hormone / receptor combination.

For example, cortisol (a steroid) molecule conveys different types of message content depending on which type of receptor it interacts with. When cortisol binds to the DNA program of the gonads, the message to direct energy away from androgen production and reproduction conveys. When cortisol binds to the DNA of a blood vessel smooth muscle cells, the message increases responsiveness to the adrenaline hormone. In other cells, it instructs DNA programs in their conservation of energy. Directing these cells to stop their cellular infrastructure investment and rejuvenation activities conserves energy. This maximizes the energy, available for survival.

All hormones message content centers around how the body directs the expenditure of available energy. Energy usage determines which enzymes activate and which ones remain or become quiet. It also determines which hormones release within the body.

The numerous, different enzymes contained within the body are analogous to molecular machinery. The different types of enzyme machines are contained within specific work areas. These different work areas can be thought of as cell factories.

The different cell factories are called organelles. Mitochondria, endoplasmic reticulum, Golgi apparatus, and nucleolus provide examples of specific organelles.

Different types of cells contain different types of enzymes (cellular machines). Many different additional enzyme machines exist within the blood stream, in the area around cells, and on cell membranes. The enzyme types within a cell depend on the products and functions of each cell type. Each cell type generates specific products.

Remember, the integrity of the following two components prove as crucial determinants for preventing the aging process: cell support structures (cell membrane, GAG integrity, and organelles), and the integrity of enzymes (cell machines). It is the overall hormone mixture (the overall message content) which determines whether energy directs toward repair and rejuvenation or into chronic survival mode.

Hormones' message content direct energy expenditure. The hormones present that direct this process reflect how wise a body directs its energy expenditures. The quality of the hormone message forms one of seven main determinants of aging quickly versus aging gracefully. If the informational content contained in the blood stream remains optimal, youthfulness continues. Youth can only be maintained when the cells receive proper direction on the wise use of their available energy

Wise use of energy involves adequate energy appropriation towards cellular maintenance, repair, toxin removal, and adequate cellular product formation. All of these processes depend on cells receiving appropriate informational direction. Cells direct energy toward rejuvenation and cellular infrastructure investment when they are given the appropriate informational substance message. Only the correct informational message will direct them to do so. The types and amounts of informational substances determine how the body spends energy. Hormone quality has a significant effect on both healing and in slowing the rate of the aging process. The science exists to assess and improve the body's hormone profile.

How Delayed Informational Substances Effect Energy Management

Testosterone is of the steroid hormone class. Its excess or deficiency serves as an example of appropriate versus inappropriate hormone directions by an informational substance. The steroid hormone class is part of the delayed onset type of informational message content. Because it is a delayed type of informational substance, testosterone alters the types and amounts of cellular energy available by its influence over a cells DNA program. The DNA program, activated or silenced, determines the maintenance and rejuvenation activities within the cell. Testosterone's presence directs anabolic activities. Scientists denote the cellular buildup message content as informational substances that are anabolic. Anabolic means to build up. In contrast, catabolic processes means to use up. Before one can understand where the message of testosterone fits, an overall picture of steroid message content is helpful.

Within the steroid class there are three basic types of metabolic activities controlled at the level of the DNA.

1. **Water and mineral content of the body**
2. **Cell survival (deferred cellular maintenance)**
3. **Cellular infrastructure investment and rejuvenation activities**

The steroid testosterone activates rejuvenation and infrastructure investment. Cortisol provides an example of the steroid class that directs body energy into maximizing the survival response. Part of the survival response makes fuel available by its release into the blood stream for survival needs. Stress, whether real or imagined, involves a catabolic process because fuel is made available by dismantling body cell structures where fuel is stored. Body structure builds itself from minerals, sugar, fat and amino acids. Cortisol frees up the last three of these raw fuel sources by directing body structure to dismantle. In addition, with the help of cortisol, aldosterone controls mineral and water balance (see the Kidney chapter in *The Body Heals*). Furthermore, aldosterone controls the rate at which steroid-producing glands manufacture other steroids like testosterone. Steroids are some of the central 'players' in how the DNA programs' of cells direct the expenditure of energy. Thyroid hormones and Vitamin A-complex also work in this capacity (at the DNA level).

The testosterone cellular message is one of cellular buildup and restorative integrity activities in male and female owners. To avoid confusion, testosterone will be discussed as representative of anabolic steroids. The anabolic class of steroids is known as the androgen class, collectively, and includes testosterone, dihydrotestosterone, DHEA, androstenedione, and progesterone. Many of these can be peripherally converted to the others to varying degrees. This allows for an increase in initially secreted potency without the masculine message in women.

In male and female owners, testosterone-like steroids direct buildup of the integrity of cellular components, by directly switching off or on DNA programs (genes). Testosterone delivers to the cell the message that cellular infrastructure investment and rejuvenation are important. This message results in increased repair rates, strong bones, increased organ size and function, increased red blood cell production, increased immune cell production and function, increased bulk to muscles, and increased mental functioning abilities.

Certain energetic and lifestyle qualities promote testosterone production and secretion. Certain other energetic and lifestyle qualities decrease its secretion and production. Good information coursing through the blood stream is important. Testosterone represents one of many necessary informational substances that help revitalize cells.

The intent of this subsection was to introduce the reader to the importance of containing sufficient anabolic message content. Without anabolic message content, the cells lack direction to invest cellular energy in rejuvenation activities. Rejuvenation activities lead to healing. Healing requires an understanding of the three roles that the steroids message serves within the body. The quality of representation of these three roles of steroids determines the "steroid tone".

A Deeper Understanding of "Steroid tone"

"Steroid tone" serves as a useful construct to help predict the youthfulness of an owner's cells. Optimal steroid combinations and relationships promote cellular youth. Unhealthy steroid mixtures diminish cellular function. Cellular dysfunction accelerates the aging process. Cellular health improves as "steroid tone" improves. The appropriate amounts of steroids in the proper proportions create a high "steroid tone". Optimal steroid mixtures direct cells to perform at maximum energy efficiency. Precise combinations of testosterone, DHEA, progesterone, cortisol, and aldosterone direct energy efficiency.

Maximum function and efficiency at the cellular level equals healthy owners through correct steroid mixtures. These appropriate steroid mixtures direct cells towards the efficient use of resources. Wise use of body energy equates cellular efficiency. Only when cellular efficiency occurs, is youthfulness possible.

Highest Quality of Steroid Types and Proportions Instructing DNA Programs = Optimal "steroid tone"

Optimal "steroid tone" only remains possible when the catabolic message content balances with the anabolic message content.

Steroids prove as powerful hormones because they turn the DNA programs on and off. The cell's health depends on the quality of informational directions (hormone types and amounts) that they receive. All other hormone types (immediate response type), if they act at all, act indirectly on cellular DNA activity. Immediate response hormones, in general, only direct what already exists within a cell.

Delayed hormone types determine what exist within a cell because they turn on and off the DNA programs. All protein synthesis requires a specific DNA segment's (gene) activation that codes for each of them. Only when unique

steroid message content instructs the required DNA will that proteins manufacture occur. Proteins comprise the metabolically active constituent of body structure. Examples of metabolically active molecular components composed of protein are: enzymes, cell receptors, 'furnace components', membrane mineral pumps, actin and myosin.

Different body barriers exist that limit where the immediate response-type hormones deliver message content. Conversely, the delayed-type hormones can go anywhere within the body. It is only the steroid class, Vitamin A and thyroid hormones that can go everywhere.

A youthful, physically fit owner, operates in optimal hormone balance. Some owners are youthful physically at age 80 while others are prematurely aged at 30. One makes their choice by the sum of their daily decisions and lifestyle behaviors that either promotes wellness, or accelerates the rate of the aging process.

If one desires youthful vigor, the enhancement of "steroid tone" constitutes a major principle. **Healthy owners have optimal "steroid tone", without exception**. Optimal "steroid tone" requires balance between the steroid forces that oppose one another (catabolic versus anabolic forces). High quality steroid mixtures direct cells to spend energy wisely between cellular maintenance, rejuvenation, product formation (unique to each cell type), and appropriate rest.

Stress unbalances "steroid tone". Stress increases the release of certain survival steroids inherent in the stress response. Under stress, the body perceives a survival threat and directs energy into survival activities. These same steroids direct body energy away from cellular maintenance and repair activities. Chronically stressed owners exist in a chronic survival pathway. The activation of these pathways predictably decreases their "steroid tone". When "steroid tone" decreases. health also decreases. Health decreases because stress hormones direct energy away from cellular maintenance, build up, waste removal, and repair activities needed to maintain the youthful state. The youthful state gradually diminishes as the stress steroids proportion increases above normal because the quality of steroid message content has deteriorated

One of the stress response steroid hormones is cortisol. Cortisol proves necessary in small amounts for proper cell function. In normal amounts, cortisol has a direct influence on many cell processes such as: immune regulation (turning down tone of one arm while raising the tone of the other arm), maintenance of blood pressure (especially in moving from sitting to standing), limiting the inflammatory response from the mechanical strains inflicted on muscles, ligaments, and joints, and in the counter-regulation of insulin's message. In these situations, the cortisol proportion of "steroid tone" is normal.

When chronic survival messages (stress) occur cortisol levels increase. The chronic increase of cortisol secretion creates an imbalance of steroid content within the blood stream. This leads to more survival message content (cortisol) and less rejuvenation message content (testosterone). The higher cortisol content lowers the proportional contribution of other steroids in their direction of energy.

When the body stays in survival mode, energy channels away from rejuvenation activities and into mounting a stress response by lowering the "steroid tone". By definition, "steroid tone" remains high when rejuvenation activity stays high. "Steroid tone" becomes low when rejuvenation activity stays low. "Steroid tone" provides a construct to help conceptualize the adequacy of the body steroid mixture, carrying information within the blood stream, for maintaining youthfulness.

When steroid mixtures deviate from optimum, the consequences to the message content effects "steroid tone". Without optimum types and amounts of steroid mixtures, cellular injury and breakdown occurs. Developing one's knowledge of how breakdown occurs, and ways to promote healing, proves imperative.

Cells need the correct informational message to heal. The function of cells depends on the hormone instructions they receive. Steroids turn on and off DNA programs within the cells and, therefore, comprise a primary consideration to maintain youthfulness. "Steroid tone" attempts to quantify the importance of the quality of instructions that cells receive from steroids.

Six Determinants of "steroid tone"

1. Health of the adrenal glands and gonads
2. Genetic inheritance
3. Environmental adrenal and gonad toxin exposure history
4. Nutritional adequacy for manufacturing the right steroids
5. Emotional lifestyle quality
6. Secretogogue influence on the adrenals and gonads. (Amount of anabolic enhancement from the secretogogues)

Five of the six determinants of "steroid tone" remain under the influence of the owner and respond to healing strategies. These are discussed in *The Body Heals* in more detail. Here, the focus concerns the missing educational content within medical schools. Along these lines, a few of the salient points are emphasized below.

Female owners need more information about how the modern medical complex depresses their "steroid tone". After this, the discussion will concern the "steroid tone" of both sexes. Following this, the importance of sufficient aldosterone will be explained.

Health of Adrenals and Ovaries Influence the "steroid tone" of Females

As females age their "steroid tone" depends more on functional adrenals. Females make less androgen in their ovaries than males make in their testes. Their ovarian-derived androgens fall off more quickly than a man of the same age.

Healthy ovaries manufacture estrogens cycled with progesterone in a balanced and cyclical fashion. Significant amounts of androgen (androstenedione and testosterone) are also manufactured. Different female owners have different rates of decline in their ovary-produced steroids.

The adrenals maintain the backup system for androgen steroid production in females. The female, like the male, needs adequate androgen production to maintain her "steroid tone". Only by maintaining "steroid tone" can the youthful human form be realized. While the adrenals remain healthy, they capably produce androgen-like steroids. DHEA (an androgen steroid) secretes only from the adrenal glands. Significant androstenedione production also occurs within the adrenal gland. Cortisol, the stress steroid, production takes place in the adrenal glands. Adrenals produce the steroid, aldosterone, which proves vital for mineral and water balance. In addition, the aldosterone secretion rate determines the rate of production for all other steroids produced within the adrenals and the gonads (ovaries and testes). A low aldosterone production rate will diminish all other steroids' production rates.

With these facts in mind the next level of "steroid tone" understanding is: "steroid tone" = adrenal (androgen steroids + stress steroids - excess stress steroids + aldosterone steroids) + ovary or testicle (androgens + progesterone + estrogens [but not excessive])

Very few physicians receive training for how to assess steroid output (24 hour urine and sex hormone binding globulin levels). Fewer practicing physicians attempt to replace lost androgen production that results from the post-operative state of a hysterectomy. After uterus removal, even if the ovaries remain left in place, they tend to die off in their steroid production role within two years. This fact results from the dependency of the ovaries for over 80 percent of their blood supply derived from the uterus. How many female owners receive false reassurance about their ovaries following their hysterectomy? It should be acknowledged that some females possess remarkably strong adrenal glands that adeptly pick up the slack in steroid production following hysterectomy. However, the majority does not evidence this ability within their adrenals.

A progressive decline in muscle mass, increased tendency for weight gain, decreased libido, decreased mental acuity, and premature osteoporosis all result from this omission in the treatment plan. These consequences result from a decline in "steroid tone".

Abnormal types of estrogens and progesterone substitutes make the androgen deficiency worse (chapter 11). These substitutes describe the standard of care for hormone replacement therapy amongst mainstream physicians. Most of these estrogen prescriptions are made from the urine of pregnant horses. Alternatively, some prescriptions are made synthetically from yams or soy by a chemical process and the same chemical mixture results. These abnormal mixtures of estrogens are not healthy. Nor are they adequate substitutes for the human estrogen-message content.

The optimal estrogen-message content occurs when healthy ratios of three different estrogens (estriol, estradiol, and estrone) exist. Optimal estrogen ratios occur within healthy females. Common prescriptions of estrogen substitutes contain an overabundance of alpha estradiol, which amplifies the message of cell division by a factor of thirty, within estrogen-responsive tissues. The estrogen responsive tissues include the breast, uterus, cervix, vulva, vagina, ovaries, and fat cells (located within the breast, hips, and thighs).

These prescriptions also contain horse estrogens (equilin and equilinin). Horse estrogen sends out horse estrogen messages. The estrogen-responsive tissues within the human female receive the unnatural horse estrogen message. The human female's body was not designed to receive horse-specific estrogen-message content. As quoted previously, Uzzi Reis, MD OB/GYN, author of *Natural Hormone Balance for Women*, says it very well. He asks, "Are you a horse? Do you eat hay? Then why take horse estrogen?"

Part of the female "steroid tone" derives from estrogen. Each estrogen-type possesses a different shape that determines its message content. When this natural shape is altered, the message contents changes. Over twenty different types of natural estrogen occur in plants and animals. Also, unnatural environmental contaminant, the estrogen mimics, creep inside owner's bodies and add abnormal message content. The estrogen mimics pummel most owners with inappropriate message content (chapter 7).

An imbalanced message content caused by the wrong types and amounts of estrogen delivers, a confused message to estrogen-dependent tissues. The precise shape of natural estrogen has been altered, which diminishes health. Properly proportioned amounts of human estrogens convey a precise message to the target cells that prove necessary to maintain health.

Hormone replacement strategies that contain abnormal progesterone substitutes, further compromise "steroid tone". Only one real progesterone molecule occurs naturally. The precise shape of the real progesterone molecule contains the message content needed for true health.

Altered or synthetic progesterone lowers "steroid tone" further by interfering with the biosynthesis of other steroid hormones. Other steroids require progesterone as their building block. Progesterone substitutes retard this process. The process becomes retarded when progesterone substitutes fool enzyme machines that need real progesterone to build other steroids. The altered shape of synthetic progesterone cannot serve as a building block for the other needed body steroids.

Natural progesterone cannot be patented, and therefore, it remains less profitable for manufacture by pharmaceutical companies. Complications occur with the use of progesterone substitutes. They always have side effects (a different shape changes the message content). This fact alone leads to imbalances in "steroid tone". Progesterone proves necessary for building many other steroid hormones that are needed within the body. These other steroids elevate "steroid tone" and a healthy body manifests.

An analogy given by the late progesterone expert, Dr. John Lee, MD, states that progesterone is the basic 'chassis' for many other steroid designs. Dr. Lee pointed out that the progesterone substitute situation is like auto manufactures that use a common chassis for multiple car types. If the chassis fails to properly develop, the assembly process for the remainder of the automobile halts at different points along the assembly line. Where this occurs depends on where the defective chassis lesion occurs. This leads to a marked slowing in finishing different automobile types at the auto factory.

Similar to automobile assembly, abnormal progesterone substitutes can jam the steroid assembly process in female ovaries and adrenals. The 'assembly lines' jam up within the enzymatic machinery of the cells because synthetic progesterone contains an altered shape. The altered shape often proves close enough to penetrate into the assembly line (enzyme machine) but not close enough to build from it.

No new steroids can be built because the substitute steroid is not the correct shape to be processed into other urgently needed steroids. It is close enough in shape to natural progesterone to get into the enzymatic machinery. Once these substitutes engage within the enzymatic machines, they compete with the small amount of natural progesterone for the manufacture of other steroids.

Steroid mismatch, quantified in severity by a diminished "steroid tone", leads to a poor quality of life. This fact describes the first part of a complex problem. Part of the solution involves obtaining an accurate steroid hormone profile. The 24-hour urine test quantitative and qualitative proves as a start for addressing where one stands in his/her "steroid tone".

The unfortunate female that continues to take abnormal hormone messengers often feels lousy, while on an accelerated path to old age, as well. One of the central problems with altered mixtures of steroids (prescription estrogens and progesterone substitutes) concerns the fact that they interfere with and diminish the androgen component of "steroid tone". The lower "steroid tone" that results puts the female in androgen steroid deficiency. The androgen message content needed to rejuvenate her cells isn't available. A deficiency in the androgen message content allows DNA programs to respond inappropriately in regard to cellular maintenance and rejuvenation activities.

The adrenals and gonads perform independent tasks to maintain "steroid tone". Adrenals have unique hormone products that will be discussed in detail here. This will be followed by a discussion of the adrenal contribution to the androgen class of steroids (build up and maintenance) by the synthesis of DHEA. The adrenal contribution to "steroid tone" depends on the health of these glands. This is the first determinant of "steroid tone" and the adrenal component of this will be reviewed first.

Manufacture sites for the different components of "steroid tone"

Adrenal component:	**Gonad Component**
DHEA	estrogen
Estrogens (nl only)	progesterone
Cortisol (normal levels only)	testosterone
Estrogens (nl levels only)	androstenedione
Aldosterone	
Progesterone	
Androstenedione	

Each of the above steroids delivers precise message content, inherent in their unique shapes, which the cells need in appropriate amounts to direct energy expenditure efficiently. Any of the above steroids causes problems when it proves excessive or deficient. The emphasis on excessive cortisol and estrogen only serves as a reminder for the frequentness of their abnormal increase. When correctly proportioned, the cells receive the message to spend energy wisely, which allows for youthfulness.

There are six determinants of "steroid tone". Five of the six the owner has control over.
All of these determinants are discussed in *The Body Heals*. Here the emphasis concerns the missing educational content and why re-including it proves important for healing.

"Steroid tone" (A brief overview of some of its determinants)

Health of Adrenals and Gonads

The adrenals and gonads contribute to "steroid tone" by their unique contributions and overlapped contributions. This subsection will explain:
1. How chronic stress lowers the adrenal contribution to "steroid tone"
2. "steroid tone" from adrenals and gonads depends on the adrenal manufacture of aldosterone.
3. Types of adrenal androgens manufactured compared to the gonads
4. Overlap between estrogen and progesterone produced in the adrenals and gonads
5. Introductory remarks about powerful androgens manufactured in the ovaries and testes.

The contribution of the adrenal gland to "steroid tone" will be the first consideration in this subsection. The adrenals' part of the first determinant of "steroid tone" provides a good place to start the discussion. It concerns the effect of chronic stress on steroid output of the adrenals.

Chronic Stress, Adrenals, and "Steroid Tone"

Survival describes the primary role of the adrenal glands. Survival of chronic stress comes with a high price on "steroid tone". Physiologically, standing up proves stressful. A tremendous change in gravitational force occurs when going from sitting to standing. Without a concerted interplay between cortisol and adrenaline, this would not be possible. Cortisol, secreted by the adrenal cortex, puts blood vessels in a responsive state each morning before waking up. Adrenaline, made by the inner part of the adrenal, also increases when one stands upright or feels stress. The body design allows for a certain average level of cortisol manufacture. The body design can handle occasional stress, as well, without detrimental effects.

The human body needs about 20-25mg/day of cortisol for the maintenance of high "steroid tone". Orally this translates to about 40mg/day because of the liver first pass effect that deactivates cortisol. The first pass effect describes the fact that most orally ingested substances pass into the liver, and a certain proportion is deactivated, before entering the blood stream.

A cortisol deficiency results in a fall in blood pressure, following into unconsciousness. Sufficient adrenal output of cortisol facilitates correcting a falling blood sugar, as well. Therefore, cortisol-deficient owners often present with hypoglycemia, sugar cravings, and low blood pressure.

The more insulin secreted, the higher the amount of cortisol needed to counteract insulin's message to take sugar molecules out of the blood stream. Remember, abnormal insulin need arises primarily after growth hormone secretion falls, leading to the consequent fall off of IGF-1, as well. This primary defect sets the stage for more insulin need (insulin resistance).

These unhealthy bodies survive during the between meals state by a more violent means of elevating blood fuel (Dr. Herb Joiner-Bey's phrase). Cortisol proves as the major player in these bodies. Epinephrine and glucagon deliver no message content without enough cortisol messages preceding it, which directs the DNA programs to manufacture each of their receptors. This fact explains why cortisol deficiency presents with low blood pressure and hypoglycemia.

Cortisol also serves to tone down hyper-vigilance of the lymphocyte arm of the immune system. In health, this results in the prevention of inappropriate activation against body tissues manifesting as autoimmune disease and allergies. Less well recognized is the fact that rising cortisol stimulates the phagocytic arm of the immune system. These two facts, taken together, help explain the common right shift (increased lymphocytes with decreased leukocytes) found in the White blood cell (WBC) differentials of autoimmune disease patients before appropriate steroid replacements are given.

When the secretion of cortisol rises higher than normal, the body directs energy away from cellular maintenance to accommodate the stress reaction, whether it proves real or imagined. Deferred maintenance occurs when the body temporarily lowers "steroid tone" to survive a perceived threat. The human body can handle occasional deferred maintenance. Survival of a perceived threat involves the redirection of body energy into fuel release (catabolic) and out of rejuvenation pathways (anabolic).

The job of steroid hormones is to reroute body energy as the situation merits. When a survival situation occurs, more cortisol (catabolic), and less androgen (anabolic), release. Consequently, "steroid tone" decreases.

Deferred maintenance in a car proves similar. An owner can overlook the scheduled oil change once in awhile. But continued neglect on this maintanance will cause wear on the engine's functions. When the body perceives one stress after another, the aging process begins. Health requires adequate time for continual repair and cellular maintenance activities.

The stress response discussion can become complicated with the addition of the numerous physiological particulars and associated hormone cascades and feedback loops. Summarize mentally; when the body perceives a survival threat, a rapid response time is essential to quickly maximize the physical strength. The body is smart enough to know that an 'oil change', 'cellular garbage removal', 'spark plugs changes', etc. use energy poorly when survival becomes the issue. If this threat becomes chronic, deferred maintenance delivers consequences to the physical body.

Hormones carry the messages that direct energy expenditure. For this reason, cortisol production increases drastically when stress occurs. High cortisol production directs energy away from rejuvenation activities, and into maximum energy for physical strength and alertness, so the body can survive the perceived stress.

Beyond the stress response, an additional adrenal steroid hormone, aldosterone, proves fundamental to longevity. Aldosterone proves important to the overall strength of certain cell types. **In many ways, the aldosterone level supremely determines "steroid tone".**

Aldosterone – Maintenance of "Steroid Tone"

The adrenal glands respond to a narrow control range of salt and water balance that is largely controlled by the amount of aldosterone message content. The adrenal cortex secretes aldosterone within the glomerulosa layer. Potassium level, stress (ACTH level), and angiotensin type two, provide the three determiners for how much aldosterone the adrenal gland releases.

The secretion of aldosterone directs three main events directed by its instruction of various cell DNA:

1. Increased sodium retention relative to potassium removal from the body.
2. Increased cellular charge (increased power to the cell force field) of cardiac and brain cells
3. Increased steroid biosynthesis within the adrenals and gonads.

All steroids manufacture rate within the body depend on adequate aldosterone levels. Shared roles exist for the adrenals and gonads in relation to their steroid production roles. Steroid production rates within both of these glands will determine "steroid tone". Conversely, they prove different in the unique steroid products that they each produce. Aldosterone manufacture takes place in the adrenal glands. The amount of aldosterone produced, determines how much of the other body steroids are manufactured. When aldosterone production goes well, the benefit of increased "steroid tone" occurs. When aldosterone production goes poorly, the liability of decreased "steroid tone" occurs.

Androgens – Contribution to "Steroid Tone"

The adrenals and gonads share in the manufacture of androgen steroids (the builders and maintenance stimulators). By far, the major androgen manufactured within the adrenal is DHEA. This overlap of androgen production between the adrenals and gonads forms a backup system for the maintenance of "steroid tone". Healthwise, it proves advantageous to have both glands contributing to "steroid tone". High "steroid tone" promotes these activities in an efficient and youthful manner. However, in a culture that removes female ovaries on a regular basis, the backup system proves better than nothing

The contribution of DHEA to "steroid tone" begins to rise at age 7 and peaks around age 25. This level proceeds to decline throughout life and reach about 10% of peak levels in the last year of life (natural demise). DHEA levels decline more quickly in people with high insulin states. High insulin requires an increased cortisol message to counteract the message of insulin that would lower the blood sugar too far. The adrenal then needs to direct the manufacture of more cortisol preferentially. High stress seems to also cause DHEA levels to fall in order to accommodate an increased cortisol biosynthesis rate. Cortisol and DHEA are manufactured from cholesterol stores within the adrenal.

There are several different types of androgens made in the body. DHEA is only one of several. Each body tissue has its own preferred androgen that maximizes its anabolic response. When cells receive their preferred androgen, they invest appropriately in repair and rejuvenation. When directions come from their preferred androgen, the body will remain vigorous and vital.

Lung tissue seems to prefer DHEA (anabolic message) that needs to be balanced with the right amount of cortisol (catabolic message). Blood vessels seem to respond with rejuvenation to their preference for DHEA and only small amounts of cortisol as the counter balance message. Muscle cells seem to prefer testosterone for maximal activation in rejuvenation and growth. Skin benefits maximally from dihydrotestosterone (DHT). The heart needs balanced input from testosterone, thyroid, cortisol, and DHEA for continued vitality.

The brain, while healthy, concentrates DHEA at five to six times the plasma level of this anabolic steroid. This fact has led some researchers to declare DHEA the youth hormone. It would be more accurate to say DHEA is one of the youth hormones and qualify it within the concept of balance. Owners can only have steroid balance when their "steroid tone" remains high.

Progesterone and Estrogen – Contributions in Men and Women to "Steroid Tone"

Adrenal glands make progesterone and estrogen. Adrenal production of these hormones can become very important in the menopausal years of a woman. Menopause creates a drastic reduction of ovary activity for steroid production. The adrenal gland source for these hormones is important throughout life for men. Men need the message content of these hormones for their "steroid tone", just like women, but in lesser amounts. Healthy adrenals supply men and women with adequate amounts of these steroids.

Obese male and female owners convert their testosterone into estrogen within their fat cells. Zinc deficiencies rev up this process by activating aromatase activity. Aromatase is the enzyme, within fat, that converts testosterone into estrogen. Breast enlargement in these male owners commonly arises as a consequence of this phenomenon.

Gonads - "Steroid Tone"

An owner realizes optimal "steroid tone" when his/her adrenal glands and gonads remain healthy. Even if these glands have been damaged, health can be regained with an accurate real hormone replacement program. A real hormone replacement program requires an accurate "hormone report card" before the physician can advise an owner in the continuum from health to diminished function. Part of the "hormone report card" involves an assessment of "steroid tone". The doctor best ascertains an owners' message content status by the results of a **well-run 24-hour urine test.**

Both the six links in the ovary or testicle system and the adrenal system need to be intact for healthful "steroid tone" to come from the gonads and adrenals. The adrenals can help failing gonads. Function of either system needs to be determined by an accurate assessment of "steroid tone". Sometimes supplementation proves necessary in the owner with failing glands in order for their rejuvenation program to begin. This program will help these owners heal from the effects of low "steroid tone".

Nutritional Adequacy and "Steroid Tone"

Physical signs occur in people who eat processed foods. Puffy, bloated faces, sagging skin, and loss of muscular definition exemplify the consequences of nutritional deficiencies that processed food causes. Fast food restaurants provide an excellent place to make these clinical observations.

Before this manual, unless you were an Asian who imbibed in good quality ginseng, less androgen would be manufactured with each passing year. Less androgen manufacture leads to lower "steroid tone" and the ungraceful decent into old age.

Poor nutrition causes gonad and adrenal cells to possess a decreased ability to free up cholesterol and move it inside the mitochondria. The mitochondrion is the site within the gonads or adrenal glands cells where cholesterol converts into early steroid precursors. Cholesterol needs to move into the mitochondria for the first step of steroid manufacture to occur. Once cholesterol moves inside the mitochondria, it converts into the various early steroid hormone precursors. The end product within the mitochondria is pregnenolone, a necessary starting molecule from which to build all other steroids. After pregnenolone forms inside the mitochondria from cholesterol, it undergoes conversion to other steroids outside the mitochondria.

This internal conversion from cholesterol to pregnenolone proves more difficult as the owner ages.

There are four reasons the conversion of cholesterol to pregnenolone develops a roadblock with age:

1. **Aldosterone content within becomes diminished secondary to a processed food diet.**
2. **Necessary vitamins and cofactors for biosynthetic reactions of these conversions diminish.**
3. **Cholesterol content diminishes within the adrenals and gonads**
4. **The common method of taking pregnenolone supplements has possible detrimental side effects.**

This **fourth** additional point needs emphasis before proceeding with the remedies for the other three causes of diminished steroid biosynthesis. This factor exposes many short-sighted and half-thought out approaches for steroid replacement. Pregnenolone supplementation can partially bypass the need for these mitochondria first step reactions. The side effect of taking pregnenolone as a supplement for waning steroid production concerns that it contains cortisol-like message content of its own.

Increased cortisol message content is warranted in certain clinical situations. In most situations, when it occurs within one's blood stream after oral ingestion, it will contribute to decreased overall "steroid tone". "Steroid tone" becomes negatively influenced when cortisol message content rises above a very low threshold. In the normal state, pregnenolone fails to enter the blood stream in increased amounts. Instead, it converts within the adrenals and gonads into other steroids.

To counter-act these problems, pay attention to the first three nutritional factors of adrenal and gonad support. The **first** of the three nutritional factors affecting the health of these glands involves the owner's history of diet preference. This determines the aldosterone level of most owners. Aldosterone levels respond to either a 'real food' diet or a 'processed food' diet. As aging proceeds, eating processed foods leads to an eventual depletion of one's mineral balance.

Around middle age, owner's bodies become deficient in mineral balance secondary to the chronic ingestion of processed foods. Processed foods have the wrong mineral proportions.

The right mineral proportions prove necessary for high "steroid tone". Real foods (unprocessed and natural) contain a much higher proportion of potassium and magnesium content. Real food sodium content proves many times lower than processed food.

The opposite situation of mineral balance exists in owners who arrive at middle age with a history of a preference for processed foods (dead food). This food type contains a diminished potassium and magnesium content that results from food processing. Processed food usually contains high amounts of sodium. Many middle-aged owners, who eat processed foods, prematurely suffer the consequences of a decline in their "steroid tone" (see mineral table).

The central steroid defect that results from a chronic 'dead food' diet concerns their diminished aldosterone production required for normal blood pressure.

Some bodies still try to produce appropriate aldosterone in this chronic situation of a dead food diet, but high blood pressure predictably results. The dead food diet contains high sodium and low potassium content. The human body was designed to ingest the reverse of the processed foods diet's mineral content. Sodium retention, beyond healthful amounts, causes fluid retention, which elevates the blood pressure.

The other group of owners exist in bodies that sense inappropriate sodium content. These bodies normalize blood pressure by reducing aldosterone levels. The price paid by these owners regards their diminished steroid synthesis rates as a consequence of their diminished aldosterone levels.

The owner who takes an active role in the procurement of a real food diet (chapter 8) derives an advantage. Conversely, the 'dead food' (processed) diet accelerates the path to an old body in two major ways. First, diminished aldosterone or elevated blood pressures describe the choices given to the body that feeds on dead food. When a body chooses the lower aldosterone route, "steroid tone" suffers and the owner ages faster. Alternatively, when a body chooses to maintain "steroid tone" by keeping aldosterone elevated in the presence of a processed food diet, the blood pressure elevates. When the blood pressure elevates, the owner becomes older by a failure to honor the second principle of health, avoiding hardening processes (the seven principles of health are discussed in *The Body Heals*).

The **second** reason that the steroid production rate begins to fall with advancing age concerns the deficiency in vitamins and cofactors. Vitamins and cofactors prove necessary for the manufacture of many different steroids. These prove as additional nutritional dependent factors that effect "steroid tone". Enzymatic machinery must be in good working order to allow efficient steroid biosynthesis rates. Individual enzymes (cellular machines) need specific trace minerals and cofactors in order to perform in the creation of the different steroids. Only when steroids are manufactured at appropriate rates can "steroid tone" remain high.

An analogy concerns the automobile that has a full tank of gas, but all the oil has drained out. In addition, the spark plugs and carburetor have been removed. These missing components act like the cofactor and vitamins that steroid-producing enzymes (machines) need to make the necessary steroids. When a cofactor deficiency occurs, steroid production diminishes. When steroid production diminishes, "steroid tone" falls.

A partial list of vitamins required for the manufacture of steroids is: Vitamin A, pantothenic acid, folate, most of the B Vitamins, and Vitamin C. Under healthful conditions, the adrenal gland has the highest tissue concentration of Vitamin C. This fact might provide a clue as to why Vitamin C remains so important in the owners continued survival for the prevention and from the stress of illness. The stress of surviving an illness requires an increase in steroid production. The need for Vitamin C goes up with stress and illness.

The accessories, in the car engine analogy, lend themselves to help understand the reason that dietary attention and discretion become so important as owners navigate their search for health and happiness. Youth can survive for a while without the critical nutrients needed by cellular machinery. Youthfulness that endures cannot. 'Father time' observes old cellular parts struggling to work beyond their normal life span without sufficient molecular replacement parts. The body can only acquire certain molecular parts through dietary intake of the molecules needed.

Food processing destroys important nutrients required for the production of enzymes. At least five B vitamins are contained in whole grains that decrease by half within one week of grinding it into flour (half life = time for half to be gone). Oxidation of these unstable and bulky molecules occurs after the grinding process. Vitamins are positioned precisely within the seeds' molecular architecture to confer stability. When grains or seeds are ground into flour, this process destroys the protection provided by the architectural framework. The grinding process exposes these unstable molecules to the oxidative forces, in turn diminishing their nutritional value.

Oxidation takes place in vitamin-fortified foods exposed to heat, air and sunlight for the same reasons. Just because manufactures add vitamins to the box or can doesn't mean they are still intact when the owner ingests it. In contrast, real food still contains vitamins and minerals that the creator intended.

Vitamin supplements are more stable, but absorption characteristics differ widely from brand to brand. Vitamins and vitamin-fortified foods are deficient in some of the vitamins that are removed when food is processed. Folate, pantothenic acid, and lipoic acid, are especially susceptible during food processing. Compounding the deficiency problem concerns the fact that many vitamin-fortified foods and supplements prove deficient in these three vitamins. **When one of these is missing, it is as if a malicious conspiracy exists within the food industry to make owners weak and old.** The weakest link in a chemical reaction sequence will stop a body process. In a pantothenic acid deficiency, carbohydrate and fat combustion greatly curtails. With a lipoic acid deficiency, carbohydrate can only convert to lactic acid, which builds up in the tissues, and presents as sore and achy muscles. Adrenal and gonad tissues need tremendous amounts of fuel for energy. When these vitamins become deficient "steroid tone" diminishes.

The adrenals and gonads need additional trace minerals for their role in the maintenance of "steroid tone". Minerals like zinc and magnesium need adequate stomach acid for absorption. **Many western owners receive prescription medicines that block acid production. In spite of a healthful diet, these owners could become deficient in many of these critically needed minerals.**

A diet containing sufficient organic and unprocessed whole grains, vegetables, eggs, fish, meats, nuts and fruit promote "steroid tone". A real food diet promotes "steroid tone" by the fact that it contains the proper proportions of minerals and vitamins to promote the health of steroid-producing glands as well as other body tissues.

Many plants also contain antioxidant (anti-rust) molecules that confer particular benefits to specific tissues. Examples include lycopene, found in tomatoes for prostate health, bioflavonoids, found in berries for blood vessel health, acanthocyanadins found in bilberry for retina health, silymarin, found in the milk thistle for liver health. Careless food processing techniques destroy much of the anti-oxidant content and hence their potential benefits.

The lower the antioxidants in the diet, the more need for anabolic steroids to direct increased repair. Increased repair becomes necessary when diminished protection from the oxidants occurs. When oxidant damage occurs, more need to elevate "steroid tone" arises to compensate for the increased injury rate. Increased "steroid tone" compensates for the increased injury rate, because when "steroid tone" stays high, anabolism remains high. In order to derive the intended benefits of sufficient "steroid tone", purchase only quality supplements or real foods that comes from fresh organic sources.

When certain tribes throughout the world are studied, scientists observe that they enjoy remarkably good health and greater freedom from the ravages of chronic disease. These tribes share a common denominator of a diet high in plants that have high progesterone or progesterone precursors (Lee, 1993). Some of the plants known to contain relatively high amounts of progesterone or progesterone precursors are: pomegranates, European mistletoe berries, panax ginseng, Mexican wild yams, halotorrhea floribunda, and possibly soy products.

The **third** reason that the steroid production rate diminishes around middle age is best explained in the context of cholesterol lowering drugs. This discussion is found in the physician's side bar in chapter 14.

Chapter 13: Follow the Blood Fuel, and you will Understand Diabetes and Heart Disease

The Liver Determines Fuel Availability

Inappropriate fuel types in the blood stream cause diseases like diabetes, heart disease, strokes, and peripheral vascular disease. These diseases can have their origins in the liver. When the liver treats fuel types inappropriately, the blood vessels begin to break down. Two common examples of inappropriate fuel types released by the liver occur that eventually cause blood vessel injury. First concerns the high blood sugar of diabetes. The second mechanism involves the high rate of liver synthesis and release of LDL cholesterol into the blood stream, found in most heart disease victims and in those who suffer from the major form of diabetes (type II). In both cases, excesses of these fuels injure the blood vessels' inside surface. In both cases, the liver creates and releases these fuels inappropriately, and this causes the excesses found in these diseases. The cause of inappropriate release of fuel excesses results from the liver receiving the wrong hormone-type messages.

Healing involves attention to lifestyle, adequate nutrient intake, and hormone balance at the level of the liver. Recall that instead, owners are often told the hopeless mantra about the cruel hand that genetics has dealt them. The typical approach sells drugs and procedures. Healing involves

improving the types and amounts of hormones that instruct the liver on whether to store or release fuel.

Like other organs, the liver dutifully follows the message content it receives. Healing involves an assessment of the proportions of the hormones that deliver message content at the level of the liver cell. Only when the proper amounts of hormones instruct the liver, will these diseases begin to heal.

The overall hormone message delivered to the liver determines whether the liver takes fuel out or puts fuel into the blood stream. Five main hormones determine how the liver directs fuel: insulin, glucagon, growth hormone, cortisol, and epinephrine. The message content arriving at the liver determines whether the liver will manufacture fuel in storage forms (glycogen and LDL cholesterol) or release them as readily combustible types for use in the cellular power plants (mitochondria). If the liver turns into storage mode, it does this by removing fuel from the blood stream. The liver synthesizes LDL cholesterol particles with storage in mind. Even though the liver eventually releases them, their design is such that they head for the storage destinations: the macrophages that line the arteries and the fat cells.

The opposite situation occurs when the liver releases sugar and fatty acids into the blood stream. The sugar released readily accesses the cells when adequate IGF-1 circulates in the blood stream. Once inside the cells these fuels either combust in the power plants or serve for structural components in the cell. Four out of five of the above hormones encourage this type of fuel release from the liver.

It helps to arrange the hormones interacting with the liver in the antique weight scale analogy. This arrangement reveals that only insulin falls on the side of the scale tipping it in the direction of storing fuels (glycogen and LDL cholesterol). At the level of the liver, the other four hormones counter storage and encourage the 'power plant' accessible types of fuel release by the liver into the blood stream.

The insulin predominant hormone situation allows a tremendous increase in fat and cholesterol biosynthesis rates because insulin behaves like the liver's "fuel tank nozzle" connection. It preferentially desires to fill the liver cell fuel tanks first because its initial site of release, the pancreas, dumps it straight into the liver via the protal vein. This anatomical fact means that whatever the insulin secretion rate, the liver will always receive the highest amount of insulin-message content. When the liver cell fuel tanks fill up with carbohydrate (about 400 grams when adequate potassium remains available), insulin instructs the liver to make the extra sugar into fat and cholesterol. This explains why one needs insulin for fat cell growth and in the storage of liver glycogen.

Counter-regulatory hormones can overpower insulin's ability to direct carbohydrate and fat storage in the liver (each to varying degrees). Counter-regulatory hormones direct the liver to dump stored fuel into the blood stream for usage in a cell's power plants or its structural architecture.

When between meals, mentally or physically stressed, the counter-regulatory hormones levels elevate. Ideally, the body accesses the fat stores during intense and prolonged exercise. Exercising muscles and the heart prefer fat as their fuel source. The red blood cells and nerves rely exclusively on carbohydrate for their energy needs. Carbohydrate storage is limited to about 1500 calories in the liver and about 500 calories in the muscles. When the glycogen stores burn up, as in the case of prolonged exercise, the body needs other fuel sources for energy. A 150 pound athlete with 15% body fat has access to 22.5 pounds of fat times 3500 calories per pound of fat (about 80,000 calories). The proper counter-regulatory hormones allow access to the tremendous fat fuel storehouses.

Remember, all raw fuels (sugar, fat, and amino acids) must convert to the simplest fatty acid, acetate, before, combusting in the presence of oxygen, within the mitochondria. Fat needs the least processing for conversion into acetate and, therefore, serves as the preferred fuel of most body cell types. Notable exceptions occur in the nerve and red blood cells.

Nerves and red blood cells, exclusively, need sugar for all their energy needs. This fact explains the desirability of adequate counter-hormones that direct the additional release of fat. Processes that conserve glycogen for the nerve and red blood cells enhance endurance because nerve and red blood cell's optimal function are preserved when their sugar supply remains available. This happens when the muscles and heart have access to more fat for their energy needs. Conversely, exercising owners that insist on promoting high insulin states compromise their red blood cells and nerves due to sugar stores being consumed more quickly. When insulin excess occurs in the liver, it competes with the ability of the liver to dump fat into the blood stream and create more sugar from amino acids. The sugar stores dry up with the same level of activity because less fat is available. Exhausted sugar stores in the exercising athlete are commonly known as "the wall". The wall will arrive more quickly when insulin needs remain high (insulin resistance).

Longevity and exercise performance critically relate to the balance of hormones that instruct the liver. When these hormones improve, not only exercise ability but also heart disease, blood vessel disease, and diabetes risk, and their complications diminish, as well.

Insulin Causes Fuel Storage as Fat or Glycogen

The counter-hormones, glucagon, growth hormone, cortisol, and epinephrine, all cause the liver to release and synthesize readily accessible fuels into the blood stream.

Initially, insulin will only direct the liver to remove sugar from the blood stream for storage as glycogen (if sufficient potassium remains available). It can store about four hundred grams of sugar in this manner. Sedentary owners have livers that are almost always full of stored sugar. In this case, insulin directs the liver to make the excess sugar into fat and cholesterol, which are packaged for the fat depots. These depots occur in the fat cells and in the macrophages that line the arteries. At the level of the liver, insulin is the only hormone that promotes storage of fuel. The other four hormones oppose the message content of insulin at the level of the liver.

Glucagon counters insulin by four ways in the liver. First, it stimulates the liver to change available amino acids into sugar (gluconeogenesis). Second, it stimulates the release of stored sugar (glycogen) from the liver into the blood stream. Third, it stimulates the release of stored liver fat into the blood stream. Glucagon's message content makes body fuel available. Fourth, the glucagon message content decreases cholesterol and fat synthesis from carbohydrate. When cholesterol and fat are manufactured at slower rates, LDL cholesterol levels in the blood stream, will go down.

Growth hormone (GH) has some of the same effect on the liver as glucagon. **Two important longevity-promoting exceptions deserve emphasis.** First, GH inhibits the conversion of amino acids into fuel. Scientists call this a protein sparing effect. When growth hormone levels remain sufficient, it counters the ability of glucagon to convert protein into sugar. The advantage of having high growth hormone levels relative to the other counter-regulatory hormones is that it conserves protein. This fact proves important for athletes because muscles are made from protein. In contrast, all other counter-regulatory hormones to insulin catabolize protein stores.

The second different effect of growth hormone's message content regards its ability to direct the liver to release insulin-like growth factor (IGF-1). When this hormone circulates outside the liver, it acts like insulin by facilitating the muscle cells to take up fuel (sugar). Remember that in healthy owners, insulin-like growth factor (IGF-1) occurs at levels greater than 100 times that of insulin in the blood stream. This liver-secreted hormone reduces the need for insulin and does not stimulate the liver to make fat and cholesterol. A longevity advantage occurs when IGF-1 levels remain high. High IGF-1 levels depend on three basic things: an adequate release of growth hormone, a healthy liver capable of high rates of IGF-1 manufacture, and adequate DHEA or testosterone levels to stimulate the liver cell DNA programs to direct the manufacture of IGF-1 (simplified for now because IGF-1 manufacture also depends on sufficient thyroid and cortisol but decreases when estrogen levels rise).

Growth hormone's effects on the body need to be understood in a tandem-like fashion. Once one understands the tandem of growth hormone release followed by IGF-1 release, he/she can avoid the confusion discussed in the scientific literature. Medical physiology textbooks describe growth hormone as a diabetogenic (promotes blood sugar elevation) hormone. This describes a half-truth except when the liver is diseased, growth hormone production becomes abnormally high or excess estrogen occurs.

Abnormal increases in growth hormone levels can occur with the disease acromegaly and with high dose growth hormone replacement therapy. However, healthy livers with adequate androgen message content promptly release IGF-1, sugar and fat when growth hormone levels rise within normal parameters. The IGF-1 released lowers the amount of insulin required to bring fuel into the cells.

(Physician side bar) **Normally, growth hormone will counter a diabetes tendency by its message that directs the release of IGF-1.** IGF-1 behaves like insulin in the circulation. This happens because of the tandem effects of growth hormone release followed by the liver simultaneously releasing IGF-1, sugar and fat. Medical physiology textbooks focus on the fact that growth hormone initially causes the release of sugar into the blood stream. However, the tandem of IGF-1 release that normally follows causes the peripheral uptake of sugar out of the blood stream (i.e. outside the liver). It is the tandem of growth hormone release followed by IGF-1 release that prevents the overall rise in blood sugar. The insulin-like effect of IGF-1 explains why growth hormone, in normal amounts, lowers insulin requirements in patients who have a normal liver and DHEA and/or testosterone level. It also explains the observation why normal DHEA levels lower insulin requirements. Insulin requirements lower because normal DHEA levels instruct the liver DNA programs to increase the amount of IGF-1 manufactured. IGF-1 releases when growth hormone levels elevate. The IGF-1 released, acts like insulin in the cells outside of the liver (the periphery). In the periphery, IGF-1 directs many cells to take sugar out of the blood stream. When adequate IGF-1 secretes, the insulin needed to normalize the blood sugar decreases. Some physicians feel that insulin, outside of the liver in the healthful state, is unnecessary beyond very low levels.

IGF-1 has the additional benefit of facilitating the uptake of cell nutrition and minerals. IGF-1 occurs at 100 times greater the amount of insulin in the circulation when an owner remains healthy. This makes sense since about 100 times more insulin-like activity needs to exist to direct the proper nourishment of the cells outside the liver and fat. The highest pure insulin-type receptor concentration occurs on the liver and fat cells at about 200,000 receptors per cell. Because of the anatomy of the pancreas secreting into the portal vein that leads straight into the liver, whatever the insulin release rate, the liver always receives the highest message content of insulin. High insulin release rates favor the liver sucking excess nutrition out of the blood stream because of this anatomical fact.

High levels of IGF-1 diminish the need for insulin in the cells outside the liver and fat. Conversely, low levels of IGF-1 require an increased insulin secretion because a sugar load will require more insulin to return the blood sugar to normal following a carbohydrate meal. However, healthy owners have more than 100 times IGF-1 in their blood stream as compared to insulin. Unhealthy owners have liver strain because more insulin forces the liver into sucking excessive sugar out of the blood stream. The extra insulin also increases the rate of LDL cholesterol synthesis. The imbalance between insulin levels and IGF-1 levels creates a situation that favors increased body fat formation and hungry body cells. **Yet, this important relationship between excess insulin need being explained by falling IGF-1 levels, remains a secret.**

Cortisol is the next counter-hormone to insulin's message content. Cortisol powerfully counters insulin in its ability to remove sugar molecules from the blood stream.

Cortisol directs the liver to release stored liver sugar and fat into the blood stream. It also instructs the fat cells to release fatty acid fuels into the blood stream. In addition, it acts on the protein stores of the body and causes them to release amino acids into the blood stream (catabolism). The liver then sucks up the released amino acids for processing into sugar. The process of gluconeogenesis denotes the conversion of liver-sequestered amino acids into sugar.

Extremely high cortisol release tends to deplete the body protein content. The metabolically active component of the body consists of protein. Diminished protein content logically extends to the need for fewer calories per day. It also causes smaller muscles and organ size because this is where the protein comes from. High amounts of cortisol release occur with stress and when growth hormone levels fall off. Remember, only growth hormone protects the body protein content during times of stress (fasting, exercising, between meals, worry, etc.)

(Physician side bar) Cortisol instructs the liver cell DNA. The liver cell DNA, when instructed by cortisol, leads to the formation of certain cell receptors. The cell receptors are needed to recognize hormones that are not as powerful as level one-type hormones. Only level one-type hormones, like cortisol, directly instruct the DNA programs. The cortisol directed receptors manufacture that proves necessary to recognize adrenalin (epinephrine) and glucagon. These are level three and two hormones respectively (**Appendix B**). The liver will be unable to recognize the message content of epinephrine and glucagon without sufficient cortisol. Cortisol deficiency sets up a situation of the 'lesser hormones' not being able to deliver their message content (elevate the blood sugar in this case). The only other counter-regulatory hormone to insulin, growth hormone, will cause the release of IGF-1. This situation exacerbates low blood sugars when the liver fails to release enough sugar between meals. Here lies a little recognized mechanism for how low blood sugar occurs between meals.

Low blood sugars (hypoglycemia) are the hallmark of diminished adrenal reserve (chapter 10). The adrenal gland manufactures all body cortisol. Deficient cortisol, in the setting of high insulin, will lead to diminished blood sugar levels. Unfortunately, many of these hypoglycemic-prone owners are prescribed frequent feedings. This approach leads to weight gain and a compounding of problems with the passage of time.

However, a **24-urine test** will document diminished adrenal cortisol production. Occasionally, the additional test of Cortrosyn challenge (beyond the level of this discussion) of the adrenal reserve function will be needed to elucidate borderline cortisol reserve.

The implementation of several considerations heals diminished adrenal function. First, dietary changes for correcting carbohydrate and mineral imbalances contribute to a strong start. Second, the results of the 24-hour urine test document the scope of the steroid imbalance that includes cortisol deficiency. In some cases replacement with real steroid hormones becomes necessary. In others, diet and life style changes suffice. Customizing replacements to actual needs prevents side effects from cortisol replacement. In addition, changing the carbohydrate and mineral content of the diet prevents side effects. The replacement program often includes other adrenal steroids as indicated by the 24-hour urine test. When these factors are considered together, side effects are reduced or eliminated.

Epinephrine is one other counter regulatory hormone that opposes insulin. Epinephrine acts like cortisol in its ability to free fatty acids from the fat stores. However, its release powerfully inhibits insulin secretion. Ephedra acts in a similar manner to epinephrine. This fact explains its weight loss effect.

Blood pressure elevations from either one are unusual. In contrast, norepinephrine powerfully raises blood pressure.

Growth Hormone, the other counter regulatory hormone, acts mostly in the liver in its opposition to insulin. However, in one important way, both insulin and growth hormone share a common message theme. These two hormones both have in common the conservation of body protein. Insulin conserves body protein following meals while growth hormone conserves body protein between meals (fasting and exercising).

The Liver Controls the Body Fat Content

Diabetes and heart disease are often diseases that are secondary to the liver receiving poor informational direction. 90 percent of all diabetics suffer from excess insulin need (insulin resistance). Most heart disease owners also have excess message content from insulin (increased insulin release rates). When excess insulin causes these diseases, they begin with poor message content at the level of the liver. The poor message content arises from excess insulin. The liver cell dutifully follows the message content it receives. Insulin in the liver opposes growth hormone, epinephrine, cortisol, and glucagon message content. The balance of message content between the hormone insulin and the other four counter hormones comprises a major determinant in the risk for that owner developing these two diseases.

The complete cholesterol profile that typically occurs on an annual basis provides clues as to the summation of message content in one's liver. Some owners may have a normal blood cholesterol profile, but an obese body. **Only 50 percent of heart disease victims have abnormal cholesterol. The other fifty percent have normal cholesterol.** The fact that most heart disease owners are obese, points to the fact that they have too much insulin because it is always a pre-requisite for body fat (chapters 2, 7, 9 and 14). With more insulin, more message-content exists to create and maintain fat and cholesterol. High insulin leads to macrophages that line the inside of arteries being stuffed full with LDL cholesterol. Fat-laden macrophages eventually plug an artery even if the blood cholesterol remains normal.

Whenever one receives suboptimal lab results or they become obese, several things need to be considered and investigated. With this consideration and some life style changes, the excess insulin caused diseases often diminish. Altering the message content that the liver receives proves critical. When these primary factors remain ignored, symptom-control medicine becomes the only choice.

Healing from heart disease or diabetes involves alleviating one or more of these message abnormalities at the level of the liver:

1. **Unfavorable insulin and glucagon ratio of message content in the liver**
2. **Potassium deficiency leading to insulin resistance connection**
3. **Growth hormone connection**
    a) **Excess**
    b) **Deficiency**
4. **Cortisol excess**
    a) **Normal pancreas**
    b) **Wounded pancreas**
5. **Thyroid status**
6. **Growth hormone when the liver is unhealthy**
7. **Excessive proinsulin levels**
8. **Excessive estrogen levels**
9. **Low androgen levels**

A key difference occurs between the disease processes of diabetes and heart disease. The difference concerns the elevated blood sugar within the diabetic. However, these two diseases share a common pathology. 90 percent of diabetics have elevated insulin secretion rates and the majority of atherosclerotic heart disease involves elevated insulin secretion rates, as well. In most adult onset diabetics, their insulin need has finally elevated to the point (genetically determined) where their pancreas can no longer handle the increased demand and the blood sugar rises.

Five basic reasons exist for elevated insulin need. Insulin need rises when body mass goes up, IGF-1 levels fall, total body potassium decreases, chronic stress predominates and/or carbohydrate consumption increases. When a pancreas cannot meet the insulin demanded by the excessive presence of any one or more of the above conditions, the blood sugar will rise. By definition, when blood sugar rises beyond 140, diabetes is diagnosed. However, the same process of elevated insulin plugs up the blood vessels of the typical heart diseased owner. The pure heart diseased owner, who remains non-diabetic, can still make enough insulin to keep his blood sugar normal. **Here lies the common fundamental common link between adult onset diabetics and most atherosclerotic heart disease victims: elevated insulin secretion rates due to increased insulin need. Unfortunately, very few ask why insulin need increases and instead run straight for symptom-control methods.**

Many heart disease patients start out with normal blood sugars and only after many years their pancreas becomes exhausted. This commonality between these two diseases explains why mainstream medicine finally acknowledges that at the time of diagnosis of adult onset diabetes, heart disease is presumed to already exist. **90 percent of diabetes, and the majority of heart diseased owners, have elevated blood insulin secretion rates. They both involve excessive insulin need.**

The high insulin levels that occur in both diseases lead to increased blood fat abnormalities. However, in the case of the adult onset diabetic, the amount of insulin needed exceeds the ability of their pancreas to excrete enough insulin. Adult onset diabetes results when any one or more of the above five processes causes the pancreas to exceed its ability to excrete enough insulin. In all five situations, higher insulin output is required (insulin resistance). High insulin levels direct the liver to make excess LDL cholesterol. The excess LDL cholesterol released into the blood stream causes the vessel walls to collect LDL cholesterol in the macrophages (**especially when inflammatory conditions prevail**). The elevated blood sugar of diabetics provides an additional mechanism that injures the blood vessel.

Mainstream medicine tends to focus on normalizing the blood sugar with the price paid in the form of health consequences from the increasing insulin message content. Conventional physicians are taught to peripherally address the increased insulin-caused cholesterol and fat-making side effects, with cholesterol lowering drugs. They are also taught to prescribe blood pressure medication for the high blood pressure caused by excess insulin or mineral imbalance (chapter 4). Healing requires that insulin levels come down rather than pummel the liver with poison.

That insulin feeds fat formation in one's arteries proves particularly disturbing when one realizes how mainstream medicine treats many adult onset diabetics. They sidestep the central determinant: insulin excess that arises from its increased need within the body. The majority of diabetics receive treatment that involves methodologies, which raise insulin levels even further. This may normalize blood sugars, but it will only make the fat accumulating in the arteries worse. Clinically, the higher insulin levels show up as a worsening cholesterol profile. The cholesterol profile worsens with these treatment strategies because the higher the insulin, the more the liver receives message content to make cholesterol and fat from the sugar it sucks out of the blood stream.

Mainstream physicians are taught to remedy the worsening cholesterol profiles with the common class of liver poison, the statin drugs. Statin drugs inhibit the cholesterol making enzyme, HMG CoA reductase. Biochemistry textbooks discuss the fact that if the insulin message content decreases, this enzyme turns down its activity level naturally. In addition, the enzyme HMG Co A reductase turns down its activity further when glucagon levels within the liver elevate (see below). These facts explain why the high protein/fat and low carbohydrate diet often leads to a lower cholesterol level.

Rather than educate physicians about this buried and ignored fact, the symptom-control approaches remain the standard of care. These common symptom-control approaches always have side effects and have nothing to do with how one heals (the second part of the inflammation secret, in chapter 14, describes these side effects in more detail).

(Side bar for physicians) Another common symptom-control approach to treating adult onset diabetes involves the metaformin-like drugs given to increase insulin sensitivity. Their most common side effect, metabolic acidosis, provides a clue for how the increase in insulin sensitivity comes about.

Red blood cells and exercising muscles provide reliable sources for the constant creation of lactic acid. Normally, the liver removes this to keep the blood pH balanced. Anything that poisons the liver will decrease the liver's ability to perform this important task. In addition, a decreased conversion of lactic acid to pyruvate, a sugar intermediary, will lower the gluconeogenesis rate as well. A lowered gluconeogenesis rate will decrease the rate at which the liver can dump sugar into the blood stream and lower the amount of insulin needed. This is probably not the primary effect for how these drugs lower insulin requirements.

Remember, the more IGF-1 available, the less insulin is required. Also, remember that the bulk of IGF-1 binds to a carrier protein called insulin-like growth factor binding protein (IGFBP). Associated with this complex of IGF-1 and its binding protein is the acid labile subunit (ALS). A rise in acid content within the blood stream will allow ALS to undergo a conformational change, which frees up and allows IGF-1 to help insulin with fuel delivery (an increase in insulin sensitivity).

> An additional insight occurs that regards the natural process of increases in insulin sensitivity when the blood turns acidic. It has long been recognized that anaerobic exercise (weight lifting) raises growth hormone levels many more times than does aerobic exercise. Here again, it is the rise in lactic acid levels that seems to increase growth hormone secretion. Drugs like metaformin tend to raise lactic acid levels, as they pummel the liver, and this fact recreates the rise in lactic acid seen with anaerobic exercise. As growth hormone levels rise, the secretion rate of IGF-1 rises as well. In addition, the IGF-1 within the blood stream becomes more helpful with sugar removal because the ALS fragment has undergone a conformational change. Rather than the mainstream textbooks and eduction system helping physicians to understand the important roles that growth hormone and IGF-1 have in insulin sensitivity, they receive piecemeal information. Piecemeal-educated physicians enable drug sales to increase, but the overall healing rate decreases.

Passive patients require these symptom-control approaches but what about those owners who desire healing? The first step in healing an insulin-excess disease involves understanding, which Type an owner might have. Contrary to the mainstream medicine approach to adult onset diabetes, numerous additional causes for this disease process exist. Before healing can occur, the afflicted needs to know which process causes his/her disease.

All eleven combinations of factors effect the message content at the level of the liver by their unique effect on the amount of insulin-message content present. **Remember, obesity has a powerful association with both heart disease and diabetes. The eleven combination groupings below help explain why. When one understands why they have a disease, they can begin to heal. Healing is facilitated when one's physician inquires into which type of liver message abnormality promotes a given owner's disease process.**

Insulin and Glucagon Message Content in the Liver

It is more accurate to say that the activity of the cholesterol- manufacturing enzyme in the liver, HMG Co A reductase, is determined by the ratio, in amount, between glucagon and insulin. A high protein/good fat and low carbohydrate diet will tend to increase glucagon levels relative to insulin. Similarly, stress management and regular exercise will tend to improve this ratio (see Exercise and Muscles in the *Glandular Failure* book). This explains why, owners that eat steak and eggs, while simultaneously decreasing carbohydrate will tend to see a drop in their cholesterol (chapter 14). Other factors exists that influence blood cholesterol level, but this ratio remains all-important in most owners. Without placing appropriate attention on an improved insulin and glucagon ratio, healing a blood cholesterol problem remains difficult.

Diminished Potassium Leads to an Increased Insulin Need

It was explained earlier that a fall in total body potassium leads to insulin resistance (more insulin is needed for the same sugar load). Increased insulin means that more fat and cholesterol-making message will arrive at the liver. Diminished body potassium has detrimental effects to the insulin and glucagon ratio. This mechanism of altered blood fat creation from the liver is rarely recognized in America today.

This basic defect arises because owners who subsist on a processed food diet chronically stuff their cells with the wrong mineral ratios. The body was designed to intake at least three times as much potassium as sodium (see mineral table). Around middle age the kidney begins to falter in its ability to conserve potassium and excrete excess sodium.

The potassium deficiency of middle age means less of this mineral becomes available to bring the blood sugar down following a carbohydrate meal. In order to bring one sugar molecule inside a liver cell for sugar storage purposes, sufficient potassium must be available. This also remains true for all cells except in the brain and red blood cells. Inadequate potassium eventually causes the pancreas to secrete extra insulin. Even though insufficient potassium inhibits insulin release initially, eventually, the body senses the delay in the blood sugar fall after eating and more insulin releases into the portal vein. This will be met with resistance because the basic defect involves not enough potassium to uptake the sugar into the liver cells. It is slightly more complicated than this because of the IGF-1 that is released between meals. Potassium deficiency impedes the storage of sugar as glycogen because a fixed amount of potassium, per gram of glycogen in the liver needs to be present. The liver manufacture of fat and cholesterol does not depend on potassium levels.

The extra insulin that occurs in these situations will activate the fat-making machinery in the liver preferentially. This happens whenever the liver receives excess insulin message content. In contrast, the healthy body has ample potassium to facilitate the rapid liver uptake of sugar out of the blood stream to make glycogen following a meal. It also has sufficient IGF-1 to facilitate sufficient organ and muscle uptake of sugar, which lessens the liver proportion of sugar removed out of the blood stream. Between meals or with exercise the liver stored potassium and IGF secrete together. With adequate potassium, IGF-1 can promote the uptake of nutrients. Potassium and other nutrients are needed for cell energy and rejuvenation (i.e. strong, large muscles). With insufficient potassium, the blood sugar normalizes more by the liver than by the peripheral cells ("hungry cell syndrome").

The dependency of insulin on adequate body potassium exposes a defect in the high protein diet proponents. It clarifies how the fruit and vegetable proponents have a piece of the puzzle that pertains to diets that work. When both of these pieces correctly re-unite, a superior diet and cholesterol profile becomes possible.

The high protein diet premise improves by adding in the optimal ratio of potassium to sodium mineral content. This drastically lowers the insulin-message content needed by the body. A lower message content of insulin will improve the ratio between it and glucagon. This will allow less cholesterol and fat synthesis in the liver. Diminished cholesterol and fat synthesis leads to improved blood cholesterol. When less insulin becomes necessary, the pancreas strain diminishes. In the case of diabetes, the need for extra insulin becomes less likely.

Growth Hormone Connection - What Message the Liver Receives and its Effects on Diabetes and Heart Disease

Growth Hormone Excess

Excessive growth hormone (GH) tends to promote diabetes when its level exceeds the ability of the liver to secrete the consequent insulin-like growth factor (IGF-1). Within the liver, it promotes the release of sugar and fat into the blood stream (a diabetogenic effect). The second effect concerns the simultaneous release of insulin-like growth factor (IGF-1). IGF-1 acts like insulin out in the periphery, muscle, and organ cells. IGF-1 helps insulin take sugar out of the blood stream. The diseased liver cannot release sufficient IGF-1. This defect occurs at varying degrees of severity. Elevated GH with a diminished IGF-1 release will cause the blood sugar to rise. When the blood sugar rises, the pancreas attempts to normalize it by secreting insulin. When blood sugar rises beyond the pancreases' ability to manufacture the insulin necessary to counter act the excess growth hormone, diabetes results. Growth hormone excess can occur either in acromegaly or with high dose growth hormone replacement protocols. It is the increased insulin, in the above scenario that leads to altered blood cholesterol profiles. When this occurs, heart disease, and eventually diabetes, becomes more likely.

Within this subgroup of owners that may develop diabetes are those with a wounded pancreas. Their high IGF-1 levels are their only protection from full-on diabetes. Sometime in adulthood, as the

IGF-1 levels fall, these owners develop diabetes. They can usually be recognized clinically as those atypical-looking diabetics that have large muscles and diminished body fat for their age. These signs constitute a rare type of physique for any diabetic and should alert the clinician to look into their fasting insulin, C-peptide and IGF-1 level. Also, serum iron studies identify those owners whose pancreas was damaged by its accumulation. Again, these rare types of diabetic patients have as their fundamental defect, a wounded pancreas, and as their salvation, the particularly strong ability to make IGF-1.

This type of diabetic patient benefits from insulin treatment because insulin deficiency, and not IGF-1 deficiency, drives their disease process. In contrast, the typical emaciated insulin-dependent diabetic usually suffers from IGF-1 deficiency first that eventually exhausts his/her pancreas (beta cell burnout), and diabetes develops. Measures that raise IGF-1 early in the disease process, could save some of these owner's pancreases from total burn out. Physicians would first have to know to check a fasting IGF-1 level. Sadly, this is not usually part of the mainstream education content.

Growth Hormone Deficiency

For different reasons, problems with blood sugar control occur when growth hormone secretion rates prove deficient. Blood sugar will tend to rise because less liver direction occurs to release insulin-like growth factor (IGF-1). IGF-1 levels occur at levels greater than 100 times those of insulin in the blood stream of a healthy owner. IGF-1 helps insulin with taking nutrition out of the blood stream and into the cells. With less IGF-1, more insulin must be secreted for the same sugar load. The increased demand for insulin can exhaust the pancreas of some owners, and diabetes develops. Sedentary lifestyles promote decline in growth hormone secretion rates. Conversely, owners that exercise have higher growth hormone levels. That means less insulin will be required because of the increased liver stimulation to secrete IGF-1. Less insulin creates less message content in the liver to make fat and cholesterol. Athletic training will decrease cholesterol levels for these reasons.

Clinically, growth hormone deficient owners express as one type of Syndrome X patient. Their fundamental health defect results from a fall in their IGF-1 levels. Healthy people have over 100 times the IGF-1 compared to insulin within their blood streams. The liver is large and the pancreas is small. The smaller pancreas, when forced to increase its insulin production rate many fold, eventually exhausts itself. A small fall in IGF-1 levels requires a marked increase in insulin production to offset the deficiency in the total amount of "fuel nozzle" hormones for the body cells outside the liver and fat. IGF-1 levels fall from three basic mechanisms: liver injury, decreased growth hormone secretion rates, and diminished DHEA and testosterone levels, which direct the liver DNA to make IGF-1. Growth hormone tells the liver to secrete IGF-1. Chronic mental stress, occurring with a sedentary lifestyle also lowers IGF-1 levels secondary to other reasons (see below).

Excess Cortisol Levels - The Message the Liver Receives Depends on the Health of the Pancreas

Excess Cortisol

Excess cortisol creates obesity and/or borderline diabetes. In either case, the blood vessels sustain damage. The phenotype distinguishes which process occurs. The 24-hour urine test confirms the physical exam and blood findings. With increased cortisol, owners with a normal pancreas tend to become obese. With the passage of time, they will tend to appear cushingoid (moon face, buffalo hump, stria on the abdomen, panus formation on the abdomen, and muscle loss). If the cortisol level elevates high enough, they can reach the upper limit of their pancreas for its insulin production capacity.

Diabetes results. It is the insulin that makes them fat. It is the cortisol that elevates their blood sugar and sucks down their body protein content (catabolic effect).

Mainstream physicians are generally groomed to think that cortisol directly makes these owners fat. This is not true. First, the elevated cortisol directs the liver to begin creating and dumping sugar into the blood stream. This results from the fact that cortisol levels increase when the body thinks an emergency exists. When modern stress causes increased cortisol release, no physical challenge ever comes and the body eventually recognizes the increased blood sugar as inappropriate. When the body recognizes the increase in blood sugar as inappropriate, insulin levels rise. When increased insulin secretes into the portal vein, the liver receives a higher message content to make fat. Increased fat synthesis leads to weight gain.

The second group of increased cortisol producers is often missed clinically because they lack body fat, and this fools physicians. Any owner who has heart disease and appears on the emaciated side of physical body habitués deserves a deeper inquiry. Although they have increased cortisol output, they could have a 'wounded' pancreas. Wounded pancreases cannot increase insulin production to match the increased sugar output of high cortisol. Instead, these owners rely on their IGF-1 to eventually bring their sugars back down to normal. Increased blood sugar proves only transient, but the return to normal levels delays. The prolonged increase in blood sugar has oxidizing effects on the blood vessels (increased glycation rate, otherwise known as an increased rate of blood vessel "rust" formation). The normal fasting sugars are almost always normal, but the glucose challenge tests are not. These owners acquire blood vessel injury from the episodic elevations of their blood sugar levels, following the cortisol surges or carbohydrate binges. Increased blood vessel injury occurs from the "rust" processes that high sugar levels cause in the vessel walls. **These types of patients provide another situation for which insulin shots will prolong life because their insulin deficiency is at the root of their disease process.**

Further complicating these owner's health problems concerns the fact that they also crave sugar. They crave sugar because they lack sufficient insulin. Sufficient insulin is required so that the blood fuel can stay constant between meals. Normally, between meals, the release of growth hormone occurs when blood fuel first begins to fall. The arrival of growth hormone at the liver that is stuffed full of glycogen, which insulin directed following the last meal, causes sugar, fat and IGF-1 to release. The IGF-1 delivers the fuel to the hungry cells in the between meal state. However, in these types of afflicted owners, their insulin release was inadequat, following their last meal, so their glycogen stores prove insufficient. **Here lies the mechanism for another type of hypoglycemic-prone owner.** These types present clinically as emaciated in their muscle mass and have very low body fat. They get hypoglycemic because they lack sufficient insulin to instruct the adequate storage of sugar within their livers to get them through the between meal state.

Thyroid Levels

Thyroid levels form a determinate of how fast the cell power plants can utilize blood fat. Owners with low thyroid levels have a diminished ability to utilize fuel in their power plants (mitochondria). Their livers become feeble because of the diminished thyroid message content at the level of the liver cell DNA programs. Scientific experiments on dogs that had their thyroids partially or totally destroyed clearly showed the pathologic changes at the level of the liver. Without adequate thyroid, the liver becomes pathologic because it lacks appropriate instruction at the level its DNA programs.

The thyroid hormone also determines how many mineral pumps are present within the 100 trillion cell membranes. At rest, the largest amount of calories burn from recharging these 100 trillion cell batteries through activity of the mineral pumps. The thyroid message partially concerns itself with telling the body cell's DNA program to manufacture more mineral pumps.

The more mineral pumps that exist, the more calories burned while an owner rests. Scientists call this the basic metabolic rate. The metabolic rate depends on two things: the amount of mineral pumps and the strength of the furnace flame within the mitochondria. Weight gain propagates until someone helps the thyroid hormone levels to increase toward normal levels. Nuclear fallout, spent rocket fuel, and other contaminants around the world, have poisoned millions of owner's thyroid glands. Rather than educate physicians properly about the need to check the thyroid more completely, countless owners receive false reassurance that their thyroid hormone level checked out fine (chapter 7).

Growth Hormone and the Unhealthy Liver

Unhealthy livers are unable to release adequate insulin-like growth factor (IGF-1) when growth hormone instructs them to do so. **The growth hormone can be diabetogenic in these situations.** Injured liver cells still make fuel available when directed to do so long after their ability to make proteins curtails. The liver manufactures the blood stream amount of insulin-like growth factor (IGF-1). Many different mechanisms occur that contribute to an ill liver (see appendix). Some of these include poor nutrition, excessive liver toxin exposure (alcohol, prescription drugs, putrefaction of the colon contents with liver reabsorption), poor trophic hormone levels (cortisol, thyroid, androgens, etc.) and excess iron storage.

It is interesting that many medical textbooks emphasize that growth hormone is diabetogenic (promotes diabetes). Sensationalizing this rare possibility leads to yet another example of how physicians' thinking gets groomed into the more profitable ways to treat disease. Instead of saying that growth hormone is diabetogenic when the liver is sick, or the amount of growth hormone exceeds the

ability of the liver to produce IGF-1, they propagate a half-truth. To tell the whole truth would facilitate a curiosity for the importance of IGF-1 for blood sugar control.

Insulin - Pro-hormone Levels

Insulin is first made within a 'package', the pro-hormone, that converts to insulin before release into the blood stream. Certain situations create an increased release of the pro-hormone form of insulin (in the package). This occurs when the pancreas strains to increase insulin production in response to some other body condition (obesity, high carbohydrate diets, insulin resistance). When this occurs, the liver's ability to remove sugar from the blood stream diminishes per amount of pancreas secretion. The pro-hormone seems to retain some of its message content for the ability to make the liver create fat from sugar. This also happens in the growth of fat cells.

High Estrogen Levels will Increase Insulin Need

There has been a flurry of media attention toward supposed new evidence about increased estrogen levels and the increased risk for heart disease. All along, the evidence for this predictable association has been buried in the medical textbooks.

This chain of events starts with high estrogen levels that lead to increased growth hormone release while estrogen simultaneously curtails the liver's ability to release insulin-like-growth factor type 1 (IGF-1). However, growth hormone arriving at the liver still manages to trigger the liver release of sugar and fat into the blood stream. The decrease of IGF-1 and the increased growth hormone message causes the sugar release to be uncompensated. This exaggerated blood sugar elevation occurs because high estrogen inhibits IGF-1 release but promotes growth hormone release. In this situation, the blood sugar will rise higher than it does with normal estrogen levels. The body eventually senses the increased blood sugar levels as inappropriate and insulin secretes.

The increased insulin secretion rate causes the liver to receive increased message content to manufacture sugar into fat and cholesterol. Fat and cholesterol secrete into the blood stream as LDL cholesterol. The blood has more LDL cholesterol and the triglyceride levels will be higher when measured. Triglyceride levels are only the summation of all the fat in the blood stream (the fat content of HDL, LDL, and VLDL cholesterol). Both high triglycerides and LDL cholesterol associate with an increased risk of heart disease.

Low androgen levels

Many diabetics' diseases trace back to a fall in their androgen levels for one reason or another. Early on in their disease, if their physician recognizes this deficiency, when it occurs, total pancreas burn out can be avoided. In addition, many of the complications of diabetes such as: blood vessel pathology, colitis, and digestive tract dysfunction, are made worse when androgen levels stay low.

Prediction: in the near future more attention as to whether insulin-dependent diabetes resulted from liver injury first or pancreas injury first, will come into the mainstream. The liver injury first variety has a component of causality in low androgens. Pancreas strain occurs whenever androgens fall because IGF-1 levels consequently fall off as well.

(Side bar for physicians) The important role of IGF-1 and the amount of GAG formation on the lining of the blood vessels, colon, and stomach, was previously mentioned. Briefly, IGF-1's presence in these tissues controls the important step of sulfation for these molecules' creation. In fact, the older literature called IGF-1, sulfation factor. A fall of the androgen-message content in the body directly causes IGF-1 to fall off throughout the body.

A deficiency in this layer paves the way for an increased injury rate in these tissues. Add in the unmanaged high blood sugars of the uncontrolled diabetic, and the injury rate accelerates. Restoring the androgen level to normal would make sense as an additional step beyond blood sugar control alone.

Chapter 14: Inflammation and Heart disease: The Second Part of the Secret

The Big Difference Between Liver Manufactured Fat and Dietary Fat is the second part of the Secret

After this, a discussion follows for how excess insulin often associates with, and contributes to inflammation, within the blood vessels

The body packages fat with varying amounts of cholesterol, but technically, cholesterol really denotes a modified fat molecule. Fat and cholesterol need to associate with protein in order to float in the blood stream. The variable that determines fat availability to the metabolically hungry cells concerns, which carrier protein types add to it that allow it to solubilize within the blood stream.

A distinction occurs for the difference between carrier proteins occurring between the liver's manufactured fat, and fat from the diet. Diet-derived fat has less potential to accumulate in blood vessel walls. The carrier protein of dietary fat contains a protein package that has less potential to plug up a vessel. Where fat originates provides the crucial difference between transport packages. When fat-cholesterol-protein complexes originate in the digestive tract following a meal, the metabolically hungry cells easily absorb them. Remember, insulin is the fuel storage hormone. When insulin directs the liver to make cholesterol-fat-protein complexes, they are designed for storage and not immediate fuel needs. One more way the body proves smart and consistent.

The insulin message content concerns itself with fuel storage in the body. The majority of fuel storage occurs as fat. Normal amounts of diet derived fat form complexes, which rapidly assimilate into the metabolically hungry cells (skeletal muscle, cardiac muscle, kidney, etc.). In contrast, liver-manufactured fat contains a design that does not readily clear from the blood stream except by fat and macrophage cells.

In other words, insulin directed fat-cholesterol-protein complexes are less able to serve as fuel. They contain designs that follow from the direction of insulin, the fuel storage hormone. Again, the body is smart and consistent. The consistent message of insulin causes greater amounts of stored fuel (glycogen and fat). The insulin directed fat-cholesterol-protein complexes are designed with fuel storage in mind.

The Unique Way Fat Absorbs from the Diet Illuminates the Fallacy of the 'Fat is Bad Campaign'.

A physiologic fact clarifies the lack of 'stickiness' of diet-derived fat on vessel walls. Dietary fat and cholesterol absorb via the lymphatics, which differs from all other nutrients. This means that lymph vessels receive the highest vessel concentration exposure of dietary cholesterol and fat. Atherosclerosis (the growth of fat within vessels) of lymphatic vessels is unheard of. Even more damning concerns the fact that lymph fluid moves in a sluggish manner, compared to blood flow within the arteries. If there were anything 'sticky' about diet derived fat, it would be more pronounced in the sluggish lymph vessels.

The difference between the types of cholesterol-fat package that blood vessel walls encounter compared to the cholesterol-fat-package that lymphatic vessels transport following a fatty meal explains this fact.

This difference explains the true cause for the majority of heart disease: excess insulin. The insulin-directed, liver manufactured cholesterol-fat packages collect in blood vessel walls within the macrophages. Anatomically, the lymphatic vessels do not encounter insulin-directed and liver-manufactured cholesterol-fat packages. These vessels only encounter diet-derived cholesterol-fat packages. These apparently do not deposit along lymph vessel walls.

If only medical schools taught that the body is smart and consistent. Insulin-directed fat and cholesterol particles possess structures designed with storage in mind. Long-term storage sites for these types of particles exist in the liver, blood vessel macrophages, and fat cells. Conversely, diet-derived fat and cholesterol particles, the chylomicrons, have a design that readily allows removal by the body cells, and they store short term or combust as fuel.

> **Even though lymph vessel's fluid flows in a sluggish manner and encounters very high levels of diet-derived fat and cholesterol, they do not plug-up. Anatomically, the small intestine delivers fat and cholesterol into the lymph vessels following a meal. The protective factor for lymphatic vessels involves the fact that they have no exposure to liver-manufactured cholesterol-fat-protein complexes (LDL). Intestinal lymphatic vessels eventually drain into the left neck area, the thoracic duct. In this location, the fatty parts of digestion dump into the blood stream.**
>
> **In contrast, other products of digestion such as protein, carbohydrates, minerals, and vitamins, etc., dump directly from the intestinal cells into the portal vein. The portal vein collects all intestinal blood and nutrition (except fat and cholesterol) from the digestive tract and takes it straight to the liver.**

The blood vessels clog up whenever insulin levels rise to the point of directing the liver to excessively manufacture the 'sticky' type of cholesterol-fat packages (LDL cholesterol). Some of this LDL cholesterol absorbs into the macrophages that line blood vessels. Macrophages denote immune system scavenger cells that, under well-fed circumstances, bed down on blood vessel linings and stuff themselves with LDL cholesterol.

When the liver creates excessive amounts of fat-protein-cholesterol complexes (LDL cholesterol), they incorporate into macrophages in abnormal amounts. Excessively stuffed macrophages with LDL cholesterol, grow and grow. Year after year, they continue to accumulate LDL cholesterol and eventually form giant cells called foam cells. Foam cells denote the earliest lesions recognized by scientist as the beginning of heart disease.

Some of the places that macrophages bed down and become foam cells occur in the coronary arteries, hearing apparatus, kidney vessels, peripheral leg vessels, and retina. These tissues prefer fat for fuel. The LDL cholesterol accumulation trouble compounds with a sedentary owner.

High insulin levels in sedentary owners allow LDL cholesterol to continuously collect in the macrophages. These cells permit fat to collect due to lack of exercise. After many years, this vicious cycle allows fatty streaks to grow enough to block blood flow. Blood flow can suddenly worsen in these narrowed areas when other factors promote blood clots to form. When severe enough, the constriction causes cell death to areas beyond the blockage.

The other common mechanism for the sudden loss of blood flow involves vessel spasms in the narrow area. These two climaxes describe the typical scenario for the number one killer of Americans past middle age, heart disease. The earlier available information on this subject has been disjointed and fragmented.

High insulin-producing bodies manufacture more fat and cholesterol. Insulin-directed cholesterol-fat packages are designed for storage depots. These packages designed for the storage depots of the body, are slow to drain off out of the blood stream. These individuals have an increased risk for this type of heart disease when they are living sedentary lifestyles, have unmanaged stress, contain mineral imbalances, suffer a fall in IGF-1 levels, and/or consume high insulin-promoting diets. All five of these risk factors increase insulin levels (increased insulin need). Increased risk arises from the increased tendency for macrophages to ingest more LDL cholesterol than is healthy.

The relationship between high insulin levels because of falling IGF-1 levels, high stress levels, reversed minerals ratios diet, high carbohydrate intake, and sedentary lifestyles are the crux of the problem for the majority of all heart disease victims. The other risk factors for heart disease development accelerate this primary disease producing mechanism in the blood vessels. Rather than focus on the hopeless mantra about some owners' genetics, empowerment comes from a focus on how dietary and lifestyle changes prevent the problem.

Some owners have a greater tendency for heart disease based on primitive survival strategies. A survival advantage was obtained in prehistoric times when a body could store fat in times of plenty, in order to survive periods of famine. Owners that made more insulin evidenced a survival advantage. The food supply was never predictable so there was no accumulation of blood vessel fat.

In contrast, the modern day food supply fails to be interrupted and these same survival equipped insulin-producing machines create excess fat. Add in the greatly increased insulin requirement that becomes necessary to handle a chronic processed food diet. This occurs secondary to its diminished potassium content. Also add in the overactive mental stress-caused increased insulin need. These same survival equipped owners are now fat producing machines.

An owner still has the ability to turn off his/her fat-making machine. The liver fat-making machine turns off by consistently choosing a low insulin requiring diet, obtaining ample potassium, minimizing sodium, doing aerobic exercise, correcting the other fat promoting hormones, and

stress management (as suggested in earlier chapters). Instead of helping owners understand this, they are led down the erroneous path of what is for sale by the complex.

Unfortunately, for the average owner, little incentive exists to share (publish and sensationalize) these basic scientific understandings. The 'fat is bad campaign' largely cotains hype that allows the relationship between insulin and blood vessel disease to remain a secret. Knowledge about the insulin secret jeopardizes the more lucrative approaches for treating blood vessel disease. However, the lucrative approaches contain side effects and toxicities that, if commonly known, would create even more reluctance for these symptom-control methods. Symptom-control, so prevalent within the mainstream paradigm, has nothing to do with healing. Passive owners remain stuck with symptom-control and all its unfavorable side effects. However, what about those owners that possess the focus to commit to a path of healing?

> (Physicians side bar) Inflammation and Heart disease: a Holistic Perspective
>
> The amount of insulin within the body determines the amount of fat-maker message. Hormones, like insulin, carry information to the body cells. Hormone information always concerns how cells direct energy expenditure. Insulin carries information that tells the cells to store energy. Most body energy storage occurs as fat. Cholesterol is one type of body fat. The enzyme in the liver that makes sugar into cholesterol turns up its activity when insulin levels rise. Insulin levels rise following carbohydrate meals or excess mental stress (among several other promoters). Rather than tell doctors and the public about this simple cause and effect relationship, the story of the wonders of the statin drugs bombards media outlets.
> Statin drugs poison this liver enzyme's ability to listen to the insulin message. The trouble with poisons concerns their inevitable side effects and toxicities. One nasty side effect from

these medications concerns the depletion of Co enzyme Q10 in the body. The heart needs the lion's share of this important nutrient. Deficiency here causes one type of heart failure.

Another emerging understanding for how statin drugs lower heart disease risk involves their ability to subdue inflammation. Rather than come clean and educate physicians about the most likely mechanism for how this occurs, the statin selling companies perpetrate the story that it remains largely a mystery. The argument for it being a mystery, diminishes once a few critical clues add back into the discussion. Additionally, their rosy innocence fades as well, because their likely downside emerges.

The **first** clue involves the long-known association between heart disease and the Type A personality types. Type A personality types are classically described as hard driving, over achieving, and always worried about their next deal. Physiologically, these emotions when chronically expressed lead to a constant stress hormone response. The stress response was designed to survive physical stressors. In order to survive a physical stress, the massive dumping of fuel into the blood stream makes sense because exercising muscles consume the fuel. Additionally, physical stressors often lead to trauma. This explains why the acute phase reactants predictably elevate with the onset of the stressor. The acute phase reactants prove appropriate with trauma, but deleterious with mental stress. C-reactive protein is only one acute phase reactant. Others include complement, interferon, fibrinogen, ferritin, ceruloplasmin and amyloid. Fibrinogen directly increases the clotting tendencies of blood. Ferritin elevations increase iron absorption into the body tissues.

The trauma associated with physical stressors underscores the desirability for new blood cells' manufacture where-with-all. However, with mental stress, once iron absorbs into the body, it proves very difficult to remove. This detail may help explain the emerging realization that many heart disease patients have elevated ferritin levels. It further explains a potential reason that chelation therapy maintains its devotees, despite the ongoing criticism. Specifically, EDTA binds and removes iron from the body. This fact may prove as the number one benefit for this approach.

Lastly, concerning the acute phase reactants elevation in the setting of mental stressors, involves its inappropriate effect toward an increase in angiogenesis propensity. The angiogenesis propensity increases when the acute phase reactants elevate. This again makes sense with physical stressors because these traumas associate with the need for new blood vessel formation.

Chronic mental stress promotes two powerful processes that promote the angiogenesis critical to tumor growth: increased insulin needs and the heightened angiogenesis propensity described above. **These facts, taken together, provide a likely mechanism for why overweight and stressed individuals suffer increased morbidity and mortality from cancer.**

The **second** clue involves the emerging research results that document that the statin drugs lower C-reactive protein levels. Once one recalls the connection between HMG Co A reductase activity and steroid synthesis rates, a more holistic picture emerges. Anything that subdues the ability of the adrenal glands to make steroids, will also diminish the magnitude of cortisol released for a given stressor. In turn, less cortisol release subdues the acute phase reactants' release. C-reactive protein is only one of the acute phase reactants. The normalization of acute phase reactants, in the chronic mentally stressed state, leads to less inflammation for the reasons described above.

These facts initially sound too good to be true. This old adage once again proves useful because the downside to this scenario provides insight into the advantages of counseling Type A personality-type owners about the bigger picture of cause and effect relationships.

In order to better appreciate the downside of the statins, one needs to recall the typical body habitus of the Type A personality owner. The majority of them are large in the waistline, or at the very least, they have increased visceral fat. Currently, a waist measurement above 40 inches is felt to predict these metabolic syndrome types at risk for accelerated aging and blood vessel disease. Over fifty years ago, obese individuals were found to have increased stress steroids in their urine.

Uniting these two facts together it becomes more likely to understand one of the metabolic syndrome individual's driving forces, an exaggerated stress steroid release rate for a given stressor. Another way to look at this is, in the setting of chronic mental stress, those prehistorically equipped survival machines selected for down through the ages have become the metabolic syndrome victims from chronic sedentary-type stressors. What was once a survival benefit derived from mounting a strong fuel release and acute phase reactant release (both secondary to a strong cortisol release) in the setting of physical stress, now has become a curse, promoting excessive body fat accumulation and blood vessel inflammation.

With mental stress, the increased blood fuel has nowhere to go, and hence, increased insulin amounts eventually release to normalize the blood sugar. Unfortunately, insulin released into the portal vein heads straight for the liver. HMG Co A reductase turns on with increasing insulin and off with increasing glucagon. Because the liver (also fat cells) cells have 200,000 pure insulin-type receptors per cell, insulin increases profoundly effect the cholesterol profile.

The very survival of the statin drug-selling rosy picture depends on eviscerating certain scientific consequences that result from a diminished glandular ability. When healthy, the adrenal glands, make both catabolic and anabolic message content. A higher anabolic message content leads to a faster repair rate. The lower the antioxidants, the more repairs needs to occur. Here lies the likely additional risk of chronically consuming statin drugs in place of healing lifestyles; they contribute to the lack of repair from ongoing wear and tear that the blood vessels encounter. Disrepair causes inflammatory damage despite their benefit from decreased cholesterol and acute phase reactants levels.

Any drug or toxin that inhibits the steroid manufacture ability within the adrenals or gonads, will also decrease the repair rate that logically follows from diminished anabolic message content. Here lies another downside that remains ignored until one begins to examine the interrelatedness of steroid synthesis rates and HMG Co A reductase activity.

> In one way or another, blood vessel disease results from the repair rate not keeping up with the injury rate. Statin drugs may in fact lower the injury rate by diminishing the acute phase reactants' caused inflammation and cortisol-related blood sugar spikes. The lessened blood sugar spikes lead to decreased insulin need despite a sedentary and stress-filled lifestyle. A subdued stress response means that less acute phase reactants release, as well. However, what is not being said concerns their probable negative influence on the repair rate of blood vessels. The repair rate of blood vessels depends on androgen levels, like all other DNA-containing body cells. Since science has already documented subdued acute phase reactants with statin usage, it remains quite likely that other steroids' synthesis rates decrease, as well
>
> The likely consequence of diminished testosterone, which results from statin drug usage may help further elucidate the ongoing suspicion about their contribution to heart failure. Many in the holistic community attribute this tendency to the diminished Co enzyme Q10 levels that logically follow. However, maybe a fall off in testosterone in some chronic stain users, contributes to their pump failure as well.
>
> Following serial 24-hour urine measurements for steroids would provide a logical next step for testing the severity of diminished anabolic message content. If each doctor in the holistic community began collecting baseline 24-hour urine specimens for steroids, and followed them serially, a new level of understanding would emerge about the association of a heightened stress response, increased insulin need, and elevated acute phase reactants in the development of blood vessel disease.

On the Other Hand: Chemically-Reactive Fats in the Diet Cause Heart Disease

The consumption of unhealthy fats are not allowed in high fat diets if one wishes to be free of blood vessel disease. The people free of heart disease, while they indulge in a high fat and low carbohydrate diets, are not the ones that consume high amounts of chemically reactive fats. Chemically reactive fats have the scientific name, partially hydrogenated vegetable fats. This distinction about good fat and bad fat is often overlooked and leads to confusion in the minds of clinicians as well as owners, in regard to the safety of high fat diets. Diets made up of real fats are safe, while diets made up of large quantities of chemically reactive fats are not. Chemically reactive fats contribute to oxidation (rust) in the blood vessels.

The chemically reactive fat groups are chemically altered polyunsaturated fats. The chemical process of hydrogenation has altered them. The hydrogenation process causes a twisting deformation that is an unnatural occurrence in real fats. Numerous baked goods, margarines, breads, snacks, and chips have altered fats added to them. The hydrogenation process provides one example where altered fats add firmness to the product. These polyunsaturated fats are chemically altered and become more twisted when they stack together. Fats in the body need to be stacked together in the cellular membranes (the lipid bi-layer). The twisted configurations of chemically altered fat means they form awkward fat conglomerates (irregularities) that line the cell membrane.

Endothelial cells fit together like tiles on the interior blood vessel lining. These cells, like all cells, have a cell membrane made up of fat interspersed with proteins. The polyunsaturated partially hydrogenated fats are also chemically reactive with many oxidizing agents that may be in the blood stream (aluminum, fluoride, oxygen radicals, carbon monoxide, ozone and other smog components, etc.). When these fats oxidize, they promote '"Velcro"' formations on the inside wall of the blood vessel. This formation summons the macrophages to lay down a temporary patch job that sometimes is never repaired. When LDL cholesterol is high, these macrophages collect fat and eventually grow into foam cells.

A component of blood vessel health depends on whether the inner lining layer (the tiles) of the blood vessel wall composes itself with the chemically altered polyunsaturated fats (hydrogenated fats) or healthy fats. The diet determines this content. Diets consisting of fast food fats, margarine, fried foods, baked goods, and commercial breads will add twisted fats to the lining layers of that owner's blood vessels. Owners whose diets contain real fats, have surfaces in the blood vessel, which are composed of the less chemically reactive fats (real fat).

Picture two beautiful flowerbeds. In one, short stocky stems grow, and in the other, fragile, slender stems grow. The contrast between the two types of stems allows an analogy that elucidates the body fat composition-type problem.

Short stocky stems are analogous to blood vessel friendly fats (olive oils, fish oils and canola oils). They are more durable. Good fats lining one's arteries only become possible when the owner makes good diet choices when consuming fats. Fragile long stems are analogous to chemically altered polyunsaturated fats (found in junk food, processed food, and fast food). They are more vulnerable to numerous oxidizing agents that occur in the blood stream.

Visualize a dog (oxidizing agent) that sequentially runs around in each type of flowerbed. The short stocky stems would sustain less damage because of the differences in structural characteristics between the two flowerbeds. The oxidative vulnerability in the blood vessels is analogous to what happens in the blood vessel lining cells when unhealthy fat is eaten. The vulnerability of blood vessel lining cells to trampling by the "dogs" being unleashed in the blood stream, are determined by the composition of the "stems". In a dirty environment, where air pollution, water pollution, and food contaminants prevail, the blood vessel lining cells overexpose to oxidizing agents (rust producers). The rust producers are analogous to the dog running around in the flowerbed. Real fats versus altered fats are analogous to the durability of the stems in the flowerbed. The more chemically reactive (altered) the fats become, the more they create rust ("Velcro" formations). The more the lining cells in the blood vessels compose themselves with real fats, the more durable they become when confronting oxidizing agents.

This consideration gradates the relative risk of different types of dietary fat and their potential to produce disease. The amount of abdominal fat is a clinical marker for diet or lifestyle determined high insulin levels. Men who have a greater abdominal measurement than hip measurement evidence high insulin levels. Women who are greater than 80% their waist compared to hip measurement evidence high insulin as well. Until insulin levels become optimal, by diet and lifestyle changes, health deteriorates.

The higher the oxidant exposure load that operates on a daily basis, the more important it becomes to minimize consumption of the chemically reactive fats. Owners who are chronically exposed to air pollution, water impurities (fluoridation), and impurities in their food, will have an increased rate at which their chemically reactive fats oxidize. Chemically reactive fats oxidize when exposed to harmful pollutants. Improving dietary fat choices and avoiding environmental 'rust' producers benefit healing.

Additional Hormones that are Beyond the Diet, but Influence Digested Foods to Deposit as Fat

Most owners who take active steps in their daily exercise and dietary decisions will notice a dramatic fall in their blood cholesterol. Their glucagon and insulin ratio have been favorably altered. Adequate message content from other body hormones are also important - androgen (from adrenals and gonads), estrogens, thyroid hormone, IGF-1, and cortisol. When these are correctly proportioned, blood fat-cholesterol-protein complexes will benefit.

These considerations can be assessed (except for IGF-1) through a complete 24-hour urine test that includes a quantitative and qualitative analysis of what hormone levels are manufactured. Healthy owners have optimal amounts of critical steroid and thyroid hormones that pass into their urine over a 24-hour period. Unhealthy owners pass sub-optimal amounts of critical androgen steroid hormones and possibly excessive amounts of estrogen and stress steroids. If thyroid function is inadequate, the urine is often the most reliable way to detect the deficiency. These hormone considerations become important when lifestyle and dietary modification fail to improve the cholesterol profile.

The need for a 24-hour urine collection illustrates what science has revealed versus what is practiced. Hormone levels can fluctuate widely in the blood stream. Some hormones have life spans measured in seconds. Most have life spans measured in minutes. When a blood sample is taken, the amount of hormone measured in that sample reflects that blood's informational content at the instant the venous sample is drawn. This method provides an accurate measurement only if the hormones in question are relatively stable in the blood stream.

Throughout the day, most hormones vary widely in the blood stream. The different informational substances convey a precise message to the body cells. Different activities of daily living obligate the release of different hormones that communicate to cells on how to spend their energy. Each of the varied life situations requires different informational direction of the body energy quotient. Therefore, the hormone levels and types during stress, pleasurable activity, fasting, or post-exercise, will predictably be different. Different activities and emotional states require a change in the blood stream information to accommodate the change in body energy direction required.

An accurate method to assess hormone tone and pressure would incorporate the basic scientific understanding that over a typical 24-hours, an average amount of hormone output will occur. Urine measurements are useful only when the hormone of interest exits the body via the kidney. This is true for thyroid and steroid hormones, and includes the different breakdown derivatives of these different hormones. Urine that is collected in a typical day can more accurately measure the types and amounts of hormones present. This sophisticated approach toward an assessment of the hormone status is more appropriate.

Most of the larger hormones composed of amino acid sequences (peptides or proteins) do not pass in the urine. Therefore, the urine is not the place to check for these hormone-types. This class of hormones must be measured in the blood stream. Insulin, glucagon, IGF-1, and some of the larger pituitary and hypothalamic hormones provide examples of this class. If a more accurate method for the assessment of hormone status exists, patients have the right to know about this option.

(Side bar) Many physicians are unaware that they are victims of an education that has removed some basic scientific understanding that conflict with profit. There have been numerous instances where a patient brings in a well-run 24-hour urine analysis only to be scoffed at by their conventionally trained, but limited second opinion physician. Owners are advised to have a little fun with these types of practitioners. Asking them to explain all the big words that describe the different breakdown products of certain hormones is a start to this fun adventure. At this point, a good physician will admit that he doesn't understand the results and will look into it. Unfortunately, many physicians that are confronted with what they do not understand habitually resort to attempts to discredit approaches that inquire above their education level. When one confronts the later type of practitioner, it may be time to begin thinking about a new doctor.

Chapter 15: The Glandular Failure Epidemic

Millions of middle-aged boomers find themselves with old feeling and appearing bodies. Many try creams and potions. Others try extreme diets and workout schedules. All of these approaches have merit. None of them work when their glands fail.

Youthful feeling and appearing bodies need proper glandular secretions. Glands secrete the message content into the blood stream that tells the bodies cells how to spend their energy. Scientists call the message content secreted into the blood stream by these glands, hormones. Optimal hormone secretions direct the youthful regeneration message to continue. Middle age has a large component of causality in failing glands. Failing glands secrete less rejuvenation message.

Simple science discussed here. Yet, mainstream medicine, paradoxically, spends little effort evaluating where one's glands' function lies. Because of this blind spot in the mainstream scientific standard of care, glandular failure is the epidemic of the boomer generation.

Glandular failure results from many causes. Some of them are: poor genetic constitution, poor nutrition, numerous environmental toxins that concentrate in one's glands, poor exercise habits, surgical removal of certain glands, fake hormone replacement, certain prescription medications, viral infections, and prolonged stress, to name a few. This book has been about how one identifies whether glandular failure operates in their aging process. It also identifies what causes their particular glandular problem from the list mentioned above. In addition, the safest solutions are reviewed. The good news is that scientifically validated solutions exist, which heal the problem. Healing has one side effect.

Doctors, like myself have very little realization that our complex-funded educations have eviscerated certain key scientific facts from our training. It seems rather fantastical at first. However, as the years ticked by in my medical practice, I began to notice many patients' claims presented sound evidence that something had been removed from my education about how things in the body really worked.

I have devoted the last several years to studying what many different medical textbooks really say about longevity. One big determinant of longevity concerns the quality of one's glandular secretions. This self-study program has led me to conclude that many doctors receive a 'piecemeal education'. Without their knowing it, piecemeal-educated physicians, dutifully practice symptom-control medicine. In this way, the medical industrial complex maintains its huge profit. Many doctors will find this assertion painful. I, too, have found it painful to realize the years I invested from my life, were devoted to learning a biased presentation of what science really knows. Beyond me, however, exists the suffering patient. As physicians, we are called upon to rise above our egos and do what is best for our patients.

Another realization has occurred to me. The certified experts, who the complex endorses to suppress rebels like me, are the ones that learned early on to keep their mouths shut. The medical educational process does not allow for dissension while one receives his/her education. More shackles to honest practice are applied by the medical legal rule, the standard of care. Otherwise known, by some physicians, as the keeper of the herd mentality. The many inconsistencies that patients provide, while one receives their training and also in practice, better stay ignored lest one will find their career ambitions blemished. We all need to stay mindful of this truism the next time a media outlet expounds upon a certified expert's news sound byte regarding some supposed new wonder drug or procedure. Most of these speeches utilize science poorly. Many times the research funded by the complex presents in a half truthful way. Half-truths that are epidemic in the mainstream literature do not reflect good science. Unless we stay aware of this fact, we are doomed to become victims of our profit-driven health care system.

Victim or healed, it all starts with personal choice. Some are passive in their disease process. For them, all that is possible are the symptom-control approaches with all their associated side effects and toxicities. This book is a waste of time for passive patients. Stay with your mainstream doctor. However, many other patients exist that truly desire healing information and accept the responsibility that comes from this decision. Responsibility allows focus. Focus leads to results. Small incremental results lead to healing.

The glands that need to heal

Pituitary
Thyroid
Adrenals
Gonads (ovaries or testes)
Liver
Pancreas

What do glandular failure owners look like? The appearance of the afflicted depends on the glands that fail. For example, the classically obese middle aged owner often results from a falling liver secretion rate of insulin-like growth factor type one (IGF-1). Mainstream medicine almost universally ignores this basic medical fact. Part of this perpetuated ignorance follows from the mysterious lowering of the normal value for this important hormone within the blood stream. Also a part results from disconnecting, in physician's minds, IGF-1 from its important blood sugar-lowering role as a helper to insulin. Additionally, insulin's fat-maker role in the body is almost completely ignored as well. The lower our IGF-1 level, the more insulin we need to deliver fuel to the body cells. The higher our insulin secretion rate, the fatter we will become.

Another prominent example that something is wrong with some of our glandular secretions concerns those owners that have joint pain. Rather than teach physicians this basic medical fact, they dutifully prescribe symptom-control painkiller prescriptions. In addition, physicians are taught to fear part of the hormone secretion problem, diminished adrenal function. Again, this is unnecessary and unscientific.

A final example concerns wrinkled and sagging skin. The mainstream is found touting the need to protect oneself from the sun. All the while, the primary determinant of nice skin, proper glandular secretions, remains largely ignored.

All three of these and more glandular failure signs are discussed throughout this text. In addition, the nutritional molecular building blocks that both the glands and body cells need to follow through on the message from the gland's secretion are reviewed. After all, there exists a beautiful interplay between proper nutrition and the glands that secrete message content. Proper attention to both of these processes puts the owner of a body on the longevity tract of life.

Chapter 16: Nutritional Deficiency Caused Fuel Burning Problems

Often times, blood vessel disease develops as the direct result of varying types of nutritional deficiency. Most blood vessels will heal when nutritional deficiencies correct. The deficiencies injure blood vessels through "rust" promotion, hardening processes, or opportunistic mechanisms. Usually all three mechanisms are set into motion by nutritional imbalance (*The Body Heals*).

Increased Blood Fat from Nutritional Deficiency

It has been asserted in the popular media that niacin supplementation may lower blood cholesterol. A more accurate statement would be to say that niacin is one of five nutritional cofactors that need to be present for optimal blood fat to occur. When all five of the cofactors are present, the body can absorb blood fat and burn it in the cellular power plants. When fat processes in this way, it creates the energy packets (acetate) that are needed for cell power plant function. This combustion process of acetate ends with the release of carbon dioxide and water.

When the other four cofactors are not present, many owners are condemned to failed attempts at natural healing. These owners often return to symptom-control medicine ("the complex"). The necessity of these factors is well documented in the medical biochemistry textbooks, but the discussion occurs in a convoluted fashion. Knowledge of these fundamental 'must have' nutrients provides another way to heal. Pantothenic acid, carnitine, riboflavin, and Co enzyme Q10 are required for fat combustion in addition to niacin.

Without these factors, there is the tendency for blood fat to rise (LDL cholesterol) despite efforts to optimize insulin, cortisol, epinephrine, thyroid, estrogen, IGF-1, and androgens (chapter 7). Owners who eat a low carbohydrate diet, exercise aerobically, and participate in stress reduction measures may not improve their health if one or more of these cofactors is absent. These motivated owners fail to achieve their desired blood fat and weight loss because no one has counseled them on these basic nutritional cornerstones.

Living in these nutritional 'traps' becomes analogous to the creation of a smaller 'drain' for fat to exit once it has entered their blood stream. The drain enlarges when the cells have the nutritional mechanisms to combust it (explained below). Optimal combustion of fat cannot occur without all of the necessary cofactors. When fat fails to combust, it builds within a cell and eventually spills backward into the blood stream. Increased fat is analogous to a drain that can no longer dispose of its contents. One of the contents in the blood stream is fat. The inclusion of these factors in the diet, or, in some cases, receiving them intravenously, will allow a 'bigger drain' to form. The drain in this analogy involves the increased rate of fat removal made possible when the cells have the nutritional ability to process fat into carbon dioxide and water.

Owners who lack these five nutrients cannot properly access fat for the production of energy packets. This causes their cells to have power plant (mitochondria) problems because fat is the preferred fuel for many cell types. In fact, all raw fuel (protein, fat, and carbohydrate) must first be converted to the fatty acid, acetate, in order for it to burn within the

cell power plants. Because fat is the easiest to convert to acetate, it constitutes the preferred power plant fuel of most body cells. The brain and red blood cells provide notable exception to this preference because they can only burn sugar for fuel.

Many owners do not receive sufficient amounts of these nutritional cofactors from their food. Multi vitamin pills may not solve this problem. When food is cooked and processed, the five nutritional cofactors are destroyed. Absorption of nutrients constitutes a critical factor in the health of an owner. Disease processes and medications effect what absorbs and remains in the body. Empowerment comes from understanding why these factors play such a crucial role in the interrelationship between cellular power plants and energy extraction.

Carnitine is made from the amino acid, lysine. Vitamin C, Vitamin B6, and SAMe (S-adenosyl methionine) are all needed for its manufacture. Note that SAMe is critical to its manufacture and becomes rapidly depleted without adequate folate, Vitamin B6, Vitamin B12, serine and methionine, the methyl donor system (chapter 4). For each carnitine manufactured, three SAMe molecules are used. Meat contains various levels of carnitine. **Severe carnitine deficiency shows up as fatty liver disease, kidney hemorrhage, and some forms of heart failure.**

Carnitine, as a carrier molecule, delivers fat to the cellular power plant furnace for combustion. The liver, kidney, and heart cells need, tremendous amounts of energy to perform. The cells cannot use the potential energy contained in the fat molecules without transportation by carnitine. Endurance athletes supplement with carnitine for increased performance.

Niacin (Vitamin B3) is the second factor necessary to burn fat in the creation of energy packets. Two other cofactors, riboflavin (Vitamin B2) and pantothenic acid (Vitamin B5) need to be considered with niacin. These three cofactors must be present in optimal amounts just inside the outer furnace (mitochondria). When all three are present, the combustion of fat traps energy packets (ATP). When any one of the three diminishes, there arises a progressive disability to trap energy. Heat is created instead of energy packets.

Pantothenic acid deficiency diminishes the rate of combustion of fat in the power plant. Fat can only be utilized when it is broken down two carbons at a time, and attached to a pantothenic acid-containing molecular machine, Co Enzyme A. This process cannot occur until carnitine delivers fat to the outside compartment of the cell furnace, the mitochondrion. This acid forms the essential ingredient for the manufacture of Coenzyme A. Coenzyme A is the carrier molecule that allows the orderly combusting of fat energy, two carbons at a time (as acetate). A deficiency in either carnitine or the above cofactors disables the refining process to acetate. When fat is the raw material for fuel combustion, these cofactors are required or body fat will accumulate in the blood stream. Pantothenic acid deficiency leads to a marked slow down in one's ability to burn fat calories.

The type of fuel that the mitochondria accept for combustion is restricted to one processed fuel type only, acetate. Certain nutritional cofactors are necessary in order to make acetate from the raw fuels of protein, carbohydrate, and fat. Many owners have power plant problems because no one counsels them about what these cofactors entail. The refined fuel requirement is similar to power plants in the physical world. These structures can only combust one specific fuel type for operational purposes (natural gas, coal, radio active material, or fuel oil, etc.). Whether raw fuel starts out as protein, fat or sugar, it needs to be processed into acetate (the simplest fatty acid) before it can be combusted in the mitochondria. Acetate is the only fuel that the body power plants can utilize aerobically. When acetate burns in the presence of oxygen, carbon dioxide gas, water, and energy packets, are created. The cell

power plants only accept acetate for burning within the mitochondria.

Coenzyme Q10 (ubiquinone) is the last nutritional Cofactor. It is similar to niacin, riboflavin, and pantothenic acid, but Coenzyme Q10 allows for additional trapping of more energy [ATP] within the cell. **Co enzyme Q10 is special in that it is made from the same enzymatic machinery as cholesterol.** Without adequate Co enzyme Q10, the cells are compromised in their ability to generate energy packets and make more heat energy instead. This energy is waste. Without Co enzyme Q10, energy packet (ATP) formation diminishes.

Extreme energetic compromise occurs when the heart is without sufficient Coenzyme Q10, because it constitutes a vital component, within each of its cells 2000 mitochondrion. It is necessary to effectively trap energy within the power plant.

Heart cells contain around 2,000 mitochondria. This many mitochondria make sense since the heart's pumping action requires tremendous amounts of energy to sustain the force of each beat. Adequate Co enzyme Q10 is a determinant of the performance of a heart cell. Lowered work ability leads to lower cardiac function. The heart has the highest needs for coenzyme Q10 in the body. Huge amounts of energy packets are needed here. Each heart cell has thousands of power plants (mitochondria) that need all five cofactors to maintain healthy cell function.

Popular cholesterol-lowering drugs known as the statin class, inhibit Co enzyme Q10's production. The body's sufficient attainment of this nutrient is further compromised because coenzyme Q10 is unstable within most processing techniques for food.

The suspicion exists that people on these drugs tend to die at about the same rate as the untreated groups, but for different reasons. This is more alarming when adding in the suspected increase in cancer rates for owners who take these drugs.

The explanation could be from the fact that initially, cancer cells have an inferior ability to generate energy compared to healthy cells. When the body is healthy, this is a major advantage, within the immune system, for destroying cancer cells at an early stage. Most immune systems continuously destroy cancer cells by generating high energy bursts and targeting these packets at cancer cells. This exposes a link as to why those taking statin drugs could be at increased risk for cancer. These drugs tend to deplete the body content of coenzyme Q10, and hence, cells like immune system cell-types have diminished ability to out perform the cancer cell in energy generation.

The above facts do not mean that statin drugs are never indicted for the prevention of heart disease. **One example of their need results from the many owners who insist on taking a passive role in their disease process. For this group, their doctor has very few alternatives.** Those owners willing to take responsibility for their health can use therapies without these side effects. These remedies can often times avoid statin drug usage and its potential side effects. The inclusion of high quality coenzyme Q10 would be a big help in the clinical situations where the statin drugs are needed. This need does not often occur in a motivated patient.

These factors need to be present nutritionally in order for fat to be utilized in the production of energy work packets. The utilization of sugar as fuel has other requirements.

Accessing Carbohydrate Energy for Cellular Needs

Carbohydrates can only be burned anaerobically (without oxygen) when any of five nutritional cofactors are deficient. This leads to massive increases in lactic acid production and fatigue. Fatigued cells have difficulty defending from "rust" and hardening processes. In the blood vessel lining cells, this leads to an increase in "Velcro" formation.

When any of the five nutritional factors are deficient, certain cells have no way of obtaining the necessary sugar-derived fragment, acetate. This fragment can only be combusted within the mitochondria in the presence oxygen. Nerve cells provide an example of a cell type that completely depends on sugar for their acetate needs.

In order to burn sugar (carbohydrate) to carbon dioxide and water, the cell needs five types of nutritional molecules in sufficient amounts, plus adequate oxygen in the combustion chamber. Lipoic acid, riboflavin, niacin, pantothenic acid, and thiamine, in the presence of adequate magnesium, constitute these factors.

The first part of sugar breakdown occurs without oxygen and a three-carbon fragment, pyruvate, is formed. Only when there is adequate oxygen and the five above factors, can this molecule enter the power plant for further energy release. With a deficiency, pyruvate breaks down to lactic acid. The liver usually clears this acid from the blood stream, but when formation becomes excessive, it builds up in the muscles to prevent death.

The enzyme, pyruvic dehydrogenase, and these five factors, cut the 'head' off and make a two-carbon molecule, acetate. Pyruvate needs to stabilize before it degenerates into lactic acid. The stabilizing and carrier molecule is Co enzyme A (formed from pantothenic acid). The larger share of energy contained in a sugar molecule cannot be utilized unless all of the factors are present.

There are many owners in pain and experiencing chronic fatigue only because their cells have a decreased ability to burn sugar energy in a healthy way. The smallest physical exertion condemns these owners to bed rest. Their tissues are full of lactic acid and this creates pain. These patients need to find a competent, nutritionally oriented physician or they will continue to suffer. Not all chronic fatigue and muscle aches are from this cause, but a significant percentage is due to nutritional deficiency.

Amino acids can be used as fuel only after the liver converts them into sugar in a process called gluconeogenesis. All amino acids contain at least one nitrogen group (the amide). This group must be removed and eventually converted into urea in the liver, for excretion by the kidneys. Adequate urea helps the kidneys concentrate their waste and conserve water. Cortisol, epinephrine, and glucagon hormones encourage gluconeogenesis. Epinephrine and glucagon have little effect without adequate cortisol. Insulin and growth hormone oppose gluconeogenesis. Amino acids are another source of raw fuel that needs refining to acetate before becoming combustible.

SECTION 5: Methods for Dumbing Down Doctors

Methods for Dumbing Doctors Down

1. Fear tactics: Ephedra
2. Evisceration tactics: vitamins and minerals
3. Half-truth tactics: Growth hormone is diabetogenic
4. The knee-jerk reaction tactic from neurolinguistically programming the doctor: prolactin and steroids
5. Blind alley tactics: estrogen and CAD risk
6. The Corrupt presentation of a studies results tactic: SSRI antidepressant vs. St. Johns Wort vs. placebo
7. The upwardly mobile textbook writer tactic: insulin
8. When in a corner, act like it was your idea all along: homocysteine and fish oils
9. Use the media to lie: the high protein diet and kidney damage
10. Use the legal system to protect a good thing: cholesterol-lowering drugs and fake hormone replacement
11. Teach the Doctor the wrong mechanism for how a medicine works
12. "The need for further study" mantra has replaced commonsense
13. Get ready for a patented erection enhancer medication tactic
14. Periodically, change the name of a term so that doctors fail to realize important connecting concepts.
15. Arbitrarily measure one related substance differently than another related substances to conceal the relative importance of one.
16. Use code names so that the doctor will not know he/she prescribes a known nerve toxin to which children have little defense.
17. Certified expert tactic
18. The emperor has no clothes tactic
19. Smoke and mirrors tactic
20. Evidenced-based medicine tactic

The Best Personal Protection for the last nine theoretical possibilities is to spread a truthful message as fast as possible and arrange to tell the above facts in a more damaging way (once one's head is in a vice or is found dead)

The last nine ways to silence rebel physicians are theoretical and therefore, no examples follow.

21. Make a legal example out of a doctor who dares to speak up
22. Use the media to spread halve truths about the doctor's personal or professional life
23. Kill or harm someone in the doctors' family in order to silence him/her.
24. Poison the doctor and his family in order to silence him/her
25. Frame the doctor in a way that creates negative public sentiment
26. Engage the IRS to harass the doctor
27. Arrange for an accident. If I were in Dr.'s Lee or Atkin's family, I would conduct a thorough investigation just because so many in the complex benefited from their sudden death.
28. Engage the services of certain publishers to buy up books that threaten the complex's interests. Buy them cheap and then make sure they never go anywhere. Alternatively, utilize the editorial staff to dilute down the power contained in the holistic message.
29. Invoke the National Securities Act that strips a citizen of his Bill Rights protections, and prevents him/her from telling anyone that the government hassles him/her.

    A friend of mine, who is a naturopathic physician, attended a holistic seminar where the majority were medical doctors. His comment was profound: He noted that most of the holistically oriented physicians in attendance were well into middle age. By middle age, doctors accumulate 'around the block' knowledge and some still possess the fortitude to learn anew.
    My wife's grandfather farmed his entire life. Well into his eighties, he realized that the supposed science of agribusiness was largely just a bunch of hype. He was an old man by the time

he figured out that the tried-and-true organic farming methods were best for all concerned, except the business of selling chemicals to farmers.

At first, the above instances of later-in-life wisdom seem divergent. However, in both instances the science was later found to be corrupt. Most of the time, this discovery occurs long after there is any fight left in one's spirit. The complex wins.

The title of this book and the section headings may seem inflammatory, at first. This is not the intent. Rather, I would like to express a personal opinion about my interpretation of the many inconsistencies and healing antidotes that real patients provide. I have studied many mainstream medical textbooks looking for clues for how to explain the unexplainable healing effects resulting from alternative medical advice.

After almost five years, I am truly shocked about what is pandered as the standard of care. It has taken me quite a while to figure out some of the methods that I think are used on physicians like myself. This section concerns my personal opinion on how these methods take form. Last I knew, this country still allowed enough freedom of speech to express a personal opinion on a given subject.

Yet, I realize that I need to proceed with caution because one slip, in one sentence, will land me in court with the complex. They often crush the little guy with frivolous lawsuits that cost many thousands of dollars to defend. Americans take note: This is probably the favorite tool of the complex. The complex consists of the government, pharmaceutical companies, food and agribusiness conglomerates, hospitals, insurance companies, the AMA, and mainstream medical schools. A paranoid list you say. Read on and decide for yourself. In each of the above listed components of the complex, exists a vested interest in keeping a good thing going. In order to keep their good thing going, they each need to keep doctors dumbed down. A formidable task because doctors usually possess a keen and innate intelligence.

Doctors, like myself, have very little reason to doubt our educations accurateness of presentation until patients begin providing evidence that conflict with our training. Looking back on it, I feel the complex effectively appeal to our egos. Doctor's egos inflate because they constantly, but subtly, cast disparaging remarks about the level of education in the other fields of health care. The end result causes doctors to develop a false sense of superiority. Very few ever marry a chiropractor that proves beyond a shadow of doubt that medical educations mislead. Even fewer still, encounter opportunities to work along side alternative health care providers and see for themselves the inconsistencies of their sacred dogma.

The spirit behind this section and the entire book involves helping to better serve the suffering patients out there. It has been quite painful to me that so much of what I endeavored to learn during my medical training turns out to be twisted half-truths. We all have a choice when we confront dishonesty. We can pretend it doesn't exist. We can rationalize about how challenging the dishonesty will harm our "good thing". Or we can have courage to do the right thing for our patients, and diligently pursue truth with an open mind.

1. The Fear Tactic

Ephedra or ephedrine serves as an introductory example for how the complex creates irrational fear. In order to understand ephedra beyond these effective tactics, one needs a few pieces of additional information to connect certain facts into their knowledge base.

A. Ephedra possesses epinephrine like message content.
B. Epinephrine is a mood enhancer
C. With reasonable doses, epinephrine minimally affects blood pressure
D. Epinephrine powerfully inhibits insulin release
E. In one week, more people die from aspirin like medication than have ever died from ephedra
F. Ephedra and epinephrine powerfully resolve wheezing inexpensively
G. Most patented inhalers' active ingredient is similar in structure to epinephrine and ephedra. Some people have died from these

patented medications but ephedra receives the 'lion's share' of negative press coverage. Pharmaceutical companies know that epinephrine-like molecular structure raises the blood pressure minimally, but norepinephrine-like structure raises it significantly. Norepinephrine has little effect on wheezing and allergy symptoms (see **methyl donor system discussion**).

H. Ephedra and epinephrine powerfully resolve allergy symptoms

Aspirin-like medicines are, without a doubt, more dangerous than ephedra. Acetaminophen causes many cases of liver failure that leads to the need for a liver transplant. Yet they still sell these drugs over the counter. Keep in mind all the money at stake from patients switching to various alternative methods, which diminish demand for patented pharmaceuticals given to treat the above diseases symptoms. It begins to smell of another frame job. This is my personal opinion, of course, but I challenge anyone to do the research for him or herself.

2. The Textbook Evisceration Tactic: vitamins and minerals

Biochemistry studies the chemical reactions of life. **Vitamins,** by definition, facilitate chemical reactions necessary for life to continue. It would sound far-fetched to boldly state that the newer medical biochemical textbooks, which student doctors study in medical school, have had many important concepts about vitamins and minerals removed.

Unfortunately, this is what has happened. My medical school biochemistry book (1975 edition) contained an entire chapter devoted to how vitamins work within the body. While researching my first book I bought the newer, 2000, edition, and was shocked to find the entire Vitamin Chapter removed. There were further disturbing trends in the newer text version. Such as the trend toward discussing vitamin driven reactions in abbreviated ways.

Minerals within the body need to occur at optimal ratios. Over forty years ago, the importance of optimal **potassium** intake was openly discussed. Sufficient potassium proves necessary to hold protein in cells, increase the cell's voltage, allow insulin to deliver sugar into cells, keep cholesterol synthesis at bay, store glycogen, and defend the cell from harmful ions. This information is also mysteriously missig in the newer editions of medical texts. Where did all this knowledge go within the newer textbooks with the same Publishing companies?

Zinc is another mineral that proves critical if one is to remain healthy. Its absorption requires sufficient stomach acid. How many patients became zinc deficient while on acid blocker therapy? How many doctors today are aware of the critical role zinc plays in health maintenance?

Examples of the critical role that zinc plays in the reactions of life include:

1. Serves as a cofactor for the enzyme, carbonic anhydrase, which is the major acid-alkaline control enzyme throughout the body. Whether it proves sufficient within the blood stream, stomach, urine or pancreas, largely determines the pH balance in that locale. High levels of this enzyme are found in the stomach, pancreas, kidneys, and white and red blood cells.
2. Proves critical toward inhibiting the conversion of testosterone into estrogen. How many middle aged men and women owners age prematurely because a zinc deficiency lowers their testosterone and raises their estrogen. Estrogen's role in fat growth was discussed in chapter 7.
3. Activity or silence of the genetic program depends on adequate zinc levels. Scientist call the DNA receptor that Vitamin A, thyroid hormones and all steroids use to activate or repress DNA programs, Zinc fingers.
4. Angiotensin converting enzyme (ACE) requires sufficient zinc for its activity. ACE deactivates histamine like activity occurring from a related substance called bradykinin. Mainstream physicians are groomed into thinking ACE is the culprit behind many blood pressure

elevation problems (**see Teach the doctor the wrong mechanism for how a medication works below**). However, ACE also proves necessary to keep allergic symptoms at bay. This explains why these blood pressure medications that block ACE activity produce the common side effect of dry cough. How many allergy sufferers result from zinc deficiency?

3. The half-truth tactic: growth hormone is diabetogenic

Maintaining balance between IGF-1 and insulin form an important biochemical determinant of youthfulness. It is important to avoid the popular practice of receiving growth hormone injections without a proper evaluation of the IGF-1 levels. Without a proper evaluation of one's liver's ability to increase IGF-1 levels, GH will tend to promote high blood sugars and, therefore, increase insulin output. Increased insulin output associates with all the negative effects on body physique discussed in the Syndrome X subsections.

This last fact explains the negative publicity associating growth hormone injections with breast and abdominal fat growth. Normal livers respond to growth hormone by releasing stored IGF-1, along with sugar and fat. The released IGF-1 delivers the sugar and fat released to the organs and muscles, negating the need for insulin in the fasting state. Unhealthy livers can still release sugar and fat, but release diminished amounts of IGF-1, and insulin release rates consequently need to increase to pick up the slack in the elevated blood sugar. Higher insulin release rates always arrive at the liver first (pancreas-portal vein connection). High insulin, arriving at the liver, stimulates the fat and cholesterol-making liver machinery abnormally. The extra fat and cholesterol deposits within the breast and abdomen (as well as within the arteries). All these side effects could be avoided if someone first helped the liver to heal (chapter 13).

Growth hormone and why the pituitary secretes it

The most misunderstood and neglected role of the counter-response hormones to insulin, is growth hormone (GH). This neglect occurs because its name leads owners down an erroneous mental image path. A major effect of growth hormone concerns its ability to cause the liver to release its stored IGF-1. Growth hormone also conserves the protein content of the muscles and organs, while in the fasting state or while exercising.

> (Physicians side bar) Growth hormone's protein conservation message content explains where its name originates. Protein conservation proves as a pre-requisite for growth to occur. Growth hormone, other than its stimulatory effect on cartilage cell growth, has few direct effects on the tissues. One additional direct effect concerns its ability to act like the other three counter-hormones to the message of insulin, at the level of the liver, with two important exceptions. First, involves the fact that unlike epinephrine, cortisol and glucagon, growth hormone has a powerful protein sparing effect. Growth hormone's message content in the liver inhibits the conversion of amino acids into sugar (a protein sparing effect). The second difference from the other insulin counter hormones involves the fact that GH directs the liver to release a special hormone called insulin-like growth factor type 1 (IGF-1). Like the other counter hormones to insulin, it stimulates the release of sugar stored as liver glycogen into the blood stream. Also, like the other counter hormones to insulin, it stimulates the liver to release stored fats into the blood stream for fuel.
>
> Insulin-like growth factor type 1 (IGF-1) can only release from the liver with the direction of growth hormone's presence. Mainstream medical confusion arises from the fact that the effects of IGF-1 message content directly oppose the initial fuel release effects of growth hormone. IGF-1 release occurs simultaneous to the growth hormone-directed liver release of sugar and fat into the blood stream. If one sees the overall effect in the sequential release of growth hormone followed by IGF-1, this begins to make more sense. The more

IGF-1 released, the less insulin needed. The less insulin needed, the less fat-maker message within the body.

Growth hormone stimulates the release of fat and carbohydrates from liver stores into the blood stream. The second part of its message involves the simultaneous release, from the liver, of adequate insulin-like growth factor (IGF-1) into the blood stream. The IGF-1 hormone in the peripheral tissues (blood stream) behaves very much like insulin does in the liver and body fat cells. The body needs less insulin when the liver secretes adequate IGF-1. When adequate growth hormone has stimulated sufficient IGF-1 release into the blood stream, the peripheral tissues, like muscle, are facilitated to procure fuel (carbohydrate and fat). This describes the insulin-like effect of IGF-1. However, remember that IGF-1 rises between meals, which feeds the cells in the fasting state. In contrast, insulin rises following meals, which allows the liver to store sufficient fuel to allow it to supply a constant blood fuel until the next meal.

Sufficient release of IGF-1 negates the initial increase in blood sugar and blood fat, caused by the presence of growth hormone's message to the liver. Mechanistically, IGF-1 behaves like insulin in the peripheral tissues. IGF-1's presence instructs the peripheral tissues to take up the fuel released by growth hormones presence. Many clinicians fail to appreciate this sequential arrangement, which operates in the healthy population. Both IGF-1 and insulin bind to some of the same cell receptors. This makes sense when one realizes their similar message content that regards instruction of different cells within the body to take up fuel out of the blood stream.

Different cell types have different affinities for IGF-1 and insulin. Each cell types relative affinity is determined by different cell receptor concentrations for either insulin or IGF-1. For example, the liver and fat cells have the highest amount of pure insulin-type receptors of any other cell type. There are about 200,000 insulin receptors per fat or liver cell. Insulin directs these tissues to store fuel. Here the IGF-1 does not bind well to these types of insulin receptors and, therefore, has essentially no effect in the creation or maintenance of body fat. In contrast, the IGF-1 receptors are found throughout most of the

> rest of the cells in the body. In healthy owners, IGF-1 blood levels, occur at levels 100 times that of insulin levels. This makes sense since there are roughly one hundred times the cells that prefer IGF-1 to insulin.

Many disease processes have their origins in a falling IGF-1 level. When the IGF-1 level falls, insulin needs rise abnormally (insulin resistance). Increased insulin need leads to health consequences that increased IGF-1 does not share.

A major advantage of adequate IGF-1 to that of higher insulin involves the fact that insulin levels determine the amount of body fat. Fat is the major stored fuel type because the body possesses a limited ability to store sugar as glycogen. Total storage capacity for glycogen is about 500 grams (about 2200 calories). About four hundred grams store in the liver and the other one hundred grams store in the muscles. Sedentary and well-fed owners have little opportunity to draw down these stored forms of sugar. The more sedentary and well-fed the owner, the more carbohydrate that channel into his/her liver's making fat and cholesterol. **The body is smart and consistent.** Insulin directed pathways are designed with fuel storage in mind. The major fuel storage sites occur in arterial macrophages, the liver and fat cells.

Certain genetically predisposed owners have a higher insulin secretion on a daily basis on a similar diet as compared to normal owners. The increased insulin-responding owner means these owners create more message content that directs their livers to make carbohydrates into LDL cholesterol. In these same owners, practices that increase growth hormone will result in increased IGF-1 release from the healthy liver. Increased levels of IGF-1 share essentially none of the liver stimulation effects that lead to increased LDL cholesterol manufacture. This will help lessen the need for insulin (the carrier of the fat and cholesterol maker message) secretion by facilitating the cells to uptake sugar from the blood stream, beyond the liver.

Following a meal in healthy owners use most of their insulin production at the level of their liver. This situation allows low insulin needs because these owners produce sufficient growth hormone between meals. **Insulin needs rise whenever an owner consumes carbohydrate, they chronically consume a potassium-depleted diet, experience unmanaged mental stress, and/or when their IGF-1 levels fall off (chapter 8).** Less insulin need occurs when IGF-1 levels increase because it facilitates the removal of sugar from the blood stream. Unlike insulin, which has a major effect on the liver and fat cell's ability to remove sugar out of the blood stream, IGF-1 concentrates its effect in the periphery cells (muscles and organs). IGF-1 competes with insulin as to where the extra nutrition sucks out of the blood stream. Higher IGF-1 favors increased nutrition procurement for the muscle and organs cells. Higher insulin levels favor the uptake of nutrition out of the blood stream by liver and fat cells.

Two major stimuli cause growth hormone's release. The GH releasing stimulus results from either fasting or intense exercise. Both of these conditions produce a decrease in blood fuel levels. IGF-1 releases, along with sugar and fat, from a normal liver after growth hormone levels rise.

The overall scheme involves the initiator, low blood fuel. This decrease causes an initial rise in growth hormone, which initially directs the liver to release IGF-1, sugar, and fat into the blood stream. The released IGF-1, acts like peripheral insulin in facilitating the organs and muscles uptake of the released fuel from the liver. In this way, the body has a mechanism for ensuring that appropriate amounts of fuel remain available in the blood stream between meals and when physical exertion draws down the blood fuel level.

Exercise powerfully contributes to the amount of growth hormone released and hence, IGF-1 levels. This release does much the same thing in the periphery that insulin does in the liver and fat storage cells. However, low blood sugar effects are prevented because growth hormone also directs the liver to dump sugar into the blood stream with the liver released IGF-1. The design of IGF-1 facilitates the peripheral cells' uptake of fuel out of the blood stream that, in these cases, growth hormone started. Where growth hormone production falls off and IGF-1 as well, the need for insulin production increases (insulin resistance). In these unhealthy situations, insulin must pick up the slack in the periphery (muscles and organs). This process describes only one of the mechanisms for insulin resistance (chapter 13).

Increased IGF-1 levels occur for the opposite reasons of increased insulin levels. The increase in IGF-1, in the exercising or fasting state, facilitates cellular uptake of the growth hormone-stimulated liver release of sugar and fat into the blood stream. However, the fuel storage adequacy in the liver depends on enough insulin directing the liver to suck up nutrition for storage purposes following a meal. Without sufficient insulin, there would be no stored fuel to release when GH directed the release of fuel and IGF-1 from the liver. In this way, the healthy body balances the blood fuel supply following meals and between meals. Insulin and IGF-1 remove nutrients from the blood stream following meals. Insulin directs nutrients into the storage pathways that occur in the liver and fat cells. Conversely, IGF-1 directs nutrients into the vast majority of other cell types. The healthy body, having at least one hundred times more IGF-1 than insulin in the blood stream, evidences this fact.

Increased insulin becomes necessary to shore up lagging growth hormone with its consequent diminished IGF-1 output. There are three subtle, but dangerous consequences to a body that relies on increased insulin production. First, the stimulation of the appetite center leads to an increased tendency to gain weight. Second, increased insulin stimulates the liver in its manufacture of LDL cholesterol. Third, an increased reliance on cortisol, glucagon, and epinephrine, occurs to keep the blood sugar elevated, between meals, when growth hormone levels fall.

The consequence of normalizing blood sugar levels between meals with elevated cortisol, glucagon and epinephrine concerns diminished protein conservation (muscle and organ mass). Only growth

hormone proves able to retain body protein when fasting or exercising.

Proteins constitute the metabolically active component of body tissues. Examples of metabolically active proteins are: enzymes, cell receptors, actin and myosin and mineral pumps. The metabolically active components of body tissues burn calories. Less body protein leads to less muscle mass and organ size. Less protein content also leads to a lower metabolic rate. These are some of the major characteristics of the aging process.

Growth hormone release occurs from regular exercise, low normal blood sugars, fasting, glucagon, the low secretion rate of serotonin in the hypothalamus, and when the hypothalamus neurons secrete dopamine. There are other details, but if one keeps these five determinants in mind, it encourages making better choices.

The above discussion gives a mechanistic explanation for why "couch potatoes" tend to develop insulin resistance (increased insulin need). Increased insulin resistance will eventually exhaust the genetically determined ability of the pancreas to increase its insulin production. When this happens, it exhausts the pancreas beyond its genetically determined capability, and adult onset diabetes manifests.

Making things worse is the fact that when GH secretion rates fall, the protein content in the body decreases proportionally. Sufficient GH release proves as a fundamental requirement for the conservation of body protein between meals. Without adequate GH between meals, the body increases the secretion rate of cortisol, glucagon, and epinephrine, in order to maintain blood sugar levels. All three of these hormones activate the liver machinery that converts protein stores into sugar (gluconeogenesis). Unless an owner can conserve protein between meals, while exercising, or fasting, the metabolically active components of his/her body tissue dismantle just to stay alive when these conditions occur. Death delays only from sacrificing proteins for blood fuel maintenance needs, while these owners fast, are between meals, or they attempt to exercise.

The other extreme of health contains highly trained athletes who secrete high levels of IGF-1, secondary to their increased growth hormone secretion rates. Increased growth hormone secretion occurs because exercise increases the fuel delivery requirements. GH is one of the main hormones that raise the liver secretion rate of fuel into the blood stream. More importantly, growth hormone spares body protein content from breakdown. In contrast, the other three blood fuel-increasing hormones, cortisol, epinephrine, and glucagons, make protein fair game.

As stated previously, IGF-1 levels depend on sufficient GH release. Another benefit of high IGF-1 levels involves the fact that insulin requirements diminish. The highly trained athlete needs very little insulin for efficient fuel delivery into his/her exercising muscle cells because of his/her high IGF-1 levels. For this reason, exercise lowers LDL cholesterol levels. The decreased need for insulin results in a lessened stimulus to manufacture LDL cholesterol in the liver.

It has long been known that growth hormone levels decline with age. A sedentary life style accelerates this decline. Conversely, regular exercise increases IGF-1 levels secondary to increased growth hormone release.

These facts unite several health consequences of insulin resistance into a common thread of causality. With aging, there occurs a sequential decline of growth hormone and IGF-1 levels with certain diets and lifestyles. The decline of these two hormones explains some of the insulin resistance occurring as age advances and sedentary lifestyles continue. It also explains how regular exercise remedies insulin resistance by raising growth hormone and IGF-1 levels. Applying this association could save owners the unnecessary complications of diabetes and the acceleration of their aging processes. Lastly, the fall in growth hormone levels brought about by a sedentary lifestyle explains why muscle and organ mass decrease with age.

> **Growth hormone conserves protein content. Unless owners have processes operating in their lives that encourage GH secretion, they will lose protein. Lost body protein manifests as shrunken organs, muscles, joints, and skin. All the telltale signs for the shrinkage of old age processes occurring. Insulin need increases when GH release declines and leads to decreases in IGF-1 levels. This creates more body fat. The typical middle-aged effect involves shrunken organs, joints, and muscles that hide their assault on body form amongst the increased fat.**

4. The knee jerk (Neurolinguistic Programming) tactic: prolactin and steroids

Within the master hormone gland (the pituitary), is a powerful hormone, prolactin. The ovary and testicles become inhibited when prolactin releases beyond low levels. Although many physicians have been groomed into the 'knee jerk' mental summary that prolactin stimulates milk production, the evidence clearly implicates prolactin as a powerful inhibitor of ovarian and testicle function. The confusion arises because they know that a pregnant woman's steroid production becomes very high and that her prolactin level also elevates

One solves this false discrepancy when one additional fact is included: later in the pregnancy the ovaries are powerfully inhibited by prolactin. It is the placenta, which cranks out the huge amounts of steroids that increase with the pregnant state, despite the inhibited ovaries. The presence of a placenta during pregnancy counteracts the quiescent ovaries. However, in other pathologic states, where a placenta is absent and prolactin elevates, steroid production plummets.

Four common clinical states occur where prolactin, produced within the pituitary, induces ovary inhibition without the benefit of having a placenta. The absence of a placenta will cause a decrease in the steroids produced by the ovary in these cases. Men always lack a placenta. Anytime a man's prolactin elevates, his testicles will decrease their steroid production rates.

The four states that stimulate the pituitary to release high levels of prolactin include: low thyroid function, use of birth control pills, chronic stress, and high serotonin. In these cases, the production of the ovarian and testicle's component of body steroids greatly diminishes because these situations lead to increased prolactin. Steroids are so powerful, if any one of them diminishes, the DNA content of the body will become either dormant or hyper. Most people understad, a danger to over-all health exists, when the DNA misbehaves. With an appropriate prolactin level, healing transpires.

Mechanisms for increased pituitary release of prolactin:

  A. Birth control pill usage
  B. High serotonin levels
  C. Chronic stress
  D. Low thyroid gland function

(Note that men can have the last three in the list, as well, but explaining it through a women's body facilitates understanding.)

Increased prolactin levels result from the increased estrogen in birth control pills. Prolactin inhibits ovarian hormone manufacture and release. This hormone-induced mechanism associated with obesity is generally not in operation during pregnancy. The pregnant state has the growing placenta that generates the needed steroids. The placenta manufactures androgens even though the ovary becomes relatively dormant by the fifth month of pregnancy. When female owners take birth control pills the body thinks it is pregnant and prolactin levels rise. Prolactin levels rise when estrogen levels approach pregnancy levels (as with taking birth control pills).

Potential obesity occurs because, like pregnancy, the birth control pills increase prolactin levels. Unlike pregnancy, no placenta exists as the hormone factory to correct for the inhibition of the ovaries in their steroid production. Additional potential problems exist. Birth control pills do not contain androgens, only estrogen and progestins (abnormally shaped progesterone substitutes). Androgen production can fall, some adrenals fail in the challenge to increase androgen production, and obesity ensues.

High serotonin levels can occur when one takes serotonin reuptake inhibitors (SSRI) Type anti-depressants. The elevation of serotonin within the pituitary inhibits growth hormone release, but encourages prolactin release. This fact may help explain why sexual dysfunction remains such a prominent side effect when these prescriptions are taken.

Chronic stress tends to raise prolactin levels. Prolactin levels elevate when increased cortisol release stimulates prolactin release as part of the stress response.

Low thyroid gland function will stimulate the hypothalamus to release thyroid-releasing hormone (TRH). TRH is a very powerful secretogogue for prolactin release from the pituitary.

The second knee jerk reaction: steroids are bad

Medical textbooks are curiously deficient in the discussion of interrelated consequences of a diminished adrenal reserve. Instead, their discussion focuses only on the most extreme examples of adrenal dysfunction. Examples of these extremes are Addison's disease (cortisol deficiency) and Cushing's disease (cortisol excess).

A peripheral discussion might surface regarding the role of the adrenal hormone, cortisol, and its role in the prevention of hypoglycemia. Cortisol is the major player in the prevention of hypoglycemia for many middle-aged owners. Most textbook discussions concern hormones within the adrenal gland, but fail to unite the fact that adrenal steroid hormones secrete together in a preformed ratio. A reoccurring tendency within the medical textbooks exists that completely ignores the concept that some owners may have diminished adrenal function under conditions of stress. These owners' level of dysfunction is not as severe as those of an Addisonian patient.

Doctors are taught to think about disease of the adrenal, in a piecemeal fashion. Cushing's disease exemplifies this. A hallmark of this disease is losing muscle and gaining body fat. A consistent failure exists in emphasizing the reason body fat goes up. This is not directly related to the markedly elevated cortisol levels that are present with this disease.

Cortisol initially promotes fat and sugar dumping into the blood stream. Increased body fat proves secondary to elevated blood sugar spikes. The elevated blood sugar results from the high cortisol message content which directs the liver to release sugar into the blood stream. The body eventually realizes that the blood sugar has elevated inappropriately.

Elevated blood sugars suppress growth hormone secretion but promote excess insulin release into the blood stream to counter this situation. The increase in insulin required to make the blood sugar normal leads to the increased fat manufacture rate. Remember, whatever the pancreatic insulin secretion rate, the liver always receives the highest concentration of its message content (basic anatomy of the pancreas portal vein connection to the liver). The liver and fat cells also contain the highest pure insulin-type receptor concentration at about 200,000 per cell. High insulin states, within the liver, cause the blood sugar to preferentially suck up into it. The liver turns this sugar into LDL cholesterol.

Lost protein is due two other abnormal hormonal processes that occur with chronic stress and elevated insulin levels. The first part is due to the fact that elevated cortisol levels lead to increased prolactin release. Increases in prolactin levels inhibit the gonads' release of androgens that constitute a counter weight to the high level of insulin's ability to make patients fat. Remember that the androgens promote muscle and organ growth and repair. The inhibition of the gonads is often left out of the discussion.

Also left out of the discussion concerns the additional fact that a slight elevation in the blood sugar will inhibit growth hormone release. Diminished growth hormone release will lead to a diminished ability to hold onto body proteins (chapter 7) and diminished IGF-1 release. IGF-1 helps insulin remove sugar out of the blood stream and occurs, in healthy owners, at levels one hundred times those of insulin. As growth hormone secretion falls off less IGF-1 secretes and this leads to excessive insulin need (insulin resistance). This last little detail ties in those Syndrome X (also known as metabolic syndrome or insulin resistance Syndrome) patients to a variant of Cushing's disease pathology. This specific disease example points to the incongruous discussion between the various hormone abnormalities in the way physicians learn to think about adrenal disease (chapter 13).

Cushing's and Addison's diseases provide extreme examples of adrenal dysfunction. Cushing's disease produces extremely high cortisol production rates. Conversely, Addison's disease, involves an extreme deficiency of cortisol. The deficiencies are so significant that viability can only be maintained by taking cortisol supplements.

What about those owners whose adrenal abnormality lies somewhere between these two extremes of adrenal dysfunction in stressful situations? Both of these situations have health consequences. Mainstream medicine most often recognizes only the extremes of adrenal dysfunction. Consequently, the suffering owner continues to exist and remains out of immediate danger of death. This common medical practice proves analogous to only considering thyroid dysfunction if it occurs on either extreme that puts the patient at risk for death.

Science could help those owners with (see list below, page 344) six common diseases improve their adrenal systems function. Curiously, this is not the case. Medical educations do a better job at alerting physicians to the subtleties of altered thyroid function and the diseases that follow.

Rememer, the common property of steroids, Vitamin A, and thyroid hormone must be emphasized. These hormones are the most powerful of all hormones in the body. These steroids include testosterone, estrogen, DHEA, androstenedione, cortisol, progesterone, and aldosterone. There are other steroids of less importance. The power of this group lies in the fact that only these hormone types carry their message directly to all the DNA programs throughout every cell in the body. No other hormones directly influence the DNA (genes) program.

These hormones interact with the genetic program. They directly determine which genes turn off and on. Gene activity determines which body proteins are manufactured. Healthy bodies have the exact amount of protein types needed. The only way to get the right amount of protein types is to have the right amounts of these powerful hormones giving directions. The quality, type, and amount of these powerful hormones determine how wisely the cells will spend their available energy. These hormones carry their message by virtue of their unique and precise shape. The steroids, Vitamin A, and thyroid, differ from other hormones by binding directly with many DNA receptors. They have access to every body chamber.

The unique property of these hormones allows them to be the determinants of which DNA programs activate or repress. Owners that have the proper quality, amounts, and timing of these hormones, receive a tremendous health advantage. The effectiveness of these hormones further relates into the quality and amounts of the lesser hormones manufactured. Therefore, these hormones prove the most critical of all the hormones in the body. Ways to heal begin with considering their quality within an owner.

The power of these hormones lies in their control of the genetic program. An excess or deficiency provides an abnormal message content to the DNA of the cells. When the wrong DNA programs activate or repress, the cell spends energy unwisely. Energy used foolishly on the wrong proteins, wrong repair to rest ratios, wrong immune activation level, wrong amount of cell product, etc. describes a disease process.

Though diseases have predictable results, identical excesses or deficiencies will initiate different diseases in different owners. This is only partially understood and the understood portion is complex.

Any defect within the six links in the adreal health chain causes disease (chapter 10).

In today's world of harried physicians and managed care, the owner needs to be aware of the six levels where the adrenal system can fail. Erroneously, most attention toward adrenal health inquiries limits the focus to one or two levels only. Consequently, many owners' diagnosis are incorrect and/or they receive symptom-control treatments. Thus, owners miss out on ways to heal themselves. *The Body Heals* explores the six levels of the adrenal system and how, any one of these being defective, leads to the below list of adrenal system related diseases.

Uniting high stress and a defect within the adrenal system make any of these adrenal system diseases worse.

1.	Allergies	4.	Systemic lupus
2.	Asthma.	3.	Rheumatoid arth.
3.	Colitis	6.	Crohn disease

As was explained in chapter 10, a defect at any of the six levels behaves clinically as if the adrenal system isn't functioning properly. Most physicians receive little instruction for evaluating the integrity of the entire system. The profit in treating symptoms of the above diseases overrides the incentive to educate physicians about the other side of the scientific story. Some lonely thinkers clunk along with some really good healing insights. Meanwhile the complex supports effective ways of marginalizing these scientific discoveries.

Many physicians have been effectively taught to fear cortisone treatments over the long haul. This training has been so well performed that many physicians are automatic in their response to hearing the word cortisone or steroid. This effect results from successfully confusing physicians and the public between the effects of cortisol within physiologic doses versus higher doses given to treat disease.

Further confusion results from not educating physicians in the basics of how the precise shape of the steroid delivers accurate message content. Only altered steroid shapes can get a patent advantage. However, altered steroid shapes deliver inaccurate message content to one's DNA programs. Inaccurate message content leads to side effects and toxicities

Perhaps even more damaging to overall middle-aged health concerns the fact that the optimal adrenal secretion contains preformed ratios between the different steroids listed in chapter 12. To only replace one when several prove deficient creates even more message content disharmony. The above diseases arise from an adrenal deficiency. Each unique deficiency has different proportions of the various adrenal steroids that fail to arrive at the afflicted owners DNA programs.

Without a complete inquiry into all six links, these diseases continue to smolder until they erupt. Diseases that erupt require symptom-control. Symptom-control approaches lead to side effects.

The media campaigns have persuaded physicians and owners to fear even small doses of the natural body-manufactured cortisol. This occurs despite the fact (evidence discussed more completely in Chapter 10) that the diseases mentioned above have a deficiency of cortisol function in common. These diseases often directly result due to a failure to receive adequate adrenal steroids to the DNA program.

An extension of Dr. Jefferies' work (mentioned in chapter 10) addresses the emerging realization that healthy, activated adrenals secrete a mixture of steroids in preformed ratios. This optimizes the message content of a healthy owner whenever the stress response activates. Only giving cortisol, in all instances of the above diseases, results in the potential for a lessened healing response. A lessened healing response results from the exclusion of the other adrenal steroids, which normally secrete along with cortisol.

Keep in mind that other adrenal steroid imbalances may contribute significantly to a disease process. The 24-hour urine test for adrenal steroids often proves as the best method for detecting these defects in steroid production. However, many physicians remain unable to interpret these tests. Until physicians receive education here they will remain unable to prescribe the optimal replacement of real message content.

While measuring the cortisol level of those with the potential for diminished adrenal reserve, the clinician must consider, that borderline patients tend to have deceptively normal blood cortisol levels while low stress prevails. However, during times of stress their adrenals' production of cortisol diminishes relative to need in order to remain symptom free. In these cases of diminished adrenal reserve, blood testing or a 24-hour urine test for cortisol production can be deceptively normal. Some of these patients will require an ACTH challenge test before their diminished reserve shows up on laboratory tests.

The ACTH challenge test measures the ability of the adrenals to increase cortisol production when stimulated. Since ACTH is the hormone that stimulates the adrenal to release cortisol, a challenge with this hormone should increase cortisol, in the blood stream, within thirty minutes. A normal response is two times greater than the blood level before the adrenals were challenged with ACTH.

Many owners, with diseases related to adrenal deficiency, fail to achieve this increase in cortisol production. Consequently, many of these diseases intensify when an owner experiences stress. Stress increases the need for cortisol within the cells. The cell DNA needs cortisol to survive various stresses of life. The above diseases come about when certain cell DNA programs receive defective amounts of the adrenal steroid message. If any of the six links of the adrenal system break, a deficiency results. A broken link causes a defect for all levels below it. All six links need to be intact or the above types of diseases begin to manifest.

Remember, the ability to handle stress depends on adequate increases in cortisol. Adequate increases in cortisol direct energy into survival pathways. Surgeons see first hand the importance of cortisol production in regards to the ability to survive the stress of surgery. Following the stress of surgery, a patient will die if their adrenals prove incapable of increased cortisol production. When cortisol release skyrockets into the body, potassium loss increases. Consequently, these two facts are routinely provided for post operatively. Potassium and cortisol are administered in the post-operative period. This precaution prevents severe complications in case a post-surgical owner's adrenal glands are not up to the task.

As was previously mentioned, the 24-hour urine test provides one of the best ways to screen for defects in the first four links of the adrenal health chain. The urine test misses the last two links. Unfortunately, very few physicians can interpret the complex issues that arise from the results of this test. Also, the standard method on which the 24-hour urine test is calibrated is to give the patient instructions regarding a normal stress day. This raises the question about missing those patients that only become adrenal compromised during times of stress (when an increased need for cortisol arises that they cannot provide).

Recall, chapter 10's discussion about several valuable clues that exist, which will show a deficiency in the adrenal system (all six links in the 'chain'). These clues can occur within these owners blood whenever their doctor obtains a white blood cell differential. If the eosinophils, (a type of white blood cell), are elevated, the adrenal system may be deficient. Two additional types of white blood cells, the neutraphils and lymphocytes, numbers provide additional clues. If neutrophils decrease and lymphocytes increase (a right shift), another red flag of adrenal insufficiency should go up. When either clue occurs, the physician should thoroughly check the six levels of the patient's adrenal system. A cortisol deficiency will allow abnormalities of these white blood cell types. All of the diseases (listed on page 344) have a high likelihood of increased eosinophils within their clinical picture.

5. The supposed surprise and mystery tactic: why estrogen would increase the risk of heart disease

High Estrogen Levels Can Promote Heart Disease because it promotes Fat

When estrogen rises beyond normal levels, there occurs a varying tendency to promote two of the hormonal factors creating obesity. In certain females, the ability of estrogen to raise insulin and lower androgens, describes these two factors.

Three main clinical situations promote estrogen-induced weight gain. Not all female owners will express these tendencies equally. This variability may have a genetic basis. Not all women with increased estrogen states tend to gain weight equally. High estrogen states tend to promote weight gain in many female owners. This fact will be the focus of this subsection.

The first clinical example for estrogen-induced weight gain results from birth control pills. They predictably increase insulin in the body. The first mechanism for this situation arises from an abnormal hormone tandem that high estrogen levels cause.

The first part of the hormone tandem involves the high estrogen-induced increased release rates of growth hormone from the pituitary gland. This occurs in the increased estrogen states that result from birth control pills usage. Growth hormone will initially raise the blood sugar level. It is the second hormone in this tandem, that estrogen simultaneously inhibits, which alters the normal pattern of events.

When estrogen levels remain optimal, the release of growth hormone directs the simultaneous release of insulin-like growth factor (IGF-1), the second hormone in the tandem, along with the liver stored sugar and fat. IGF-1 has powerful insulin-like blood sugar-lowering message content. This message content lowers the blood sugar that the released growth hormone initially elevated. Here, extra insulin is not needed.

Normally, this tandem hormone effect provides an effective way for the cells to receive fuel from the blood stream, between meals, without raising insulin levels. High estrogen states, although they initially stimulate growth hormone release, counteract the normal tandem by inhibiting insulin-like growth factor release (IGF-1). **The normal hormone tandem interrupts because high estrogen causes the simultaneous inhibition of IGF-1 release.**

IGF-1 is an insulin-like hormone that acts normally in the cells outside the liver and fat. Its presence lowers the amount of insulin needed by the body. The IGF-1 released assists insulin by taking sugar out of the blood stream and into the cells outside the liver and fat. When IGF-1 levels diminish, the growth hormone released directs increased sugar to be released into the blood stream. More insulin has to be secreted from the liver to make up the deficit of total "fuel nozzle" hormones. The more insulin secreted, the more message content exists to make body fat. When the liver makes fat, it secretes in the form of the deadly LDL cholesterol-type.

The second clinical situation of estrogen-caused obesity involves increased prolactin levels caused by the increased estrogen state of birth control use and/or stress-filled lifestyles. Prolactin inhibits ovarian androgen hormone formation and release. This hormone-induced mechanism, associated with obesity, generally does not operate in pregnancy because this physiologic state possesses a growing placenta. In the pregnant state, the growing placenta, more than offsets the prolactin-induced inhibition of the ovaries by serving as a hormonal factory for steroid production. Birth control usage fools the body into thinking it is pregnant. Prolactin levels rise in response to either increased estrogen or cortisol. However, in either of the above cases, no placental hormone factory exists to make up the prolactin caused androgen deficiency.

In a real pregnancy, the placenta manufactures androgens even though the ovaries become relatively dormant by the fifth month of gestation. When a female owner takes birth control pills, the body thinks it is pregnant. During birth control pill usage, prolactin levels rise because estrogen levels approach pregnancy levels. However, with birth control pill usage, there is no placenta to manufacture the androgen lost when the ovaries become inhibited by excessive prolactin.

Potential obesity problems occur because, like pregnancy, the birth control pills increase prolactin levels. Unlike pregnancy, there is no placenta (hormone factory) to correct the inhibition of steroid production within the ovaries. The potential for problems compounds due to the fact that the birth control pill does not contain androgens, only estrogen and progestins (abnormally-shaped progesterone substitutes). Androgen production can fall within these owners and their adrenals are left all alone for this task. Some female's adrenals fail at the challenge of increased androgen production and obesity ensues.

The third clinical situation of high estrogen-induced obesity is beyond the level of this discussion. For those who are curious, it involves the dramatic increase of sex hormone-binding globulin that high estrogen levels direct. Androgen that may be produced by the ovary or adrenals, in high estrogen states, gets trapped on a carrier protein in the blood stream at 98% of the efficiency level. Remember, the androgen level determines the repair rate of blood vessels. The activities of life constantly assault the blood vessels and these hormones direct their repair.

6. The Corrupt presentation of a Studies results Tactic: SSRI antidepressant vs. St. Johns Wort vs. placebo

Several years ago, multiple media outlets dutifully put the spin on a supposed definitive study about the efficacy of natural therapy with St. Johns wort and a popular SSRI antidepressant. These, in turn, were compared against a placebo. The study included moderate to severely depressed patients.

The consistent spin heard by the public was that St. Johns wort was no better than a placebo for the treatment of moderate to severe depression. The other side of the story concerns the fact that this same study showed that the popular SSRI was no better than the placebo, either. This trend emerged even though the dosage of this prescription medication was rather hefty.

This gives the average owner something to think about the next time they hear about some supposed new breakthrough or when another alternative modality gets trashed. Follow the money and you will understand loyalty. Alternative treatments, no matter how effective, cannot generate fat checks. Reality: The man with the gold makes the rules.

This fact explains why the health revolution occurs among the 'little people', one antidote at a time. The corporate giants are not interested in how one heals if it effects their ' good thing'.

7. The Upwardly Mobile Textbook Writer Tactic: Insulin

This is a hard one for traditionally trained physicians to consider with an open mind: The textbook presentation of insulin effects within the body is largely a fictional exaggeration. Mainstream doctors are groomed into thinking that insulin is the major way that the body's cells receive their nutrition. Never mind the fact that to perpetuate this fiction the textbooks have needed to be successively 'dumbed down' through various tactics. The method involves clever wording schemes, misleading diagrams, non-indexed 'widowed pearl's and numerous alias names that mean the same thing but are not commonly known. Most of these facts have been presented earlier in this manual. However, four concepts deserve emphasis here.

A. The Myth of Insulin Logic Mainstream medicine's propaganda dogma grooms physicians and patients to focus on insulin as the nutrition uptake hormone. Meanwhile, they ignore the scientific fact that IGF-1 occurs at levels greater than 100 times those of insulin in the healthy individual. The disconnection between this simple optimal ratio maintains itself by arbitrarily measuring insulin in micro units (alternatively as micro moles) and IGF-1 in nanograms throughout the medical texts. More disconnection results from the fact that numerous different names describe IGF-1. For example, the older medical literature describes IGF-1 in the following additional three ways: Nonsuppressible insulin-like activity of the blood, sulfation factor, and somatomedin C. In order for a physician to appreciate the important role that IGF-1 plays in the cells for obtaining nutrition, he/she would need to be aware of, and have time to look up, all four of these alternative descriptors for the same hormone. Reconnecting all four different names with the facts associated with them, and a common measurement method, allows the important role of IGF-1 to emerge.

Simple logic shows that there is not enough insulin to go around to all body cells. One liver or fat cell contains 200,000 pure insulin-type receptors. The 100 times more IGF-1compared to insulin makes up the volume discrepancy needed to deliver fuel uptake message content to the other body cells. Remember, whatever the insulin secretion rate, because of its portal vein connection to the pancreas, the liver will always receive the highest concentration of insulin-message content.

B. The body is smart and consistent. Hormones carry information via their precise shape, which tells the target cells how to spend their energy. Insulin-message content concerns the storage of energy. Consistent with this fact regards the stimulatory message of insulin within the liver to make more LDL cholesterol. LDL cholesterol is designed for the storage depots within the liver, fat cells and macrophages that line the arteries. To a limited extent, energy is stored, about 500 grams total, as glycogen, within the liver and muscles, if enough potassium remains available. After this, the insulin message within the liver turns on the cholesterol and fat-making machinery that changes sugar into these substances and packages them as LDL cholesterol. Remember, LDL cholesterol is constructed with storage in mind.

This fact remains consistent with the insulin message content, energy storage. Rather than teach physicians this simple relationship for how one can turn down cholesterol synthesis within the liver, they are schooled on the latest cholesterol-lowering drug that works by poisoning the ability of the liver to listen to insulin-message content. By a circuitous route (chapters 7, 8, 9 and 14), chronic mental stress elevates blood sugar levels and the acute phase reactants. One acute phase reactant is C-reactive protein and this explains why it elevates along with the blood sugar of Type A personalities. Again, rather than teach physicians the holistic importance of counseling their Type A patients about stress reduction and the importance of exercise, they are taught to prescribe these liver poisons. Liver poisons prove unnecessary when one understands the relationship of chronic mental stress elevating the blood sugar and that this requires excess insulin to remedy. The additional association for how these statin drugs really lower blood vessel inflammation was discussed in The Second Part of the Inflammation Secret in chapter 14.

C. Oh, now I hear some protest about insulin elevation in the fasting state when insulin resistance occurs. Well let's think this protest through, logically. Healthy muscles depend on adequate IGF-1 levels for their nutritional needs between meals. They also depend on adequate insulin following meals, which directs sufficient storage of sugar and fat for the next between meal states. Between meals, growth hormone releases when the brain senses a fall in blood sugar. The growth hormone released, causes the liver's stored sugar, fat, and IGF-1, to release. Sufficient IGF-1 between meals allows the muscles and organs to receive nutrition without the need for insulin. Healthy people have no need for insulin in the fasting state.

Because their IGF-1 has fallen, Syndrome X individual's need insulin in exaggerated amounts between meals. Remember, the liver always receives the highest concentration of pancreatic hormonal secretions. Liver and fat cells also have the highest amount of pure insulin-type receptors occurring at 200,000 per cell. The increased insulin output stimulates the liver and fat-making machinery. Syndrome X owners, then, have conflicting message content within their livers during the fasting state.

The first conflicting aberration concerns their diminished growth hormone output while between meals. Increased epinephrine, glucagons, and cortisol need to release in order to maintain the blood sugar level (fuel level) between meals. However, the fall in growth hormone has two health consequences. One concerns that body protein stores become fair game for dismantling when growth hormone levels fall off. Second involves the fall off of IGF-1 release. This last fact sets up the overall second conflicting message at the level of the liver. Simplistically, the conflict involves the competing message between the increased insulin needed to shore up fallen IGF-1, which also tells the liver to store fuel, and the simultaneous release of the counter-hormones, cortisol, glucagon and epinephrine, telling the liver to release fuel. Until someone helps these owners to realign the hormones that instruct their liver, these owners will continue on the accelerated path to an old body.

Popular strategies abound that purport to raise growth hormone secretion rates. All of them ignore the fact as to why the pituitary secretes growth hormone in the first place. Growth hormone secretes to protect body protein content, yet keep the blood fuel level adequate between meals or when exercising. Cognizance of this fact allows one to see that the popular approaches have their effect by peripheral pathways.

Certain amino acids are fastidiously protected from fuel combustion, within the body. Popular strategies raise growth hormone levels in some owners because these same amino acids when taken as supplements, set off the pituitary alarm that important amino acid blood levels are elevated. Examples of important amino acids that the body fastidiously protects are: arginine, ornithine, glutamine and lysine. **But what about those owners who have a pituitary defect acquired around middle age that no longer allows sufficient growth hormone release?**

Many Syndrome X owners have such a defect. They are doomed to die prematurely unless they receive counsel on how to raise their growth hormone levels. Here again popular growth hormone replacement protocols fail to inquire about liver health and androgen levels before prescribing growth hormone replacement injections. Hence, all the media attention to the supposed risk for growth hormone induced diabetes. Healthy livers that receive adequate androgen message content will curtail a diabetes tendency with growth hormone treatments (chapter 13).

IGF-1 levels depend on two basic factors. First concerns the hormonal factor. The liver needs adequate direction from thyroid, DHEA, or testosterone, and cortisol. When all three of these hormone types occur at normal levels, these hormones instruct the liver DNA to manufacture IGF-1 hormone and its binding proteins properly. Seondly, however, is the life style factor, which allows the release of IGF-1 from the liver. The lifestyle factor controls growth hormone [GH] release rates. Growth hormone releases when the blood fuel level decreases. Common situations for which the blood fuel falls are: exercise, fasting and between meals. Increased estrogen levels inhibit the release of IGF-1 by GH (chapter 13). Owners who have healthy levels of IGF-1 also have healthy levels of thyroid hormone, DHEA, testosterone, cortisol, estrogen and GH.

> The "hormone report card" evaluates these when health diminishes. Paradoxically, mainstream medicine does not routinely inquire about these important hormone considerations. The suspicion is that mainstream doctors are not taught to think about these hormone relationships. I wasn't encouraged. The science is all there, although it presents in a convoluted and disjointed fashion. As long as there continues to be divergent and multiplicitas ways to say these important facts, physicians will remain in the dark. Be kind to your physician and help him to learn anew.

High blood sugar stimulates insulin increases while low blood sugar stimulates IGF-1 release, along with sugar and fat. The opposite is also true. High blood sugar eventually decreases IGF-1 levels but low blood sugar decreases insulin release. When IGF-1 releases, there has been a preceding release of GH. The GH release response results from a falling blood sugar, which causes stored sugar to be dumped by the liver into the blood stream. The simultaneously released IGF-1 then causes the liver released sugar to be used. IGF-1 levels maintain body cell fuel levels between meals. Insulin maintains liver storage levels of sugar and fat following meals. In this way, healthy muscles have access to fuel at all times.

Maintaining balance between IGF-1 and insulin forms an important biochemical determinant of youthfulness within the muscles. It is also important to avoid the popular practice of receiving growth hormone injections without a proper evaluation of the IGF-1 levels. Without a proper evaluation of one's liver's ability to increase IGF-1 levels, GH will tend to promote high blood sugars and increase insulin output. Increased insulin output associates with all the negative effects on body physique discussed in "The Real Reason Americans are Getting Fatter chapter (chapter 7).

D. Following meals, the healthy body relies on sufficient insulin to store adequate fuel for the between meals state In the between meals state, sufficient growth hormone release tells the healthy liver to release the stored sugar, fat and IGF-1. In this way, the healthy body's cells have access to sufficient blood fuel at all times while protecting their protein content from combustion for usage as fuel.

In contrast, unhealthy people do not release sufficient growth hormone. Instead, they release excessive cortisol, glucagons, and epinephrine, between meals in order to keep their blood fuel elevated. However, body protein now becomes fair game for fuel usage and because IGF-1 levels are down, more insulin needs to be secreted between meals. Insulin secretion, in the between meals state, is abnormal. It only becomes necessary when IGF-1 levels have fallen.

(Recap - Side bar for physicians) Why would a healthy body instruct the liver to draw down the blood sugar further in the between meals state? Unhealthy bodies do this only because they lack "fuel nozzle" hormones (a fallen IGF-1 level) for their cells, as in muscle and organs. In order to keep alive, they accept the complications of increasing insulin output enough to spill over into the general circulation and allow these cells their "fuel nozzle". The major complication results from the fact that whatever the insulin secretion rate, because of the pancreas-portal vein connection to the liver, the liver receives the highest

> concentration of its message content before the other body cells can get any insulin "fuel nozzle"s. This means a contradictory message occurs within the unhealthy body's liver during the fasting state (C in above discussion).

8. When in a Corner Act Like it was Your Idea All Along Tactic: Homocysteine and Fish Oils

One way or another, heart blood vessel disease results from the repair rate of its blood vessels not keeping up with the injury rate. On their inside surface, injured blood vessels have rough areas (molecular "Velcro"). These roughened areas provide a place for the insulin-created fat particles to stick within cells called the macrophages. Macrophages are a type of immune scavenger cell that fill up on LDL cholesterol particles that follow from a high insulin-producing meal or mental stress. Macrophages also bed down on these "Velcro" areas to form temporary patches. As they serve their patching role on the inside surfaces of blood vessels, they continue to grow from ingesting more and more LDL cholesterol that follows from high insulin levels. After many years, they grow into foam cells. Foam cells constitute the earliest lesion in heart blood vessel disease. Insulin is the hormone that tells the liver to make the type of cholesterol and fat particle that the macrophages ingest (LDL cholesterol).

The injured areas ("Velcro") on the inside surfaces of the blood vessels, arise from what are called additional risk factors in the development of this type of disease. Common examples, given by the mainstream are: smoking, high blood pressure, obesity, high homocysteine levels, abnormal cholesterol profile, and diabetes. The above list can be greatly simplified when one realizes that all obesity, and about 90% of diabetes and abnormal cholesterol profiles, associate with excess insulin. If one simply remembers how to decrease their insulin levels they can eliminate these risk factors from their lives.

High blood pressure can be healed nutritionally (discussed in section two). Smoking elimination is a personal choice, but it helps when one realizes that smoke contributes to the injury rate of one's blood vessel inside surface lining. The greater the injury rate, the greater the repair rate abilities need to be. Hormone levels and nutritional status determine one's ability to repair the daily "Velcro" formation. In this subsection, an example of nutritional repair factors is discussed. These nutritional deficiencies that promote heart disease provide one example of America being the land of nutritional deficiency diseases.

Recently, mainstream media specialists admitted that only half of all heart attack victims had elevated cholesterol. Rather than retreat from their earlier 'cholesterol and fat are bad' campaign, they have woven a tale for yet even more cholesterol lowering drug sales (see Type A behavior entries chapter 14).

It took almost 30 years for the research of Dr. McCully, on homocysteine, to achieve mainstream acceptance. For many years, it was only in the alternative community that elevated homocysteine levels were felt to predict an increased risk of blood vessel disease. Meanwhile, the mainstream scientific community scoffed at this man's work. Dr. McCully even found himself dismissed from Harvard because the negative sentiment was so strong. After many years, the results of large European studies clearly showed his work was correct. The American medical power complex found itself in a 'credibility corner' and had to concede. Today, they act as if it was their research that identified this important blood vessel disease risk factor. Ponder for a moment, the needless suffering and lives lost because the profit driven medical industrial complex prevented following up on the work of Dr. McCully.

The public can learn how to better protect their health by taking note of just this one example where the dominant medical system delayed healing. Rather than wait another 30 years for additional insights about disease from the mainstream certified experts, owners need to educate themselves. Even today, surprisingly few doctors realize that in the majority of cases, homocysteine elevates when certain nutrients deplete. Instead, they are groomed into focusing on the minority with a genetic component to their elevated homocysteine elevation. This confusion propagates because this minority of patients also benefit from nutritional therapy.

Prediction: homocysteine will increasingly become viewed as a nutritional disease-associated risk marker. The diseases for which an elevated homocysteine level associates will include, not only blood vessel disease, but also some cases of high blood pressure, cancer, arthritis, multiple sclerosis and lupus. In other words, homocysteine will be increasingly used as a nutritional deficiency marker, which will recognize that the bodies repair rates are not keeping up with its injury rates.

Homocysteine elevates when there are deficiencies in one or more of the following: Vitamin B6, Vitamin B12, folate, serine, methionine and SAMe. Collectively, these nutrients are known as the methyl donor system. SAMe is used within the body at the rate of one billion times a second. Deficiencies in the above additional cofactors allow SAMe to degrade to homocysteine. Consequently, homocysteine levels rise. Deficiencies are predictable in those owners who eat food predominantly from a box, bag, can or a fast food restaurant.

The Successful Fat is Bad Campaign Tactic, but now all the sudden there are a growing list of exceptions; fish oil is one of these

My, my, the complex should really be proud of themselves for pulling off the 'fat is bad 'campaign. It is easy to expose the falsehood on the main platform on which it propagates, when one understands how fat absorbs into the body and its difference from the fat made in the liver (chapter 14).

Of interest here, regards the complex's increasing list of fats that are now supposedly O.K. Informed owners owe those doggedly stubborn consumers that kept asking intelligent questions like: if fat is so bad, why are Eskimos free of heart disease? And if fat is so bad, why do Greeks and French, who eat all kinds of fat, have a low incidence of heart disease? Another good question concerns the fact that Americans are getting fatter as they continue to eat less fat. And there is the growing realization about accelerated wrinkles in those who adhere to a low fat diet. All these conundrums explain themselves when one understands the difference between dietary fat and liver-manufactures fat. All of these topics are discussed earlier in this manual. In fact, medical physiology textbooks that are almost fifty years old, discuss the difference between dietary and liver-manufactured fat's physical properties. I wonder who removed these connecting facts about fat and cholesterol from the medical textbooks that doctors learn from?

9. Use the Media to Lie Tactic: the High Protein Diet and Kidney Damage

Almost everyone remembers the fear of kidney damage that high protein diets supposedly caused. I remember several years ago, an official spokesperson from the American Dietetic Association proclaiming on television that the high protein diet would cause kidney damage. Right then the host interrupted her and played a video of Dr. Atkins predicting her assertion. On the video Dr. Atkins wryly asked her to provide a single study that bolsters her claim". Keep inmind that Dr. Atkins' prediction of her bad mouthig occurred before the interview.

The official was dumb founded. After that, I never heard about the high protein and kidney damage assertion again. However, until that day, I had mistreated my patients by telling them the poppy cock about these supposed facts. I learned a good lesson that day about the power of media propagated poppy cock.

10. Use the Legal System to Protect a "Good Thing" Tactic: Cholesterol Lowering Drugs and Fake Hormone Replacement

Scientific fact: Insulin levels within the liver determine the activity of HMG Co A reductase. This is the enzyme that makes cholesterol. Scientific fact: When insulin directs fat and cholesterol manufacture, it is designed with storage in mind. The body is smart and consistent. Insulin contains message content that concerns energy storage. Drs.' and patients are not properly educated about these facts and misled, as well, with complex ways to say simple things.

One example concerns the hopeless mantra about the cruel hand genetics plays in certain individuals. The next step is to dutifully prescribe cholesterol-lowering medication, insulin-stimulating medication and blood pressure lowering medication. Whenever genetics gets blamed, the innuendo is that natural healing solutions are futile. No one is counseling these owners about why a body would misdirect energy into excessive storage as fat, raise the blood pressure, or need excessive insulin. Excessive fat can only come from excessive insulin. The other hormones that either hinder fat or promote its formation do so through affecting insulin levels (section 3).

Insulin need and hence its levels rise with a few main things: increased carbohydrate consumption, potassium deficiency, excessive mental stress, sedentary lifestyle, and falling IGF-1 levels. IGF-1 levels fall when growth hormone secretion falls, androgen levels fall, hypothyroidism, low cortisol levels and excess estrogen (all these are explained in section three).

In view of the above facts it would seem logical that an owner could march down to his/her doctor and show him these interconnected statements. Good luck, but more likely, the doctor is bound by the medical legal standard of care. The standard of care is determined by what the majority of doctors would do for a given condition. In the above case, it has nothing to do with the best science or the best outcome. Nope! It is all about how many votes you buy when you sell your companies' idea. The complex controls doctors effectively through the majority rules standard of care approach.

One thing an owner can bet on concerns the fear of politicians if enough angry voters get wind of these shenanigans.

Fake Hormones

Millions of women take altered message content in the form of their hormone replacement therapy. Of course, their doctors and they do not realize that their prescriptions contain altered-message content, delivered to their trillions of cells. The wrong message instructing the DNA programs leads to side effects and toxicities. Basic science says this is true. However, the discussion of these facts within the textbooks occurs in a disjointed and fragmented fashion. Textbooks written in this way keep doctors in the dark about what science really knows about hormones.

Female hormone replacement science was discussed in more detail in chapter 11. Here, the focus concerns the advantage of real hormone replacement over fake hormone replacement. Real hormones carry accurate message content. Fake hormones carry inaccurate message content to the cells. The altered message results in side effects and toxicities. Real hormones cannot be patented and hence cannot be as profitable. Hormones become fake, when the real hormone's shape becomes changed in order to get a patent. No shape change, no patent. The precise molecular shape contains the hormone message content. This is simple science being discussed here.

The miracle of convincing doctors that fake hormones are better than real hormones doesn't mean that the side effects are not real. Most doctors have been educated that fake hormones are best.

About one in nine women will develop breast cancer. A significant part of this occurrence results from fake hormone usage and excessive exposure to hormone mimics in the environment. Yet, if a woman gets cancer while on fake hormones, it is not considered malpractice. In fact, many doctors get away with prescribing fake hormones without a thorough laboratory inquiry of a patients hormone status. However, the physician that takes the time to perform a thorough laboratory inquiry into a patient's hormone status and prescribes real hormones, considers himself/herself at risk for a malpractice verdict if that patient gets cancer.

There are several possible explanations for why the standard of medical care, in regard to hormone replacement therapy, has become so ludicrous.

1. Physicians do not receive proper education about the fact that the precise shape of a hormone carries its message content. A change in the shape, in order to get a patent, changes the message content. Simple science, but not commonly taught in a way that doctors can see the problem of fake hormones.
2. The public lacks awareness that holistically trained physicians exist who can prescribe real hormone replacement therapies. The real hormone replacement therapies need to be filled by a compounding pharmacist. Compounding pharmacists specialize in real hormones.
3. The media and the medical industrial complex have a cozy arrangement. Each benefits. One from increased advertising revenue, the other from increased drug or procedure sales. One of the most effective media strategies creates fear about real hormones in both the doctor and patient's minds. However, remembering point #1 helps to show that fake hormones cannot be better than real hormones because of simple science. Only real hormones can deliver accurate message content to one's trillions of body cells.

Glandular failure describes the silent epidemic that robs countless middle-aged owners of their youthful vigor and physiques. As the different glands' secretions begin to fail, the rejuvenation message content that these hormones contain, curtails. Other glands attempt to keep the owners alive by increasing the presence of other hormones. The other hormones have side effects that would not occur if one had normal gland function. One side effect of diminished gland function is weight gain in middle age.

One crucial step in the turning off of the fat-maker machine concerns the seven hormone types, which allow or curtail fat accumulation. As long as fear propagates about real hormone replacement therapies, a powerful weight loss tool will go underutilized in those that have severe glandular deficiencies.

Almost all cases of obesity have a large glandular component. Obese people are in general not lazy, stupid, or unmotivated. At their core, obese people have a defect in one or more of their glandular secretions. The wrong hormones direct inappropriate body energy into storage as fat (chapter 7).

As explained earlier, proper nutrition, exercise training, and stress reduction measures, allow many overweight owners to be healed. Some of the weight loss effect occurs because these measures improve the glandular secretions. The above methods are important because they prove to be the safest. But how does the doctor rectify those owners whose glands have big defects? Despite their best efforts for a weight loss effect, they fail.

It becomes a personal choice about deciding to go ahead with real hormone replacement therapy. Cancer rates increase with each passing decade. Most of this increase probably stems from nutritional deficiencies, environmental toxin loads, and immune dysfunction. Yet, real hormone replacement takes the blame wherever possible.

The renaming of somatotropin to growth hormone helps to instill additional fear. The renaming of the nonsuppressible insulin-like activity of the blood to insulin-like growth factor type one (IGF-1) also helps to instill more fear still about growing cancer.

Never mind the fact that the highest insulin receptor concentration occurs on the liver and fat cells at about 200,000 receptors per cell. Breast tissue composes itself from mostly fat. Overweight females are generally considered to be at increased risk for developing breast cancer. High insulin levels are a must before an owner can gain body fat. Yet no one counsels these breast cancer victims about insulin reduction techniques. Instead IGF-1 gets the blame as a supposed risk factor for tumor growth.

If this were so, then athletic training, adolescence, and pregnancy would all be risk factors for developing cancer. In all three conditions, IGF-1 levels are several times higher than middle-aged people. However, epidemiologic studies show that each one of these situations provides protection and does not seem to be a causative factor for cancer's development. Also, as IGF-1 decreases with age, the health decreases as well.

Some overweight owners have severe glandular defects with resulting decreases in growth hormone and/or androgen secretion. Either one of these defects will lead to decreased IGF-1. When IGF-1 decreases, insulin must increase (see text). The more insulin, the more the fat-maker message within the body. A rising insulin level and a falling IGF-1 more often occurs when cancer develops rather than the reverse.

Before a prescription of either growth hormone or androgen hormones can be entertained, the liver function and adrenal function need to be evaluated and found to be normal. These types of hormone replacement will cause problems when either the liver or adrenal health are not attended to.

Many doctors fail to counsel their patients that growth hormone naturally increases when blood sugar falls. In uncontrolled diabetes and chronic grazing-type feeding habits, the blood sugar never falls so growth hormone levels fall.

Growth hormone injections need to occur when the blood sugar is already on the low side. First thing in the morning or just before exercising provide such examples.

Insulin deficiency causes one form of diabetes.

IGF-1 deficiency causes one type of Syndrome X Type Associated obesity.

Societal programming makes insulin injections seem the obvious solution.

Yet, societal programming makes growth hormone and/or androgen replacement therapy, prescribed to raise IGF-1 levels, seem risky.

Just like the insulin deficient diabetes patient, the IGF-1deficient-caused Syndrome X patient will die more quickly without treatment.

Think about the billions of dollars of lost revenue from the diminished need for prescriptions and procedures if a Syndrome X patient received proper treatment.

Truncal obesity, high blood pressure, and Type A personality should be followed with:
1. Fasting insulin and C-peptide level
2. Fasting IGF-1 level
3. 24-hour urinary steroid and thyroid profile (including estrogens for men and women)
4. Baseline PSA level for men over forty
5. Hemoglobin A1C

Growth hormone and androgens are contraindicated for most cancers. The history of cancer proves as a relative contraindication that your doctor will determine on an individual basis.

If exercise, nutritional therapy, (see text) and stress management, fail to improve the above first three-baseline labs, real hormone replacement therapy should be considered. The glandular secretions must improve before a weight loss occurs.

Some overweight owners' glands have severe defects. Obesity, heart disease, and diabetes risk, will not resolve in these cases until these defects are identified and corrected in as safe a way as possible. The initial "hormone report card" includes:

Fasting insulin and C-peptide
Fasting IGF-1
Adrenal steroids (including aldosterone)
Androgen type steroids made in the gonads
Thyroid hormones' levels (including reverse T3)

Estrogen status
Homocysteine level
Prolactin level
PSA level for men over age 40
Hemoglobin A1C

Note of caution to clinicians: over the last few years, labs routinely have been arbitrarily lowering the 'low normal' range for IGF-1 levels. Not so long ago, the normal range for IGF-1 was 250-400 ng/ml. As Americans become fatter, the normal levels of IGF-1 within the population predictably skew the 'normal'. Currently, some labs say that values as low as 80ng/ml are normal. This is ludicrous if one desires health and weight loss. The lower acceptable level for IGF-1 will probably end up being around 250ng/ml. All physically fit and youthful people have at least this value, and many have much higher levels.

The medical legal rule about standard of care makes it difficult for conventionally trained M.D.s' to practice holistically in replacing glandular deficiencies with real hormones.

Any treatment plan for a given ailment carries risk. This is true whether the plan is holistic or based in the mainstream paradigm of symptom-control. In general, holistic approaches carry less risk because they seek to heal the root cause of a problem. In contrast, mainstream medicine's standard of care protocols usually involves increased risk because they treat the symptoms of disease and not its cause. Symptom-control always has side effects and toxicities. Yet this is the legally sanctioned approach that mainstream-trained doctors are intimidated into following lest they find themselves outside the standard of care protocols. Never mind the facts contained in this and other books that suggest that the standard of care has less than perfect motives for what it touts.

As discussed previously, one in nine women will develop breast cancer. If, before cancer develops after they receive a superficial hormone evaluation and then are prescribed horse estrogens cycled with fake progesterone this is felt to be the standard of care. As long as the standard of care is upheld the risk to the doctor for a malpractice case is minimal. However, if these same women were to receive a thorough hormone evaluation and steroid deficiencies were identified and treated with real hormones, the onset of cancer would sometimes be considered due to medical malpractice (the majority rules).

Even though basic science shows real hormones to be safer than fake hormones ,the medical legal standard supports the later. It becomes a personal choice as to whether one with documented severe glandular defects decides to begin real hormones replacement therapy.

The author of this book feels that the best course involves informed consent. Informed consent, for hormone replacement therapy involves reading this authors books and others like: *Grow Young with HGH, Some Things Your Doctor may not tell You about Menopause, Natural Hormone Balance for Women, Safe Uses of Cortisol, Hormone Replacement.* The authors and the publishers of these fine books are in the back.

Informed consent also involves a balanced discussion about the medical industrial establishment's negative feelings about real hormone replacement therapies for middle-aged diseases like obesity. Patients need to be informed that mainstream medicine frowns upon growth hormone and testosterone replacement therapy for overweight owners. They purport to have ample unbiased studies that link these therapies to cancer's development and accelerated growth.

Yet, they fail to mention or consider several inconsistent details. If all the negative fear about growth hormone were true, a good night's sleep, youthfulness, fasting, and athletic training would all be an increased risk factor for developing cancer. All the above are well documented to increase growth hormone release and hence, IGF-1, as well. However, epidemiological studies have shown all these to lower the risk of cancer's development.

Each overweight owner needs to carefully consider the official view (standard of care) contrasted with the real hormone replacement viewpoint. An informed consent form needs to be signed, before beginning treatment, acknowledging the acceptance of risk for the development of cancer according to the mainstream viewpoint. Also, an agreement about keeping their doctor up to date about their condition needs to be worked out. In addition, regular follow up needs to occur.

Recognize that mainstream physicians habitually discredit that which they do not understand. In these cases show them this book or the others listed above. Kind and informed patients can help their doctors to learn anew.

Reading self-help books like these can bring about empowerment for what health care choices are available. With empowerment comes personal responsibility for what is still unknown. Health care choices currently have many unknowns.

The practice of medicine involves probabilities. I feel that it is more probable that real hormone replacement therapy prescribed for documented defects is safer than ignoring the defect, prescribing fake hormones, or engaging in symptom-control. I base my belief on the contents of my books and the others listed above. I also want to acknowledge the current state of the unknown and the consequent incomplete healing choices.

In the end, each reader prays about what the right course is for him or her to take.

11. Teach the Doctor the Wrong Mechanism for how a Medicine Works Tactic: ACE inhibitors

Yet another secret revealed: Prescription medications which raise nitric oxide levels

There is an additional insight about nitric oxide production and it's relationship to a popular blood pressure lowering medication called, the angiotensin converting enzyme inhibitors. These types of medications effect the histamine-like content of the body, which also powerfully lowers blood pressure. The mainstream textbooks say very little about this powerful association. Instead, they discuss in great detail, the blood pressure lowering effects as being the result of lowered angiotensin two levels.

It is really quite a shock to most physicians when they begin to see evidence that the touted mechanism for a drug's action is not always the only way that they have an effect on the body. The ACE inhibitors are such an example. The drug literature focuses almost exclusively on the supposed powerful role that angiotensin plays in tightening up the blood vessels. However, very little of this literature discusses the well-documented fact that inhibition of this very same enzyme raises the total body content of a histamin- like substance, bradykinin. This explains why a dry nagging cough is the number one side effect. In addition, bradykinin is well known to lower blood pressure, but it is paid for with the price of increased leakiness of the capillaries in areas like the lungs and kidney. Maybe there was a marketing problem if this mechanism was related to an increased histamine-like substance content within the body. Probably, no one will ever know for sure. Nonetheless, it is instructive to see a possible bigger problem with other drugs in how the physician gets 'groomed' into thinking about how these drugs work.

Because these drugs increase bradykinin within the body they also increase nitric oxide production. Increased bradykinin is a powerful stimulant for turning on the enzymatic machinery within the endothelial cells lining the arteries. Bradykinin and histamine share the same receptors in the body. They also act in a similar manner. They contain similar message content. Once bradykinin becomes elevated, it tends to stimulate the mast cells to release histamine, as well.

The other touted benefit of these angiotensin-converting enzyme inhibitors (ACE inhibitors), is there documented benefit in the preservation of kidney function. To understand that this benefit is both a circuitous and expensive solution in many cases, one needs to recall four things. First, ACE inhibitors conserve body potassium and this has a known kidney protective effect on the tendency to become potassium deficient. Ample serum potassium itself causes a blood pressure lowering effect. Second, this medication lowers blood pressure despite the elevated sodium in the body by the less realized mechanism of increased bradykinin within the body. Third, increased presence of bradykinin in the body, also lowers blood pressure by being a powerful stimulus for nitric oxide production.

As an aside, if a given patient was correctly counseled about a real food diet instead of a processed food diet, before kidney damage occured from chronically low potassium intake, blood pressure medication in these cases would no longer be needed.

The fourth fact to understand about the consequences of decreased angiotensin two, production is the effect this has on the adrenal glands. Rather than get lost in the inconsistent evidence that these ACE inhibitors have on aldosterone levels, it becomes more instructive to look at the consistent evidence. The evidence is consistent that decreased angiotensin two will directly correlate with a decreased ACTH output. A decreased ACTH output will decrease stimulation to the adrenal glands release of aldosterone, cortisol, and DHEA. This little detail has powerful implications for another mechanism as to how these medications lower the blood pressure. It also has powerful implications for why diseases like autoimmune disease are made worse when these owners take these types of medications. Owners with autoimmune disease are made worse because they already have a wounded adrenal system (chapter 10). The addition of an ACE inhibitor will only exaggerate the diminished adrenal function, which operates in these diseases. This also provides a clue as to why these same types of owners will be at increased risk for Neutropenia and lymphocytosis; a sign of adrenal fatigue (chapter 10).

Now it is time to turn the analysis on its head. Mentally, the biggest roadblock involves the realization that people who consume high potassium and magnesium diets, relative to total sodium intake are also going to have a high aldosterone (a increased potassium intake will powerfully stimulate aldosterone release). However, in these cases, a diuresis will ensue because total body sodium is not excessive. Stress (ACTH) alone will tend to raise aldosterone secretion rates, and in this situation of a high sodium diet, this is inappropriate. When this happens, blood pressure will rise. Blood pressure rises from the cumulative sodium retentive effects of both cortisol and aldosterone, released in the stress response. But with excessive sodium already present in the processed food diet, they inappropriately cause fluid retention. The point to consider is that, perhaps a little effort spent counseling an early hypertensive on how to change their mineral intake ratios by eating 'real foods' (see mineral table) would have some merit before condemning them to medication with all it's side effects.

ACE inhibitors have been shown to improve a patient's clinical situation while in heart failure. What is not said is that histamine-like substances have a powerful strengthening action on heart muscle. This effect is obviously one benefit of these medications. The increased histamine-like content within the blood stream will reduce the effort of the heart in getting the blood pumped with each beat. ACE inhibitors effect multiple organ systems of the body.

12. The 'Need for Further Study Mantra' has Replaced Commonsense Tactic: ElectromagneticFields

The voice of reason regularly delivers out of the complex's chosen mouthpiece. The delivery is usually smooth and intelligent. Somewhere in the discussion, the smoke and mirrors technique, which so far is tried and true in its ability to continue with the 'business as usual' effect, activates. Sure, many different words lead to its introduction but stasis occurs when the wall of further study is proclaimed.

What about the things in life that are only knowable by engaging common sense? Has our society become so deluded as to lose touch with our God-given right to think things through to their logical conclusion?

Electromagnetic fields created by power lines provide one such opportunity to engage common sense and take action. Most people know that iron polarizes (orients towards) in a magnetic field. Some have even noticed this effect while standing under a high voltage power line with their compass. Many people know that it is the iron packed into our trillions of red blood cells that carries oxygen to our cells. Few have thought about the consequences to the side of the body that happens to be opposite the electrical magnetic field created by home appliances, cell phones, electrical heaters, and high voltage power lines.

Picture the blood flowing within one's head without polarization from outside magnetic fields. A balanced release of oxygen occurs. Now picture magnetic polarization of the iron carrying oxygen to the brain. Whatever side is picked, that side will receive diminished oxygen delivery secondary to the physical laws of the universe. Rather than think these everyday things through, the power complex has neurolinguistically programmed the masses to accede to the stasis of 'future studies' mantra in place of common sense. In view of the above, does anyone doubt that there are consequences to putting one's head and blood stream into a powerful magnetic field? How much cancer and ill health derive solely from electromagnetic fields? Dr. Becker's book, *The Body Electric* does a nice job explaining electromagnetic fields.

13. Get Ready for Patented Pills for Erection Enhancement Tactic

Most doctors remember smelling salts consisting of amyl nitrate. These salts were very cheap to produce. Somewhere in the early 1980's, the gay population noted that the salts prolonged sexual performance. They became very popular. For a while, quite the media blitz erupted attempting to link AIDS to amyl nitrate use (commonly called poppers). Later, this campaign was recanted and amyl nitrate slipped out of the PDR and American Hospital Formulary. Pretty boring stuff so far, eh?

Amyl nitrate improves erections because it raises the nitric oxide level in a man's penis. Hmm... that happens to be the same mechanism that the new erection pills work through at a cost of ten dollars a pill.

14. Change the name of the same thing so that doctors fail to realize important connecting concepts: GAG and IGF-1

Dating back to antiquity, physicians noted that the aging process involved the loss of water content from the structural tissues. For the same reasons that fruit shrivels as its water content diminishes, human cells also wrinkle. In fact the same molecular compounds in fruit that powerfully suck water into a given location are also found in human cells. As fruit ripens these electrically charged molecular compounds disintegrate and water escapes. Similarly, as they age, human cells for various reasons discussed below, lose their electrically charged molecular compounds, and water escapes.

Today, modern science can explain the hormone imbalances and molecular part deficiencies that allow water to escape from one's cells. However, this science routinely presents as disjointed and convoluted discussions that fail to unite key facts. The consequence of this is that physicians and owners are not taught to think about simple healing solutions that postpone the shrinkage into old age.

Body design composes itself with an electrical molecular water-sucking grid that overpowers the gravitational forces. Gravitational forces desire to squish one's cells flat, and consequently, allow water to escape. Ubiquitous to all life forms, there exists an electrical molecular sucking grid that opposes gravity. Only when gravity is successfully opposed, can a cell hold onto its optimum water content and remain wrinkle free.

Mainstream physicians receive very little educational emphasis about how one continues to possess an optimal electrical water-sucking grid throughout their body. This fact becomes quite disturbing when one realizes that it is this grid that is found in many body locations. Some examples are:

inflates the inside of all body cells, connects and supports the outside of all body cells, lines the inside surfaces of all blood vessels, lines the respiratory tract, lines the entire length of the digestive tube, and is the substance that inflates skin cells so that they remain wrinkle free. Awareness of these facts explains why many diseases have a component of causality in the disruption of this electrical water-sucking grid. Some common electrical water-sucking grid associated diseases are: colitis, heart disease, asthma, arthritis, and diabetes.

Part of the mainstream medical confusion about the extensive involvement of this grid in so many diseases concerns the additional disturbing fact about the many disjointed alias names used to describe it. In order to appreciate that the above listed body locales all contain and rely on this electrical grid water-sucking meshwork, a physician would need to know that the following alias descriptors mean basically the same thing: glycosaminoglycans, cytoskeleton, ground substance, basal lamina, mucopolysaccharides, cell coat, cell wall, cartilage, and mucous layer, to name a few.

Ignorance further propagates because the molecular makeup of these many ways to name the same substance largely remains ignored. The most accurate chemical descriptor for the above alias names is glycosaminoglycans (GAG). GAG is made from the molecular building blocks, glucosamine and galactosamine. These basic building blocks string together to form chains and crisscrossed chains thousands of molecules long. In addition, it is the addition of various amounts of sulfate and acetate to each glucosamine and galactosamine that powerfully attracts and retains water. This property results from the fact that these two molecular additions are electrically charged and, therefore, attract water. Only when galactosamines and glucosamines contain the proper electrical charge will water content remain adequate.

Many well-meaning practitioners achieve benefits for their arthritic patients by prescribing glucosamine and galactosamine supplements. However, there is a more central determiner for how much of this electrical water-sucking grid a body manufactures. The central, more important determiner, involves the quality of one's hormones, within.

Around middle age many owners begin to suffer the consequences of diminished hormone secretion quality. Hormones deliver messages to cells that tell them what to do. The many different types of body cells are faithful servants that only do as the messages delivered by the hormones direct. Here lies the middle-aged problem: deficiency of hormone rejuvenation message content leads cells into disrepair. One of the consequences of disrepair concerns the diminished amount of new electrical water-sucking grid molecules manufactured.

The quality of the GAG layer, like other body tissue components, depends on specific hormones that direct its manufacture rate. Again, the major reason that many physicians do not understand this concept concerns the way these facts are organized within the textbooks. Additional confusion arises because of the many alias names given to a single important hormone for forming fully charged GAG throughout the body.

Currently, the medical literature calls this important GAG manufacture rate-determining hormone, insulin-like growth factor type one (IGF-1). Older literature describes this same hormone as: sulfation factor, somatomedin C, and the non-suppressible insulin-like activity of the blood stream. Some holistic physicians feel that by disconnecting important hormones, like IGF-1; by renaming and separating it from the other literature, it perpetuates physicians practicing in the dumbed-down state. The dumbed-down state of practice results when doctors are not taught simple holistic facts about how the body heals. Everyone suffers from the dumbed-down state except the industrial medical complex.

The sulfation factor name for IGF-1 describes its critical rate-determining role in the formation of fully electrically charged GAG. GAG, which is not fully charged, possesses a diminished ability to retain water.

Diminished water content leads to wrinkled cells and the shrinkage of old age. In fact, beyond the hysteria to avoid the sun and sell sun blockers, this major determiner for youthful skin remains ignored. Skin wrinkles result from the same reason that over ripe fruit wrinkles. This truism e\tends to other body cells as well. The amount of GAG in an apple or a body cell type largely determines its ability to hold onto water. Human cells require adequate IGF-1 to re-synthesize GAG as it deteriorates. Because ripened fruit lacks hormones they rot and wrinkle as their GAG content diminishes.

Remember not to confuse the IGF-1 released by the liver into the blood stream with that inside the body cells. Healthy people possess 100 times IGF-1 levels compared to insulin within their blood streams. IGF-1 helps the cells outside the liver and fat cells in their procurement of body fuel (sugar, fat and amino acids). IGF-1 and insulin are best thought of as the body's "fuel nozzle" hormones. Just as filling a car fuel tank with fuel requires a nozzle, the body cells require a "fuel nozzle", which these two hormones provide.

In contrast, IGF-1 within cells delivers a message of cell rejuvenation and repair. Part of rejuvenation and repair concerns the manufacture of fully charged GAG. Only fully charged GAG prevents the shrinkage into old age. One of the major reasons that young people have fewer wrinkles involves their greatly increased IGF-1 levels.

Around middle age, IGF-1 begins to fall off and this results in less GAG formation. The lower the GAG level the more water leaks out of the body tissues. Skin wrinkles exemplify one example of this process. Other diseases for the same reason have a component of causality from diminished GAG content in their area of pathology. For example: the thick mucous of the asthmatic, the copious mucous in the colitis patient occurring when GAG fails to form properly it breaks down at an accelerated rate into mucous, the decreased GAG of osteoarthritis, the decreased GAG in the blood vessels of some diabetics, and the decreased GAG in the blood vessels of some heart disease patients.

While the above diseases' severity cannot be entirely explained by GAG deficiency, in each case, there is a profound contribution to the course of these diseases arising from their association with diminished GAG. Since the above diseases cause so much suffering and are part of the shrinkage into old age, the determinants of IGF presence deserve attention (chapter 7). Sadly, this is not yet the case.

15. Arbitrarily Measure one Related Substance Differently than other Related Substances to Conceal the Relative Importance of One Tactic: Potassium and Insulin

These two examples have been discussed elsewhere but a brief acknowledgment here helps to be aware of this tactic. Insulin is measured in microunits or micromoles and IGF-1 is measured in nanograms. Consistently, writing the scientific literature in this way helps to perpetuate the concealment of the much greater amounts of IGF-1 in the blood streams of healthy people and the diminished amounts in unhealthy people.

All minerals in the body are measured in milligrams but routinely, potassium is measured in milliequivalents except when measuring it in the blood serum (a place where its amount is very low compared to sodium). This tendency helps to perpetuate the false emphasis on sodium and the diminished understanding that adequate potassium, relative to sodium intake, proves impossible in the processed food diet (see mineral table). Few doctors realize the importance of high potassium relative to sodium for these reasons and **"Low Voltage Cell Syndrome"** ensues around middle age.

16. Use code names so that the doctor will not know he/she is prescribing a known nerve toxin in a way that children have little defense tactic: thimerosal

Until a few years ago, much higher amounts of thimerosal were present in children's vaccines. Thimerosal is still present in the annually given flu shot at 25micograms per shot. The trouble is, many mainstream doctors are not aware that thimerosal is present in these injections. Fewer still know what thimerosal is chemically. Thimerosal is ethyl-mercury. Mercury within the brain constitutes a powerful neurotoxin.

Dental fillings contain mercury. Tuna fish contains mercury. Oil refineries and coal power plants belch mercury.

However, these oral and respiratory mechanisms of exposure are better handled within the body. Unfortunately, when mercury gains access to the body tissues outside of these protective barriers, little protection from nerve cell damage exists. The body was not designed to deal with injected mercury. The body has protective defenses for inhaled and digested mercury. Vaccines for these reasons, need to be carefully thought out in a more neutral risk versus benefits analysis.

Autism occurrence rates have sky rocketed over the last twenty years. The mainstreams certified experts act as if it is a great mystery as for why this is so. Certain pediatricians beg to differ (see ADHD discussion) and continue to provide scientific evidence that interplay exists between mercury poisoning, measles virus in vaccines, the GI tract, the immune system, errors of metabolism in certain infants, and nutritional deficiencies. None of these interrelated considerations routinely gets addressed when a mother or father inquires about them within the mainstream medical industrial complex. The mothers and fathers of the world owe several doggedly stubborn consumers a great debt; they eventually prevailed in forcing vaccine manufactures to greatly lower the thimerosal content.

17. Smoke and Mirrors Tactic

This tactic proves so effective that very few doctors realize the ubiquitousness of its presence. Pick any disease of middle age and subject the latest journal articles to one central measure: how fairly do the primary drivers of a disease process receive emphasis?

Start with obesity. How often do these medical articles emphasize any of the glandular secretions mentioned earlier in this book? Instead, they discuss, the theoretical and without clinical benefit, supposed obesity-related hormones. Meanwhile, the central determiners of obesity remain ignored. It is the central hormones causing obesity that an owner has some control over for how much or little they express. Common sense dictates that these should be vigorously followed in as scientific a manner as possible.

Most doctors fail to realize that most of these articles have designs that perpetuate confusion. Any reader can pick up the latest in mainstream medical reading material and decide for him/herself if the content confuses more than it helps.

High blood pressure provides another example of perpetuating confusion. Scientific fact: certain nutritional deficiencies or excesses promote high blood pressure in certain owner types. Some of these are: magnesium and potassium deficiencies, methyl donor deficiencies, excess insulin, nitric oxide deficiency, stiff red blood cells from specific nutrient deficiencies, and sodium excess (see text for specifics).

With the exception of the doctor giving vague advice about low sodium diets, when was the last time anyone heard of a journal article discussing these basic nutritional determinants of blood pressure? Instead, there occurs the tried and true complex descriptor of the supposed latest reason to prescribe the latest pharmaceutical darling.

Middle age is also a time of increasing risk for developing heart disease and/or diabetes. Here again, the focus tends to address peripheral determiners for both of these diseases. Rather than squarely telling owners at risk for these diseases about the common fact that both diseases generally arise because of excessive insulin need (see text for specifics) they are given vague advice. Vague advice occurs when they are told to exercise and lose weight without counseling about the central hormone and mineral aberrations that caused their disease. They are then given insulin raising, blood pressure and cholesterol lowering medications. All of these medications have potential serious side effects and do nothing to heal the cause of their problem: excessive insulin need (see text for details).

Middle-aged bodies also increasingly experience joint aches and dysfunction. Hormone imbalance and nutritional deficiencies prove major causes for allowing these destructive processes to continue. Rather than educate doctors about these basic relationships, they are schooled in the latest anti-inflammatory medication.

The 'smoke and mirrors' tactic will probably be looked back upon in history as the most effective method of retarding the health care revolution for what science has revealed, but continues to ignore, because of money. It remains effective because of human nature. Doctors are no different than any other human. They crave respect for how hard they have worked to earn the title, doctor.

Part of the reason they had to work so hard proves the hardest for them to accept. Much of the complexity contained within the medical textbooks, rest largely on the need to keep doctors dumbed-down. This is a formidable task because doctors, in general, possess a remarkable intelligence. Anyone who doubts this fact about the disorganized and fragmented thought contained in the textbooks, need only to acquire a medical textbook greater than forty years old and read the clarity of scientific presentation.

Here come the protests about how much more is known today and, of course, the text are more complex. Surprise! The older textbooks contain scientific information that has been eviscerated from today's newer versions. The removal of this information seems to me to effectively continue the downward spiral of creating dumber doctors. In its place are convoluted discussions that lead the doctors down erroneous thinking pathways, designed to sell more drugs (see text for examples).

18. The Emperor has No Clothes Tactic

This tactic speaks for itself except that very few doctors ever acknowledge their continued confusion after reading articles that are designed to confuse. Unless confusion remains rampant doctors will begin to figure out the fictional nature of how they are taught to address middle-aged disease. This text has been my attempt to point out some inconsistent details and reasons for alarm for how we are groomed to think. Today's mainstream treatment strategies for middle-aged disease clearly show that the emperor has no clothes. We can no longer look away.

19. The Certified Expert Tactic

The voice of reason and sophistication comes out of the mouth of the certified expert. Meanwhile, very few have ever thought through what it requires to become a certified expert. That 'something' is not in possession for many holistic mental giants like: Andrew Weil, Julian Whitiker, Jonathan Wright, Alan Gaby, and Steven Bratman. All of these men went to an accredited medical school but none of them went beyond their internship.

What trait is missing from the above list of holistic great thinkers? Answer: the ability to keep their mouth shut when they stumble upon a scientific inconsistency or injustice. This trait proves fatal to one's career aspirations of becoming a certified expert. Very few have ever thought through the logical consequences of a scientific system based on self-perpetuation of dogma. How clever to build into the system, out of the public's view, that in order to ever achieve expert status one must learn to keep their mouth shut or they will find themselves terminated. This book has only scratched the surface of the many scientific inconsistencies that real live patients continually provide. It has also only scratched the surface of the amount of dishonesty contained in the medical textbooks.

During the Vietnam War, the young folks trumpeted the slogan of not trusting anyone over thirty until they earned respect. A similar caution is probably in order for the certified experts, because they have often sold their souls to the complex. God bless those truly rare experts that manage to survive and please forgive my generalization.

The hope of this general statement about who passes as a certified expert involves a healthier level of skepticism for the next time a complex-endorsed mouthpiece says something that sells more drugs. It's all about money. Follow the gold and you will understand who makes the rules. The best thing we little people can do, is to begin to talk openly amongst ourselves about new healing insights, and remain ever open to the continual fact that sometimes we are wrong. Inability to admit our errors in thinking about health and disease reduces us to the level of vermin within the complex.

20. The Evidence Based Medicine Tactic

A wolf in sheep's clothing comes to mind when I think about this popular method of spreading disinformation. If you can't beat them join them, in the appearance of acting reasonably receptive to holistic ideas. Some hospitals trumpet more healing-like atmospheres on the surface of things. This is all good as long as we never lose sight of the business of medicine.

The business of medicine controls what is studied and published in the journals that doctors commonly read. This year the last journal that had some semblance of intolerance toward their reviewers beig drug funded and therefore biased in what gets published, The New England Journal of Medicine, succumbed to more lucrative articles. Across the Atlantic, until now, the more impartial European scientific community remained another throne in the side of profit-driven health care. Recently pharmaceutical companies have bought themselves largess and their research, bashing various holistic ideas, evidences the fruit of their labors.

It sounds rather fantastical at first, but think about the billions of dollars at stake, if even a small fraction of owners begins to seek out holistic medical advice. Chiropractors remember well the smear campaigns that the AMA financed in the 1960's. The AMA lost in court.

As the groundswell amongst the laypersons gathers momentum, change will come. Insurance companies, eventually respond to the will of their policyholders or they go out of business. Politicians respond to their constituents, or they lose the next election.

The stakes are high and this is why so much money flows into things like evidence-based medicine. The educational content is usually designed to steer the holistically curious, but conventionally trained physician back into the fold of the complex.

Good luck and God bless

APPENDICES

Appendix A
Stiff Red Blood Cells and Old Age

Most of the mainstream discussions about heart and cerebral vascular disease ignore the health of the red blood cells. Instead, they focus on the amount of stiffness; 'rust' formation and plaque build up within the blood vessels. All these considerations prove valid, but leaving out an intelligent discussion on what science knows about the red cells health accelerates drug sales and costs owners.

The cells that travel within these vessels (the pipes) form a very important determinant of the body's health. The cells which travel within the blood vessels can only be young and efficiently perform their purpose, when they are both flexible and without 'rust'.

Oxidation causes 'rust'. 'Rust' leads to '"Velcro"' formation. "Velcro" formation, within the blood vessel walls, causes the macrophage cells to form a patch. Macrophage cells feed on LDL cholesterol. Eventually, they grow into foam cells. Foam cells cause a clot to form when their contents de-stabilize. In the heart, or brain, this event is known as a myocardial infarction or cerebral vascular event, respectively.

The loss of red blood cell flexibility causes hardness within the body. Hard blood vessels occur after many years of high blood pressure. Unfortunately, the contribution of stiff red blood cells to elevated blood pressure tends to be ignored and again, more prescriptions become necessary.

Many chronic degenerative diseases are made worse or arise completely from these two destructive processes that damage the blood cells. Examples include: high blood pressure, fibromyalgia, complications from diabetes, peripheral vascular disease, brain deterioration syndromes, cardiac ischemia, kidney injury, and splenomegaly. When the blood cells sustain damage, restoring flexibility and function can restore them to health.

The cells that flow through the blood vessels perform some of the body's most vital functions. First, no matter where oxygen transports in the body (organs, muscle, bone, etc.), it first must be delivered by the red blood cells. The red cells deliver oxygen to the cells at the capillary level. The capillary is the level where oxygen squeezes from the red cell. The red blood cells arrive at the capillaries and literally squeeze down, as it passes through the narrow capillaries. This squeezing action releases the oxygen from the red blood cells into the body cells serviced by the capillary. This squeezing action occurs because the average capillary is slightly smaller than the diameter of a single red blood cell. Healthy red blood cells deform and squeeze through the capillary in a smooth manner. After the red blood cell traverses the capillary, the healthy red cell quickly recovers its shape.

The trillions of red blood cells within the body have the consistency of a sponge. At the level of the capillary, where oxygen unloads, a stiff sponge causes problems. When stiffness occurs, the red blood cell will tend to clog the capillary and not compress sufficiently to deliver the oxygen, nutrients, etc. which it carries.

The re-inflation of the sponge creates a vacuum effect. This vacuum causes the red blood cell to absorb waste molecules created by the body's tissue cells. The heart's beating creates the pressure wave, which propels the red blood cells forward. It is the pressure wave created by the heart that propels these sponges through these tight spaces within the body tissues. When a red cell has become stiffened or 'rusted', it has less elasticity to accomplish this important task of oxygen delivery in an optimal manner. An owner becomes more vulnerable to degenerative disease as the volume of sickly red blood cells increases within the body.

The analogy of the sponge describes a mechanism of high blood pressure. The heart pushes harder to move stiff red blood cells through the tight capillaries. To accomplish this, the blood pressure must go up. This explains why one of the most popular classes of blood pressure medicines is the calcium channel blocker. Calcium channel blockers make stiff red blood cells more flexible by increasing the red cell's magnesium level. Rather than physicians' educations providing them this fact about increased magnesium intake naturally acting as a calcium channel blocker, they are only taught about prescription type calcium channel blockers. Prescriptions always have side effects and toxicities.

The red blood cells have unique energy requirements. The red blood cells are analogous to a man buried to his neck in sand with flasks of water all around him. The water is analogous to oxygen within the red blood cell. The water content within flasks by the man's head cannot do the man any good because he lacks the appendages to get the water to his lips. The situation for oxygen usage within the red cells proves similar. Even though they transport huge amounts of oxygen, they lack the machinery to combust oxygen for their energy needs. This is true because red cells lack mitochondria. Without mitochondria, red cells are unable to burn fuel aerobically. The red cell is forced to burn fuel anaerobically, which enfeebles their ability to do normal cellular work. Cellular work within the red blood cell dramatically decreases because without oxygen, there will be less energy creation per gram of sugar consumed. Anaerobically consumed sugar creates a constant source of lactic acid as a waste product.

The fact that dead blood cells can still transport oxygen is important. This unfortunately happens in transfused blood because it's difficult to keep blood alive for longer than about seven days. The practice of transfusing dead blood into post surgical patients may be responsible for the massive organ destruction that is commonly called DIC (diffuse intra-vascular coagulation). Problems arise with dead red blood cells because without life, they are unable to generate the energy necessary to remain as flexible. Not all dead red blood cells plug the capillary, but with other dietary and lifestyle bad habits that are practiced by the donor of the blood, the risk increases (see below for details).

During the red blood cell's one hundred and twenty day lifespan, it must remain flexible. Mainstream medicine sometimes offers prescriptions, like pentoxyphyline, that have a beneficial effect on red blood cell flexibility. However, these medicines are expensive and often have side effects. In contrast, known nutritional and lifestyle choices exist that will positively effect the flexibility of red blood cells.

FACTORS THAT DETERMINE RED BLOOD CELL FLEXIBILITY

1. **Electrical cell membrane potential (the strength of the force field)**
2. **High cellular magnesium content**
3. **Low cellular calcium content**
4. **High cellular potassium content**
5. **Low cellular sodium content**
6. **Adequate cellular zinc levels**
7. **Optimal ferrous hemoglobin with minimal ferric hemoglobin**
8. **Optimal blood sugar**
9. **Healthy dietary fat choices**
10. **Quality of steroids transported within the red blood cell**
11. **Quality of enzymatic machinery within the cell**
12. **Adequate copper**
13. **The level of completeness of the methyl donor system**
14. **Adequacy of Vitamin C**
15. **Waste level within the blood stream**
16. **Thyroid status**
17. **Cholesterol status**
18. **Availability of glucosamine and galactosamine**
19. **Glutathione levels and other anti-oxidants**
20. **Level of exposure to oxidants, rust promoters, in the environment [ozone, volatile acids, inappropriate blood metals, smoking]**

1. The electrical red blood cell membrane (the strength of the force field)

Red blood cells, like other body cells, protect themselves and perform useful cellular work by the maintenance of an electrically charged membrane. However, unlike other body cells, the red blood cell is more vulnerable because its electrical charging ability is greatly reduced. Red blood cells are energetically weak. They cannot use oxygen, and are, therefore, forced into anaerobic metabolism.

One of the determinants of these cells's flexibility concerns the strength of the voltage contained in the cell membrane. Processes that weaken the voltage will make the red cell contents vulnerable to hostile invasion forces and also allow a loss in flexibility. Optimal ratios between potassium, magnesium, sodium, and calcium form a prerequisite for strong cell voltages. The red cells prove as the most vulnerable because they have diminished energy secondary to their anaerobic metabolism limitation. Processed food diets eventually prevent the red cells from having these optimal mineral ratios (chapters 4 and 8).

2. High inside the cell magnesium content

Adequate magnesium within the red blood cells causes the red blood cells to become more flexible. The blood pressure will be reduced as a result. Adequate magnesium within the red blood cell, past middle age in America, is unlikely if an owner eats a diet of processed food instead of real food.

Magnesium is also required by the red blood cells to create energy by the combustion of glucose in an anaerobic fashion. The red blood cell cannot create the energy packets (ATP and NADH, NADPH, etc.) to perform their work without adequate levels of magnesium.

The correct proportion of magnesium and potassium within the red blood cell, creates the best possible energy content within the cell membrane. In contrast, there is the additional benefit of also having a low concentration of both calcium and sodium inside the red blood cell. The red blood cells require a constant level of energy supply in order to maintain the optimal ratios of these minerals. These four minerals' concentrations form a powerful determinant to the health of any body cell. When one mineral within the red blood cell becomes deficient or excessive, their proportional relationship with one another becomes altered. When the mineral relationships alter within a cell, health consequences will occur (see ***The Body Heals***).

3. Low inside the red blood cell calcium concentration

Red blood cells contain less calcium than most of the other cell types in the body. This probably protects the hemoglobin content within the red blood cell or the enzymatic machinery that burns sugar for energy creation. As the magnesium content decreases inside the red blood cell, more calcium rushes inside. If the amount of calcium within the body cells becomes too high, the calcium tends to injure the other cellular contents. This fact underscores the need for adequate magnesium relative to calcium content within the body.

4. High cellular potassium content

The red blood cell needs potassium, like magnesium, in high concentrations inside it for many reasons. Adequate potassium within the body proves necessary for proteins to remain stable. Red blood cells will often sacrifice their potassium content for the blood stream's needs. The price paid for this donation expresses itself as a weakened electrical charge of the red blood cell membrane. A weakened electrical charge means the red blood cell has less energy for both work (flexibility) and protecting itself from the invasion of hostile ions (calcium, fluoride, etc.). However, the body prioritizes the potassium in the serum over the potassium in the red blood cell. Eventually, the deficient potassium situation recruits other body cells to sacrifice their potassium content, as well. The trouble, in part, arises because all body cells need adequate potassium in order to stabilize their protein content. Muscle cells need potassium to make larger muscle tissue. Muscle tissue is made up of protein. Therefore, owners that desire youthful vitality, need adequate potassium within their red blood cells and other body cells.

Insulin needs adequate potassium to effectively deliver fuel to the cells. High carbohydrate diets tax the potassium within the blood stream, because as sugar goes inside the cellular fuel tanks, it also must pull potassium with it (one for one ratio). The blood steam plasma must keep plasma concentrations of potassium relatively stable. In this situation, the red blood cell is forced to give up too much of its potassium. The red blood cell is first in line for donating some of its potassium, when potassium levels are low within the blood stream. Refined sugars come largely devoid of potassium content and, therefore, these types of meals can create this situation. As the problem becomes more chronic, other body cells will donate potassium to prevent further drops in the serum potassium level.

5. Low inside the cell sodium content

Stress greatly increases the tendency for sodium content to rise inside the red blood cell. This occurs until the body is near death, and then sodium content begins to fall off. The human body was not designed for chronic stress. Modern life can tend to be stressful. This fact will tend to increase inside the red blood cell sodium because stress causes sodium retention and potassium loss. The problem exaggerates for those under stress when they chronically consume a processed food diet. In these situations, the red blood cell is forced to compromise its own well being in order to improve the way the blood plasma appears. This explains why the usual blood test, which measure serum potassium, can be misleading as to the true inside the cell status for potassium content (explained better in ***The Body Heals***). Chronic stress and high sodium diets form another mechanism for the compromise of red blood cell integrity.

6. Adequate zinc levels

Adequate zinc is needed within the body cell types that make acid (hydrogen proton) or base (bicarbonate) from carbon dioxide gas. To do this, they need the enzyme, carbonic anhydrase. Carbonic anhydrase needs zinc for activity. Red blood cells, stomach, pancreas, brain, prostate, kidneys, and the testes, all need to do this. In some tissues like the stomach, this enzyme splits carbon dioxide to secrete acid. In others, like the pancreas, the opposite reaction occurs in that it secretes bicarbonate instead. In other cases, carbonic anhydrase prevents excessive body acid from accumulating, and consequently from damaging intracellular structures. Preservation of the red blood cell's architectural integrity is only possible when just the right amount of pH occurs. This enzyme proves fundamental within the body for pH balance. In the case of red blood cells it allows a continued oxygen carrying capacity. Owners' cells that lack adequate zinc levels are vulnerable to many other harmful processes.

7. Adequate ferrous hemoglobin

The iron contained on the hemoglobin in the red blood cell carries oxygen to the body's cells. When the iron contained on hemoglobin oxidizes (ferric hemoglobin), it becomes unable to transport oxygen. Less oxygen transport means less of it is available to the tissues. The body has an elaborate and multi layered system to prevent this oxidation from occurring in more than nominal amounts. Even when this oxidation occurs in excessive amounts, the healthy body has multiple systems to remedy the problem. This fact is better explained below [See the methyl donor system (13), Vitamin C (14), and glutathione levels (19)].

There are medications that irrevocably damage the red blood cell's ability to bind oxygen. Medications like sulfa drugs, acetaminophen, nitroglycerin and phenacetin, all have the potential to irreversibly form sulf-hemoglobin. Mal-digestive states can also allow hydrogen sulfide gas (rotten egg smell to farts) to become absorbed into the blood stream and combine with the red blood cell. When this happens, hemoglobin will never carry oxygen again. If one is suspicious, they can order a sulf-hemoglobin level and see what percentage of their blood proves unable to carry oxygen.

8. Both a high and low blood sugar can injure the red blood cell's flexibility

Uncontrolled diabetes (high blood sugar) has long been known to cause the red blood cells to become stiff. This constitutes a powerful mechanism for the etiology of the microvascular complications from diabetes. Conspicuous examples of the cell hardening are demonstrated when stiffened red blood cells become wedged in the capillaries of a diabetic's foot or retina.

Hypoglycemia has an adverse effect on red blood cell function. Low blood sugar renders the red blood cell vulnerable to penetration from ions like calcium. These ions will irreversibly bind with cellular contents such as proteins, causing deformation. Deformation of cell proteins causes diminished function. When the low blood sugar becomes severe enough there also arises the possibility of killing some of one's red blood cells off and, therefore, decreasing their flexibility permanently. Realize that dead red blood cells still carry oxygen. However, numerous hostile forces within the blood stream rapidly damage dead red blood cells.

9. The adequacy of healthy fat choices in one's diet

The fats contained on and within the red blood cell prove unique when compared to most other body cells. They are more similar to the brain's fat make up. These types of fats require huge amounts of the vitamins and nutrients contained within the methyl donor system (see 13 below and chapter 5). When these vitamins and nutrients are sufficient in supply, the fat content of the red blood cells and nerves optimizes. Optimized fat makeup constitutes a powerful determinant of red blood cell flexibility and nerve cell health.

When an owner eats processed foods, around middle age, varying levels of nutritional deficiency begin to occur. In many ways the red blood cell is more vulnerable than other body cells because it has a more limited ability to repair itself once damage has occurred. The red blood cell's limited ability to repair itself arises from three main sources. First, because it lacks a cell nucleus it cannot manufacture new proteins once protein damage occurs. Second, because it lacks mitochondria, energy generation becomes greatly reduced, even in the best of circumstances. Reduced energy generation leads to less ability for the work of repairing damaged fat. Third, the blood stream is a hostile environment in many life situations, and the red blood cell fat is potentially exposed to these forces at a high rate of occurrence. Damaged fats, on the surface of the red blood cell, accumulate and compromise the flexibility of the blood cell. Certain dietary habits and nutritional deficiencies provide another mechanism to injure the flexibility of the red blood cells.

10. The quality of the body steroids forms a determinant of flexibility

Many of the body steroids are transported intermingled with the fats of the red blood cell membrane. High levels of cortisol tend to decrease flexibility, while high levels of estrogen increase it. Many steroids rely on an interaction with the red blood cells as part of their delivery strategies to their target cells. In fact, enzymatic machines, within the red blood cell exist, which convert the original steroid hormone to more powerful and different steroids. One such enzyme, 17Beta dehydrogenase, acts upon some steroids, like estrogen.

11. The quality of the enzymatic machinery within the red blood cell

While the red blood cell was being constructed within the bone marrow, the cell's enzymes (cellular machines) were determined. The construction phase is the only time that a red blood cell contains DNA. DNA is necessary to instruct the manufacture of proteins which make up the red blood cell. The type and amount of the different enzymes that were made during this process, are largely determined by the quality of the message content (types of hormones). The type of hormone message content determines the instructions, which the DNA program within the immature red blood cell receives. Message content directs the DNA program. The DNA program activity determines which proteins are made within a cell. All enzymes are made from protein. Therefore, enzyme content within a cell is determined by what hormones instructed the various DNA programs. This is the last chance a red blood cell will ever get in regard to what it is metabolically equipped with, in order to perform, because it's own genetic program (DNA content) gets destroyed shortly after it releases into the circulation. In contrast, all other body cells have their DNA program still present. DNA content allows these cells to create new proteins, when older proteins become damaged. Owners who have poor informational direction at the level of their bone marrow, crank out inferiorly equipped red blood cells. The lack of genetic material within the red blood cell, after it releases into the blood stream, causes it to have unique needs and vulnerabilities.

12. Adequate copper proves necessary for an important enzyme's manufacture within the bone marrow during the red blood cell's construction phase.

One of the enzymes that are constructed while the red blood cell is being created within the bone marrow is called, catalase. This enzyme protects the red blood cell from oxygen radicals by neutralizing them. Some owners are copper deficient and this is a critical trace mineral that is needed to make the enzyme catalase. Deficiency of this enzyme causes the red blood cell to age quickly and lose its flexibility.

13. The level of completeness of all the molecular components of the methyl donor system constitutes a big determinant of red blood cell flexibility

One billion times a second, the body relies on the methyl donor system to prevent breakdown in molecular structure, or improve biological messengers throughout the body. Specialized fats in the brain and red blood cells, require extremely high amounts of the nutrients that make up the methyl donor system. This fact explains why people who fail to eat enough fat in their diet tend to become deficient within this system. The low fat diet adherents use up tremendous amounts of their methyl donor system nutrients to manufacture these specialized fats. This quantity of these types of fats is routinely included in a more balanced diet (chapters 13 and 14). The depletion of the methyl donor system by the low fat diet causes a deficiency of these specialized fats as well.

Choline (lecithin building block) provides an example of the debilitating effect of the low fat diet. Choline is a specialized fat building block. Specialized fats are needed in high concentrations within both the red blood cell and nervous system. Choline synthesis requires three methyl groups for manufacturing it one time. These specialized fats are needed by the gazillions within both the brain and red blood cell. Eggs are nature's best source of choline. The methyl donor system depends on numerous vitamins and amino acids. Methyl depletes at the rate of one billion times a second even when one eats ample fat in their diet. Owners that eat diminished fat need many times this amount per second or methyl deficiencies arise. Depletion of this system is sometimes the root cause of many degenerative diseases, like: high blood pressure, fatty liver disease, spontaneous kidney hemorrhages, neuro-degenerative disease, and blood vessel disease (explained elsewhere).

14. The adequacy of Vitamin C in the body

When other anti-oxidants become deficient (glutathione, trimethyl glycine, and ergothioneine), Vitamin C levels deplete rapidly. The maintenance of ferrous hemoglobin (see above) within the red blood cell, requires sufficient Vitamin C. This is the only form of iron that can transport oxygen to the body tissues. When Vitamin C depletes in this fashion the total daily requirement increases tremendously. Some clinicians claim that the signs of scurvy (Vitamin C deficiency) can develop when other anti-oxidants become deficient. The signs of scurvy occur, because the rate of usage of Vitamin C, is many times greater than normal when other anti-oxidants diminish. The major anti-oxidant within the red blood cell, glutathione, prevents the rapid depletion of Vitamin C. This simple peptide consists of three amino acids. Certain prescription medications tend to deplete, this important substance, from both the red blood cell and the liver. Certain prescriptions and nutritional bad habits tend to deplete Vitamin C more quickly (see liver chapter). When these situations occur, one's Vitamin C intake needs to increase. Ample Vitamin C within the red blood cell will allow continued ferrous hemoglobin content. Remember, ferrous hemoglobin proves the only form of iron that can transport oxygen.

15. **Waste level within the blood stream (this fact is beyond the level of this discussion see *The Body Heals*)**

16. **Thyroid status and red blood cell flexibility**

The amount of thyroid message content (hormone level) affects the amount of cholesterol inside the red blood cell. Cholesterol within the red blood cell competes with the specialized fats. Specialized fats, like phospholipid, give the red blood cell the maximum of flexibility. Just like increased thyroid states tending to lower the serum cholesterol, the same trend appears to be true with the red blood cell fat composition. High thyroid function increases the proportion of phospholipid relative to cholesterol in the red blood cell membrane. Conversely, low thyroid function retards flexibility. Thyroid hormone plays an important role within the body, in facilitating waste removal activities from the cells, including red blood cells. The colon, immune system, kidney's, lung, skin and liver depend on adequate thyroid message content for their waste removal activities.

17. **Cholesterol status** (explained in *Glandular Failure-Caused Obesity*)

18. **Availability of glucosamine and galactosamine to the red blood cell**

The availability of glucosamine and galactosamine is one of the significant determinants of flexibility of red blood cells. These substances promote the process of "gelation". This process allows the red blood cells to deform within the capillary. Jell-O is composed of both galactosamine and glucosamine.

These are obtained from grinding up and partially digesting animal cartilage. The same molecules that give jell-O its consistency also creates the flexibility of the red blood cells. Various combinations of modified galactosamine and glucosamine form the GAG content in the body.

Earlier it was explained how the GAG content determines the water content in a cell. The amount of GAG depends on the amount of insulin-like growth factor type one (IGF-1). The important role for IGF-1 in the body continues to be largely ignored because of the numerous name changes, which describe it in the literature. Name changes isolate scientific knowledge effectively.

In order for a physician to appreciate the many important roles of IGF-1 he/she would need to know the following three names describe the same hormone: sulfation factor, somatomedin C, and the nonsuppressible insulin-like activity of the blood stream.

The sulfation name describes the critical step in GAG formation, the addition of sulfate. Sulfate because of its electrical charge powerfully attracts water into a body local. Only with sufficient water can a cell avoid the shrinkage of old age.

19. Glutathione levels

This important antioxidant keeps the preformed enzymes and oxygen carrying capacities intact for the life of the red blood cell. Prescription drugs, could possibly deplete these antioxidants. One common medication ingredient, which requires glutathione for metabolism is acetaminophen. There are many other medications that deplete glutathione. Glutathione is found mainly in the liver and the red blood cells. Quality protein intake proves necessary to increase production of this important antioxidant.

20. The level of exposure to oxidants (rust promoters) such as environmental ozone, volatile acids in smog, inappropriate blood serum levels of metals and minerals (aluminum, fluoride).

The more the blood cells encounter rust promoters, the greater the need for the anti-oxidants within the blood stream. (Ideally, one should also be thinking about ways to reduce chronic exposure to rust promoters).

An increased blood fluoride and iodide levels will poison the energy metabolism of red blood cells. Increased exposure to these minerals will tend to jeopardize the red cells' energy production. Red blood cells whose energy production has been compromised are vulnerable to the rust and hardening mechanisms (#'s 1-20). Fluoride is a powerful rust (oxidizing agent) promoter ion within the body. This gives the average owner something to think about, the next time while shopping for toothpaste, and in deciding about iodized salt consumption.

The medical media's focus has largely been on the blood vessel, but the cells within it, prove important for one's pursuit of healthful longevity. The sensationalism of what is for sale by the complex, has largely excluded the important consideration, of how flexible one's red blood cells are within the pipes. The exclusion that regards the abilities of the trillions of microscopic sponges within has cost owners in America plenty. This is evidenced by both the quality of life lost and in the need for symptom-control medicine, with all it's side effects and diminished out comes.

When these microscopic sponges remain pliable, their ability to carry oxygen, nutrients, and deliver important body hormones proves sufficient. This process, can be thought of as, similar to when a sponge gets wrung from its water content. Like wise, when red blood cells, at the level of the capillary, squeeze out their contents of hormones, nutrients and oxygen, their flexibility forms a crucial determinant of how efficient one receives the molecules that are necessary for life to continue.

Processes, that stiffen the red blood cell, predictably will lessen this life giving process, and the owner will get a little bit older.

Appendix B
Hierarchy of Hormones - Informational Substances

It helps, to have a concise grouping of how the different hormones can be separated into a successive hierarchy. The hierarchy between the different hormones concerns, their degree of influence and length of action, when compared to one another. There are four basic groups, of successive levels of influence, on how the body spends energy. Hormones direct cell energy usage. The more powerful the hormone group, the more central it is, in the energy direction, when it arrives.

Sadly, mainstream medicine often focuses on the 'lesser' hormones. The lesser hormones receive press coverage, while the more powerful hormones, are only peripherally addressed. By taking this approach, to chronic disease treatment strategies, symptom-control is all that remains possible. Symptom-control medical approaches, always produce side effects, and have nothing to do with healing. By adding back, the hormone hierarchy, these errors become easy to expose.

Grouping the different informational substances (hormones) into four groups will help in understanding the interdependent relationship of the many various hormones. Also, many chronic degenerative diseases will begin to have healing solutions.

Common degenerative diseases amenable to healing once the hormone hierarchy is addressed are: adrenal gland caused asthma, rheumatoid arthritis, systemic lupus erythromatosus, osteoarthritis, adult onset diabetes, obesity, some cases of heart disease, ulcerative colitis, Crohn disease, some liver diseases, some kidney diseases, some cases of senility, and muscle wasting diseases.

All of these diseases, have an increased likelihood of a solution, when the clinician attends to these disease's treatment, in a logical progression, from the most powerful hormone imbalances down to the weakest. When supplementation strategies are needed, real hormones are used, because only they contain accurate message content. The body was designed for real hormone-message content. Whenever the altered shaped of the hormone substitutes are given in place of real hormones, there are always side effects. When the shape changes, to get a patent, the message content changes. Simple science discussed here but not commonly taught in a way that physicians can understand.

The four groups in the hierarchy of hormones are:

Group 1 - the supreme commanders of body energy

This powerful group of hormones directly switches off and on different DNA programs (genes). The DNA programs activated in a cell determine, the activity of the cell, and the degree of repair (rejuvenation). The activity and state of repair determine the usefulness of the cell. When cells are given good informational direction from the level one hormone class, they will be productive and healthy. The thyroid hormones, steroids, and Vitamin A, comprise the level one hormone class. The quality of the mixture and amount of level one hormones, which reach the over one hundred trillion cells, centrally determines health. An owner's health, is powerfully influenced, because these hormones all contain message content that instructs the DNA (genes) program activity.

The level one hormone class (steroids, Vitamin A and thyroid hormones), comprises the only hormones powerful enough to directly interact and instruct cellular genetic material (the DNA). Quality of the proportional mixture between these hormones determines the highest level of energy expenditure. At this primary level these hormones quality of presence determines whether a cell uses available energy efficiently or not. This class of hormone has access to every body chamber. All healthy owners predictably have high quality message content amongst the level one hormone class. Conversely, unhealthy owners predictably have lousy hormone quality as part of their aging process. These owners will continue to age prematurely, until someone helps these owners regain more optimal message content.

Group 2 – the amino acid chain

All hormones, message content is about directing cellular expendable energy. Level two hormones deliver a message when they bind to a cell surface receptor (their own unique type) or they bind a receptor inside the target cell. The level two hormones are only able to influence cell energy expenditure on existing cell structures and enzymatic machinery activity. They are unable to direct DNA programs in the manufacture of new cell structures or new enzymatic machinery. Only level one hormones are powerful enough to do that

Insulin and glucagon provide examples of level two hormones. Like other level two hormones, they are made up of a specific sequence of amino acids that are twisted around in three-dimensional space. The shape of these specific sequences and resulting twist contains precise message content. Insulin and glucagon are also an example of level two hormones that contain opposite message content. The message content difference between insulin and glucagon directs the target cell to spend energy in the opposite way. Consistent with level two hormones, each can only affect existing cellular enzymatic machines or structural content. Insulin turns off the enzyme machines that glucagon turns on. Likewise, the message content of glucagon turns off what insulin turns on. Each of these opposing hormones has enzyme machines that they activate. The direction of energy within a cell determines which enzymes are quiet or active. Hormones direct which way energy moves in a cell. Catabolism versus anabolism describes an example of opposite energy movement.

The liver cells prove instructive as an example for the opposite energy direction between the message content of insulin and glucagon. Insulin directs liver cell energy into fuel storage (anabolism). Fuel is stored in various locations, but insulin stimulates the liver in the manufacture of glycogen, triglycerides, cholesterol, and LDL cholesterol. Insulin also inhibits the liver from turning amino acids into sugar and fat. The more insulin in the body, the more these activities occur within the liver. Conversely, glucagon directs the liver to release stored fuel and curtails new cholesterol and triglyceride manufacture (catabolic effect). It also stimulates the liver contained enzymatic machines to make sugar from available amino acids.

Some level two hormones are further endowed with the ability to leave a 'last will and testament' before being chewed up into component parts by intracellular machinery. Intracellular machinery eventually dismantles the level two hormones. There is an intermediate step. The last will and directive of some level two hormones occurs between activating their receptor and being dismantled. The last will and directives are additional messages to the cell created by level two hormones activating level four hormones. These messages exist for a limited time. During that time, the level two hormones affect which level four hormone precursors a cell will receive message content from.

Insulin and glucagon provide good examples of how a hormone's presence determines which level four hormone precursors are formed. Also consistent is the fact that level four hormones precursors, stimulated by insulin, have the opposite effect on cell energy, when mature, as the direction that glucagon level four hormones impart (see group 4 below).

Group 3 – the subservient hormones

The level three hormones are composed of single amino acids, which have been structurally modified or are composed of short chains of amino acids. These hormones depend on directives of the higher hormones 'stage setting'. The level one and two hormones set the stage for structural integrity and enzyme machinery contained in a cell. The stage setting is centrally determined by the level one hormones at the DNA level. In turn, the level two hormones determine the activity of the setting, the enzymes. The level three hormones channel blood and fuel to the cells. However, the level three hormones depend on level one hormones directing the manufacture of their receptors. Without enough level three-hormone receptors being made, many chronic diseases begin (asthma from epinephrine receptor deficiency). The level four hormones can only affect the 'props' within the cell.

Biogenic amines, cytokines, and endothelin all belong to this class of hormones. Dietary deficiencies can effect development and manufacture of these hormones. Many different vitamins prove important for biogenic amines' manufacture. In general, the level three hormones have an effect on the caliber of blood vessels and properties of the cells in these vessels in a certain area of the body.

The level three hormones delivering message content in a certain blood vessel determines much about the oxygen availability, nutrient delivery, waste removal, stickiness of the vessel wall, clotting tendency, and immune cell behavior.

Group 4 – local acting, subservient hormones

These hormones exist for seconds, only long enough to deliver message content to nearby cells. Within seconds of their release, they are deactivated. These hormones only having an influence for both the duration and as far as the sound of their 'voice' will travel. This is in contrast to the other three levels of hormones that can travel more extensively in delivering their message content.

Some of the level four hormones, like nitric oxide gas, have powerful penetration abilities through body barriers. Although nitric oxide has powerful penetrating abilities, its message content delivery ability is limited due to its rapid deactivation. This short lifespan diminishes the distance of influence of nitric oxide's message content.

Other level four hormones, like the ecosanoids (hormonal fats) that include prostaglandins, leukotrienes, and lipoxin are also limited by their short life spans. The ecosanoids come from essential fatty acids (hormonal fat precursors). These include linoleic, linolenic, and arachidonic acid. All three of these essential fatty acids can only be obtained in the diet. The type of diet determines which level two hormones message content will predominate.

An example of the opposing possibilities of level two hormones and how they determine what level four hormones are possible occurs between insulin and glucagon. The opposite message content contained between glucagon and insulin has a powerful influence on which level four precursor hormones are possible. High carbohydrate diets tend to promote the pro-inflammatory hormonal fat precursors to line many cells. Certain low carbohydrate and high protein/fat diets promote anti-inflammatory hormonal fat precursors. The type of level two hormones limits the possibilities for which level four hormone precursors line numerous cells. Those hormonal fat precursors that line the surface of cells determine the likelihood of developing or preventing some malicious chronic degenerative diseases. Some diseases effected by the presence or the absences of hormonal fat precursors are cancer, heart disease, arthritis, depression, fatigue and immunodeficiency syndromes.

There are three principles about the ecosanoids (hormonal fats) that are important. First, only green plants can make two out of three of these hormonal fat precursors called the essential fatty acids. Animals like salmon that live in the wild eat plankton and, therefore, contain significant amounts of these two plant manufactured essential fatty acids. Farmed, grain-fed animals are raised without these essential fatty acids presence.

The green plant manufactured essential fatty acids are linolenic and linoleic acid. Free-range chicken eggs are good sources for these plants derived essential fatty acids. Wild game such as elk and deer are also sources for these two essential fatty acids. These are good sources for essential fatty acids because of the high content of green plants in their diet. Green plants are the source of the anti-inflammatory fatty acids, linolenic and linoleic acids. Non-green roots and grains are more likely to contain the pro-inflammatory arachidonic acid. Store bought chicken, meat and eggs, because the animals are grain fed, will be higher in the arachidonic acid type.

Second, eating all the right essential fatty acids can still output the wrong hormonal fats. These fats are subservient to the more powerful higher hormones. Level two hormones like insulin and glucagon determine which hormone fat precursors become created from essential fatty acids in the diet. The essential fatty acids in the diet are the raw material created for precursor hormonal fats. The balance of message content between insulin and glucagon predetermine which precursors are created.

Third, hormonal fat precursors are ideally contained on all the cell surfaces. When released, these hormones have a limited area of influence because of their short lifespan. Scientist denote this shortened hormone lifespan by the term paracrine. Paracrine hormones can only deliver message content in their immediate area of release. All level four hormones are paracrine in nature. The level four hormones are only released when triggered by higher hormones. Sub-optimal hormonal fat message content has a powerful influence on several chronic diseases.

The hormonal fats are so important that many powerful medications work by poisoning their ability to be produced. Some medications that work by poisoning hormonal fats are aspirin and related non-steroidal anti-inflammatory medications, cortisone derivatives, and the newer cox 2 inhibitors. These symptom-control approaches have consequences to the balance of fine tuning abilities, occurring in cells. All of these redirect body energy. With an understanding of hormonal fats and how to optimize their function, one can work with their body and begin healing.

Nitric oxide has a powerful ability to lower blood pressure and is also within this fourth class of hormones. It can only briefly increase blood delivery into its local area. This is how the medication Viagra works and why all the warnings about it lowering blood pressure are given. The medicine's content of nitric oxide increases blood flow to the penis. This natural blood flow regulator requires the presence of the nutritional co-factors: arginine, riboflavin, tetrahydrobiopterin, and thiols for its biosynthesis. Thiols are contained in garlic and onions. Tetrahydrobiopterin derives from folate. How many hypertensive and impotent owners originate simply from these nutritional deficiencies?

Be aware of the hierarchy of different hormone groups and what dietary factors are required for them to be produced. Owners, who have optimal balance at each level are in good health. Conversely, a lowered quality of informational content occurring at any of the successive levels or dietary deficiencies leads to health consequences. The science exists to help owners receive better hormones and good nutrition.

Appendix C
Disarm and Remove Toxins

The liver needs certain molecular parts to disarm many different types of toxins that are encountered when the owner creates or ingests them.

Toxins made by every day processes:

Natural body waste	Drugs
Ingested toxins	Cookware
Food additives	Food pollutants
Air pollutants	Water pollutants
Herbicides	Heavy metals
Toxins absorbed from an unhealthy colon	

The liver has a choice on how it will disarm any toxin. There are five common mechanisms for the initial inactivation of toxins. In general, all five of these processes facilitate the next phase of liver detoxification. In the initial stage the liver machinery creates a molecular appendage, which it can use to attach the final removal compounds to. This allows the toxin to become water soluble or inactive. The final removal compounds cannot attach until one of five initial reactions occur (molecular appendage types).

The five initial liver deactivation methods are:

1. Oxidation
2. Hydrogen addition
3. Hydration (addition of water)
4. Cleavage through hydrolysis (removal of water)
5. Removal of chloride, fluoride, bromide or iodide

The trouble with these processes concerns the fact that they each tend to create reactive intermediates. The liver needs protection from these intermediates. The protective molecules needed by the liver are commonly called antioxidants or 'rust retardants'. The better the supply of these substances in one's liver, the more protection one has from liver injury. The greater the load of toxins, the more antioxidants needed. More antioxidants become necessary because they will be used up quickly.

The basic list of needed liver anti-oxidants is:

Vitamin A	Vitamin E
Vitamin C	Bioflavonoids (berries)
Selenium	Zinc
Coenzyme Q10	Pycnogenol (grape seeds)

Lipoic acid (real foods only)
Thiols that are found in garlic, onions, and cruciferous vegetables

These anti-oxidants are the basic protectors of the liver tissue. The liver cells need the protection of anti-oxidants because of the reactive intermediates created when the liver begins the first phase of deactivating and/or removing a body toxin. There are also certain vitamins and nutrients that are needed to power the molecular machinery that performs the task of disarmament.

The basic list of these vitamins is:

Vitamin B1	Lipoic acid
Vitamin B2	Co enzyme Q10
Vitamin B3	Pantothenic acid
Vitamin B6	Folic acid

Phospholipids such as lecithin

The liver must begin the initial attachment of molecular appendages without releasing reactive molecules that can oxidize liver cells. The antioxidants prevent the oxidants from causing liver rust. These initial deactivation steps require specific vitamins to power the enzymatic machinery needed for these activities. Once the liver cell has created the various appendages on a toxin, it needs to proceed on to deactivation.

The basic choices for the final reaction in toxin removal are the addition of:
Sulfate
Glucuronic acid
Glutathione or n-acetyl cysteine
Acetate
Methyl
Certain amino acids: glycine, taurine, glutamine, ornithine, and arginine

Depending on the final solubility characteristics, the deactivated toxin will either be excreted in the bile or blood stream. When excreted in the bile it will be removed in the feces. However, poor bacteria content in the colon can prevent this and the toxin can be absorbed back into the body. Some toxins reabsorb because the wrong bacteria rip apart the deactivation appendage that the liver attached.

When a water-soluble toxin excretes into the blood stream, it heads for the kidneys that can remove large amounts of toxins. Many toxins and hormone excesses that the kidney removes must first be made water-soluble by the liver. This includes ammonia, steroids, small chains of amino acids, and heavy metal complexes (Bland, 1996).

BIBLIOGRAPHY

Abou-Seif, MA., Youssef, AA. *Oxidative Stress and Male IGF-I, Gonadotropin and Related Hormones in Diabetic Patients.* Clin Chem Lab Med, July, Vol. 39, No. 7, 2001.

Abrams, William B., M.D., et al. *The Merck Manual of Geriatrics.* New Jersey: Merck Sharp & Dohme Research Laboratories, 1990.

Adams, Patch, M.D., et al. *Gesundheit!* Vermont: Healing Arts Press, 1993.

Adams MR. Oral L-arginine improves endothelium-dependent dilatation and reduces monocyte adhesion to endothelial cells in young men with coronary artery disease. Dept. of Cardiology, Royal Prince Alfred Hospital, Sydney, Australia.

Arvat, Emanuela, et. Al. (2000) Stimulatory Effect of Adrenocorticotropin on Cortisol, aldosterone and Dehydroepiandrosterone Secretion in Normal Humans: Dose Response Study. The Journal of Clinical Endocrinology and Metabolism. Vol. 85 No. 9 pages 3141-3146

Aoki, Kazutaka, et al. *Dehydroepiandrosterone Suppresses the Elevated Hepatic Glucose-6-Phosphatase and Fructose-1, 6-Biophosphatase Activities in C57BL/Ksj-db/db Mice.* Diabetes, Vol. 48, August 1999.

Adkins, Robert C., MD. *Dr Adkins' New Diet Revolution.* 2nd ed. New York: M. Evans and Company, Inc, 1999.

_____. *Dr Adkins' Vita-Nutrient Solution.* New York: Simon and Shuster, 1998.

Ames Company. *Modern Urine Chemistry.* Elkhart, IN: Miles Laboratories, Inc, 1982.

Arndt, Kenneth A., MD. *Manual of Dermatologic Therapeutics.* Boston: Little, Brown and Company, 1983.

Ballentine, Rudolph, MD. *Radical Healing.* New York: Harmony Books, 1999.

Balch, James F. M.D., et al. *Prescription of Natural Healing.* New York: Garden City Park, 1990.

Barazzoni, R., et. Al. (2000) Increased Fibrinogen Production in Type 2 Diabetic Patients without Detectable Vascular Complications:

Correlation with Plasma Glucagon Concentrations. Journal of Clinical Endocrinology and Metabolism. Vol. 85. No. 9 pages 3121-3125

Bareford, D., (1986) Effects of Hyperglycemia and sorbitol accumulation on erythrocyte deformability in diabetes mellitus. Journal of Clinical Pathology. Vol. 39 Issue 7

Bargen, J.A., MD, et al. *Every Woman's Standard Medical Guide.* Indianapolis: American Publishers' Alliance Corp., 1949.

Bate-Smith, E.C., ed. *Chemical Plant Taxonomy.* London: Spotttiswoode, Ballantyne and Company Limited, 1963.

Bauer, Cathryn. *Acupressure for Everybody.* New York: Henry Holt and Company, 1991.

Becker, Robert O., M.D., et al. *The Direct Current Control System, A Link Between Environment and Organism.* New York State Journal of Medicine, April 15, 1962.

Becker, Robert O., MD, et al. *The Body Electric.* New York: William Morrow and Company, Inc, 1985.

Beers, Mark H., MD, ed. *The Merck Manual of Diagnosis and Therapy.* Whitehouse Station, NJ: Merck Research Laboratories, 1999.

Behrendt, H., M.D. *Chemistry of Erythrocytes.* Illinois: Charles C Thomas Publisher, 1957.

Bellack, Leopold, MD, ed. *Psychology of Physical Illness.* New York: Grune & Stratton, 1952.

Bellamy, MF et Al. (1998) Hyperhomocystinemia After an Oral Methionine Load Acutely Impairs Endothelial Function in Healthy Adults. Circulation 98:1848-1852.

Ber, Abram M.D., F.R.C.P. *Neutralization of Phenolic (Aromatic) Food Compounds in a Holistic General Practice.*

Berezina TL et. Al. (2002) Influence of storage on red blood cell rheological properties. Surg. Res. Jan 2002 Volume 102(1) 6-12

Bergman, Richard N., et al. *Free Fatty Acids and Pathogenesis of Type 2 Diabetes Mellitus.* Trends In Endocrinology and Metabolisim, 11, 2000.

Berkow, Robert, MD, ed. *The Merck Manual of Medical Information.* Whitehouse Station, NJ: Merck Research Laboratories, 1997.

Bensky, Dan, et al. *Chinese Herbal Medicine, Mateia Medica.* Seattle: Eastland Press, Inc, 1986.

_____. *Chinese Herbal Medicine, Formulas and Strategies.* Seattle: Eastland Press, Inc, 1990.

Berkow, Robert, MD, ed. *The Merck Manual.* 15th ed. Rahway, NJ: Merck, Sharp, & Dohme Research Laboratories, 1987.

Bernstein, Richard K., MD, F.A.C.E. *Diabetes Solution.* New York: Little, Brown and Company, 1997.

Bland, Jeffery S., PhD, ed. *Clinical Nutrition: A Functional Approach.* Gig Harbor, WA: Institute for Functional Medicine, 1999.

Bland, Jeffrey, Ph.D., *Nutritional Endocrinology.* Washington: Metagenics Educational Programs, 2002.

Bown, Deni. *Growing Herbs.* New York: Dorling Kindersley Publishing, Inc., 1995.

_____. *Encyclopedia of Herbs and Their Uses.* New York: Dorling Kindersley Publishing, Inc, 1995.

Bradly, James, M.D, et al.. *Dr. Braly's Food Allergy & Nutrition Revolution.* Connecticut: Keats Publishing, Inc., 1992.

Bratman, Steven, M.D., et al. *Natural Health Bible.* 2nd ed. California: Prima Health, 2000.

Brennan, Barbara Ann. *Light Emerging.* New York: Bantam Books, 1993.

_____. *Hands of Light.* New York: Bantam Books, 1987.

Bricklin, Mark, ed. *The Practical Encyclopedia of Natural Healing.* Emmaus, PA: Rodale Press, 1976.

_____,et al. *The Practical Encyclopedia of Natural Healing New, Revised Edition.* Emmaus, PA: Rodale Press, 1983.

Bruce, Debra F., et al. *The Unofficial Guide to Alternative Medicine.* New York: Macmillian, Inc, 1989.

Burr, Harold S. *Blueprint for Immortality*. Essex, England: The C.W. Daniel Company Limited, 1972.

Brand, Paul, MD, et al. *Fearfully and Wonderfully Made*. Grand Rapids, MI: Zondervan Publishing House, 1980.

Brink, Marijke, et al. *Angiotensin II Induces Skeletal Muscle Wasting Through Enhanced Protein Degradation and Down-Regulates Autocrine Insulin-Like Growth Factor I*. Endocrinology, Vol. 142, No. 4, 2001.

Caine, Winston K., et al. *The Male Body: An Owner's Manual*. Emmaus, PA: Rodale Press, Inc, 1996.

Capra, Fritjof. *The Tao of Physics*. New York: Bantam Books, Inc, 1984.

Carey, Ruth, Ph.D., et al. *Common Sense Nutrition*. California: Pacific Press Publishing Association, 1971.

Cattaneo, L., et al. *Characterization of the Hypothalamo-Pituitary-IGF-I Axis in Rats Made Obese by Overfeeding*. Journal of Endocrinology, February, Vol. 148, No. 2, 1996.

Choi, Cheol S., et al. *Independent Regulation of in Vivo Insulin Action on Glucose Versus K+ Uptake by Dietary Fat and K+ Content*. Diabetes, Vol. 51, April, 2002.

Chopra, Deepak M.D. *Ageless Body, Timeless Mind*. New York: Harmony Books, 1993.

Chambers, John (1999) Demonstration of Rapid Onset Vascular Endothelial Dysfunction after Hyperhomocystinemia. Circulation 99:1156-1160.

Childe, Doc L., *The HeartMath Solution*. New York: HarperCollins Publishers, 1999.

Christ, Emanual R. et al. (1998) Dyslipidemia in adult Growth Hormone Deficiency and the Effect of GH Replacement Therapy. Trends in Endocrinology and Metabolism 9: 200-206

Clasey, JL., et al. *Abdominal Visceral Fat and Fasting Insulin are Important Predictors of GH Release Independent of Age, Gender, and Other Physiological Factors*. J Clin Endocrinol Metab, August, Vol. 86, No. 8, 2001.

Clemente, Carmine, Ph.D. *Anatomy A Regional Atlas of the Human Body*. Maryland: Urban & Schwarzenberg, 1981.

Cousins, Norman. *Anatomy of An Illness as Perceived By the Patient.* New York: Bantam Books, 1979.

Company, Merck &. *The Hypercholesterolemia Handbook.* Pennsylvania: Merck Sharp & Dohme, 1989.

Cush, Keneth and Ralph DeFronzo (2000) recombinant Human Insulin-Like Growth Factor 1 Treatment for 1 week Improves Metabolic Control in Type 2 Diabetes by Ameliorating Hepatic and Muscle Insulin Resistance. The Journal of Clinical Endocrinology and Metabolism. Vol. 85 No. 9 pages 3077-3084

Cusi, Kenneth, et al. *Recombinant Human Insulin-Like Growth Factor I Treatment for 1 Week Improves Metabolic Control in Type 2 Diabetes by Ameliorating Hepatic and Muscle Insulin Resistance.* The Journal of Clinical Endocrinology and Metabolism, Vol. 85. No. 9, 2000.

Danese, Mark D., (2000) Effect of Thyroxine Therapy on Serum Lipoproteins in Patients with Mild Thyroid Failure: a Quantitative Review of the Literature. Vol. 85 No. 9. Pages 2993-3001

Davenport, Horace W., DSc. *A Digest of Digestion.* 2nd ed. Chicago: Year Book Medical Publishers Inc, 1978.

DeBoer, H., et al. *Changes in Subcutaneous and Visceral Fat mass During Growth Hormone Replacement Therapy in Adult Men.* Int. Journal of Related Metabolic Disorders, June, Vol. 20, No. 6, 1996.

De Leo, Vicenzo. *Effect of Metformin on Insulin-Like Growth Factor (IGF) I and IGF-Binding Protein I in Polycystic Ovary Syndrome.* The Journal of Clinical Endocrinology & Metabolism, December, Vol. 85, No. 4, 2000.

Dessein, PH, et al. *Hyposecretion of Adrenal Androgens and the Relation of Serum Adrenal Steroids, Serotonin and Insulin-Like Growth Factor-1 to Clinical Features in Women with Fibromyalgia.* Pain, November, Vol. 83, No. 2, 1999.

Diamond, John W., M.D. *An Alternative Medicine Definitive Guide to Cancer.* California: Future Medicine Publishing, Inc., 1997.

Dobelis, Inge N. *Reader's Digest Magic and Medicine of Plants.* Pleasantville, NY: The Reader's Digest Association, Inc, 1986.

Dowsett, M. (1999) Drug and hormone interactions of aromatase inhibitors. Endocrine Related Cancer 6 181-185

Dwing, *During Puberty in Male Baboons.* Journal of Clinical Metabolism, January, Vol. 81, No. 1, 1996.

Eden, Donna, et al. *Energy Medicine.* New York: Penguin Putnam Inc, 1998.

Ejima J et Al. (2000) relationship of HDL cholesterol and red blood cell filterability: cross-sectional study of healthy subjects. Clinical Hemorheological Microcirculation 22(1): 1-7

Epstein, Donald, et al. *The 12 Stages of Healing.* California: Amber-Allen Publishing, 1994.

Erickson MD, Robert A (2001) Testosterone-Its Real Impact. Journal of Longevity Vol 7 No. 9

Fawcett, JP, (1994) Does cholesterol depletion have adverse effects on blood rheology? Angiology Volume 45 Issue 3

Ferril, MD, William. *Glandular Failure-Caused Obesity* (2004) The Bridge Medical Publishers, Whitefish, Montana.

Ferril, MD, William (2003) *The Body Heals*, Bridge Medical Pulishers, Whitefish, Montana.

Ferril MD, William (1998) Molecular Mechanisms of Biological Aging. Medicine Tree

Ferril MD, William (1998) The Adrenal Mystery. Medicine Tree

Fitzpatrick, Thomas B., et al. *Color Atlas and Synopsis of Clinical Dermatology.* 3d ed. New York: Mcgraw-Hill Companies, 1997.

Fottner, C., et el. *Regulation of Steroidogenesis by Insulin-Like Growth Factors (IGFs) in Adult Human Adrenocortical Cells: IGF-I and, more Potently, IGF-II Preferentially Enhance Androgen Biosynthesis Through Interaction With the IGF-I Receptor and IGF-Binding Proteins.* Journal of Endocrinol, September, Vol. 158, No. 3, 1998.

Frankel, Edward. *DNA: The Ladder of Life.* 2nd ed. New York: McGraw-Hill Book Company, 1979.

Frost, Robert A., Lang, Charles H. *Differential Effects of Insulin-Like Growth Factor I (IGF-I) and IGF-Binding Protein-1 on Protein Metabolism in Human Skeletal Muscle Cells.* Endocrinology, Vol. 140, No. 9, 1999.

Gaby, Alan R., MD, et al. *Nutritional Therapy in Medical Practice.* Kent, WA: Wright/Gaby Seminars, 1996.

Gangong, William F., MD. *Review of Medical Physiology.* 10th ed. Los Altos: Lange Medical Publications, 1981..

_____. *Review of Medical Physiology.* Los Altos: Lange Medical Publications, 1971

_____. *Review of Medical Physiology.* 19th ed. Stamford, CT: Appleton&Lange, 1999.

_____. *Review of Medical Physiology.* 20th ed. McGraw-Hill Companies, Inc., 2001.

Gardner, Joy. *Healing Yourself.* Freedom, CA: The Crossing Press, 1989

Gdansky, E., et al. *Increased Number of IGF-I Receptors on Erythrocytes of Women with Polycystic Ovarian Syndrome.* Clinical Endocrinal, August, Vol. 47, No. 2, 1997.

Gerber, Richard MD. *Vibrational Medicine.* Sante Fe: Bear and Company, 1996.

Gerras, Charles, ed. *The Complete Book of Vitamins.* Emmaus, PA: Rodale Press Inc, 1977.

_____, et al. *The Encyclopedia of Common Diseases.* Emmaus, PA: Rodale Press, Inc., 1976.

Giller, Robert M., MD, et al. *Natural Prescriptions.* New York: Ballentine Books, 1994.

Glowacki, Rosen CJ, et al. *Sex steroids, The Inuslin-Like Growth Factor Regulatory System, and Aging Implications for the Management of Older Postmenopausal Women.* J Nutr Health Aging, Vol.2, No. 1, 1998.

Gokce MD, Noyan, (1999) Long Term Ascorbic Acid administration reverses Endothelial Vasomotor Dysfunction in Patients with Coronary artery Disease. Circulation;99 pages 3234-3240

Goldberg Group, Burton, ed. *Alternative Medicine The Definitive Guide.* Washington: Future Medicine Publishing, Inc., 1994.

Golden GA et Al. (1998) Steroid hormones partition to distinct sites in a model membrane bilayer: direct demonstration by small-angle X-ray diffraction.

Goodman, David, 'Soy toxins', press release

Goodman, Paul, *Compulsory Mis-education and the Community of Scholars.* New York: Vintage Books, 1962.

Gori, Francesca, et al. *Effects of Androgens on the Insulin-Like Growth Factor System in an Androgen-Responsive Human Osteoblastic Cell Line.* Endocrinology, Vol. 140, No. 12, 1999.

Graham, Ian M (June 11 1997) Plasma Homocysteine as a Risk Factor for Vascular Disease. JAMA Vol 27, No. 22

Grant Ph D, William (November 1998) the role of milk and sugar in heart disease. The American Journal of Natural Medicine.

Greenspan, Francis S.,MD, et al., eds. *Basic and Clinical Endocrinology.* Stamford, CT: Appleton&Lange, 1997.

Griffin, Tom, M.D., et al. *The Physicians Blueprint Feeling Good For Life.* Arizona: New Medical Dynamics Inc., 1983.

Grinspoon, Steven, et al. *Effects of Androgen Administration on the Growth Hormone-Insulin-Like Growth Factor I Axis in Men with Aquired Immunodeficiency Syndrome Wasting.* Journal of Clinical Endocrinology and Metabolism, Vol. 83, No. 12, 1998.

Gurnell, Eleanor M., (2001) Dehydroepiandrosterone replacement therapy. European Journal of Endocrinology. 145 pages 103-106

Guyton, Arthur C., M.D. *Textbook of Medical Physiology.* 7th ed. Pennsylvania: W.B. Saunders Company, 1986.

Halmos, Gabor, et. al. (2000) Human Ovarian Cancer Express Somatostatin Receptor. The Journal of Clinical Endocrinology and Metabolism. Vol. 85 No. 10 pages3509-3512

Hamel, Frederick G., et al. *Regulation of Multicatalytic Enzyme Activity by Insulin and the Insulin-Degrading Enzyme.* Endocrinology, Vol. 139, No. 10, 1998.

Handelsman, DJ, Crawford, BA. *Androgens Regulate Circulating Levels of Insulin-Like Growth Factor (IGF)-I and IGF Binding Protien-3*

Hanley, Anthony J.G., et al. *Increased Proinsulin Levels and Decreased Acute Insulin Response Independently Predict the Incidence of Type 2 Diabetes in the Insulin Resistance Atherosclerosis Study.* Diabetes, Vol. 51, April, 2002.

Hansten, Philip. *Drug Interactions.* 4th ed. London: Henry Kimpton Publishers, 1979.

Harper, Harold A., PhD. *Review of Physiological Chemistry.* 7th ed. Los Altos: Lange Medical Publications, 1959.

Harris, J.R., ed. *Blood Cell Biochemistry, Erythroid Cells.* New York: Plenum Press, 1990.

Harrington, James and Christin Carter-Su (2001) Signaling Pathways activated by the growth hormone receptor. Trends in Endocrinology. Vol. 12 No. 6 August 2001

Harrison, George R. *How Things Work.* New York: William Morrow and Co., 1941.

Hayes, Francis J., (2000) aromatase Inhibition in the Human Male Reveals a Hypothalamic Site of Estrogen Feedback. Journal of Clinical Endocrinology and Metabolism. Vol. 85 No. 9 pages 3027-3035

Heitzer, Thomas (2000) Tetrahydrobiopterin Improves Endothelium-Dependent Vasodialtion in Chronic Smokers. Circulation Research;86:e36

Heller, Richard F., MS, PhD, et al. *The Carbohydrate Addict's Healthy Heart Program.* New York: Ballentine Publishing Group, 1999.

Hendrickson, James E., MD. *The Molecules of Nature.* New York: W.A. Benjamin, 1965.

Hiramatsu R, and Nisula BC (1987 June) Erythrocyte-associated cortisol: measurement, kinetics of dissociation and potential physiological significance. Journal of Clinical Endocrinology and Metabolism. Vol. 64 No. 6 pages 1224-32

Hiramatsu, Ryoh and Bruce C. Nisula (1990) Uptake of erythrocyte-associated component of blood testosterone and corticosterone to rat brain. Journal of steroid biochemistry. Pages 383-87

Hiramatsu, R (1991) Uptake of erythrocytes-associated component of blood testosterone and corticosterone to rat brain. J of Steroid Biochemistry Mol Biol Mar 38: 383-7

Hoffman, David. *The Complete Illustrated Holistic Herbal.* New York: Barnes&Noble, Inc, 1996.

Hunt, Valerie V. *Infinite Mind: The Science of Human Vibrations of Consciousness.* Malibu, CA: Malibu Publishing Co, 1996.

Isaacson, Robert L., et al. *Toxin-Induced Blood Vessel Inclusions Caused by the Chronic Administration of Aluminum and Sodium Fluoride and Their Implications for Dementia.* Annals New York Academy of Sciences,

Jacobson GM (1975) 17 Beta-estradiol transport and metabolism in human red blood cells. J Clin Endocrinology and Metab. Feb 40 Issue 2

Jawetz, Ernest, MD, PhD, et al. *Review of Medical Microbiology.* 15th ed. Los Altos: Lange Medical Publications, 1982.

Jin, Weijun et Al. (2002) Lipases and HDL metabolism. Trends in Endocrinology Vol 13 No. 4 May 2002

Jones, T.W.H. *Dictionary of the Bach Flower Remedies.* Essex, England: C.W. Daniel Company Limited, 1995.

Junqueira, Luis C., MD, et al. *Basic Histology.* 3rd ed. Los Altos: Lange Medical Publications, 1980.

Kamat, Amrita, et. Al. (2002) Mechanisms in tissue-specific regulation of estrogen biosynthesis in humans. Trends in Endocrinology and Metabolism. Vol. 13 April 2002 pgs. 122-128

Kellner, Michael, et al. *Atrial Natriuretic Factor Inhibits the CRH-Stimulated Secretion of ACTH and Cortisol in Man.* Life Sciences, Vol. 60, 1992.

Kemper, Donald ed. *Healthwise Handbook.* Idaho: Healthwise, Inc. 1976.

Keough, Carol, ed. *Future Youth.* Emmaus, PA: Rodale Press, Inc, 1987.

Khalsa, Dharma Singh, MD, et al. *Brain Longevity.* New York: Time Warner Company, 1997.

Kirpichnikov, Dmitri, and James Sowers (2001) Diabetes mellitus and diabetes-associated vascular disease. Trends in Endocrinology and Metabolism. Vol. 12 No. 5 July 2001.

Kishi, Yutaka, et al. *Alph-Lipoic Acid: Effects on Glucose Uptake, Sorbitol Pathway, and Energy Metabolism in Experimental Diabetic Neuropathy.* Diabetes, Vol. 48, October, 1999.

Klaassen, Curtis D., Ph.D. *Casarett & Doull's Toxicology.* 6th ed. McGraw-Hill Medical Publishing Division, 2001.

Klatz, Ronald, et al. *Grow Young with HGH.* New York: Harper Perennial, 1997.

Kotelchuck, David, ed. *Prognosis Negative.* New York: Vintage Books, 1976.

Krupka RM and R Deves (1980) asymmetric binding of steroids to internal and external sites in the glucose carrier of erythrocytes. Biochim biophys Acta Vol 598 Issue 1

Kraemer W.J., et el. *Effects of Heavy-Resistance Training On Hormonal Response Patterns In Younger VS. Older Men.* Journal of Applied Physiology, September, Vol. 87, No.3, 1999.

Lacayo, Richard (April 24, 2000) Testosterone. TIME Magazine: Page 58

Lasley, Bill L., et al. *The Relationship of Circultating Dehydroepiandrosterone, Testosterone, and Estradiol to Stages of the Menopausal Transition and Ethnicity.* The Journal of Clinical Endocrinology and Metabolism, Vol. 87, No. 8, 2002.

Laughlin, Gail and Elizibeth Barret-Conner (2000) Sexual dimorphism in the Influence of Advanced Aging on the Adrenal Hormone levels: The Rancho Bernardo Study. The Journal of Clinical Endocrinology and Metabolism pgs 3561-3568

Leavelle, Dennis E., MD, ed. *Mayo Medical Laboratories Interpretive Handbook.* Rochester, MN: Mayo Medical Laboratories, 1997.

Lee, John R., MD, et al. *What Your Doctor May Not Tell You About Premenopause.* New York: Warner Books, Inc, 1999.

_____. *Natural Progesterone: the Multiple Roles of a Remarkable Hormone.* Sebastopol, CA: BLL Publishing, 1993.

Lehninger, Albert L. *Biochemistry.* New York: Worth Publishers, Inc, 1975.

_____ *Biochemicstry*. New York: Worth Publishers, Inc., 2000.

LeShan, Lawrence, Ph.D. *Psychological States as Factors in the Development of Malignant Disease: A Critical Review.* New York Journal of Medicine, August 24, 1958.

Levitt, B.B. *Electromagnetic Fields*. New York: Harcourt Brace and Company, 1995.

Ley, Beth. *DHEA: Unlocking the Secrets to the Fountain of Youth.* California: BL Publications, 1996.

Lewis, John G., et al. *Caution on the use of saliva measurements to monitor absorption of progesterone from transdermal creams in postmenopausal women.* Maturitas, 4, 2002.

Lovern, J.A., *The Chemistry of Lipids of Biochemistry Significance.* London: Methuen & Co. LTD, 1955.

Lowe, John C., et al. *The Metabolic Treatment of Fibromyalgia.* Boulder, CO: Mc Dowell Publishing Company, 2000.

Lowenthal, Albert A., MD. *Endoctrine Glands and Sexual Problems.* Chicago:_____, 1928.

Lorand, Arnold, MD. *Old Age Deferred.* Philadelphia: F.A. Davis Publishers, 1911.

Maciocia, Giovanni. *Tongue Diagnosis in Chinese Medicine.* Seattle: Eastland Press, Inc, 1987.

Martin, Janet L., et al. *Insulin-Like Growth Factor Binding Protein-3 Is Regulated by Dihydrotestosterone and Stimulates Deoxyribonucleic Acid Synthesis and Cell Proliferation in LNCaP Prostate Carcinoma Cells.* Endocrinology, Vol. 141, No. 7, 2000.

Mauras, Nelly, et. al. (2000) Estrogen Suppression in Males: Metabolic Effects. The Journal of Clinical Endocrinology and Metabolism. Vol85 No. 7 pages2370-2377.

McCarty, MF. *Androgenic Progestins Amplify the Breast Cancer Risk Associated with Hormone Replacement Therapy by Boosting IGF-I Activity.* Med Hypotheses, February, Vol. 56, No. 2, 2001.

McCarty, MF. *Modulation of Adipocyte Lipoprotein Lipase Expression as a Strategy for Preventing or Treating Visceral Obesity.* Med Hypotheses, August, Vol. 57, No. 2, 2001.

Mawatari S and Murakami K. (1999) Effects of ascorbic acid on peroxidation of human erythrocyte membranes by lipoxygenase. Ntrition Science vitaminology (Tokyo) Dec 45(6)687-99

McCann, Una D. (August 27, 1997)Brain Serotonin Neurotoxicity and Primary Pulmonry Hypertension From Fenfluramine and Dexfenfluramine. JAMA Vol.278, No 8

McEvoy, Gerald K., Pharm.D, ed. *AHFS Drug Information, 2001.* Bethesda, MD: American Society of Health-System Pharmacists, Inc, 2001.

_____. *AHFS Drug Information, 1986.* Bethesda, MD: American Society of Health-System Pharmacists, Inc, 1986.

Mchedlishvili, G, New evidence for involvement of blood rheological disorders in rise of peripheral resistance in essential hyperttension. Clinical Hemorheology Microcirculation Vol 17 Issue 1

McLaughlin, T, et Al. (2000) Carbohydrate Induced Hypertriglyceridemia: An Insight into the Link between Plasma Insulin and Triglyceride Concentrations. The Journal of Clinical Endocrinology and Metabolism. Vol85. No. 9 pages 3085-3088

McIntosh, M., et al. *Opposing Actions of Dehydroepiandrosterone and Corticosterone in Rats.* Proc Soc Exp Biol Med, July, Vol. 221, No. 3, 1999.

Mellon, Cynthia H. and Lisa D. Griffin (2002) Neurosteroids: biochemistry and clinical significance. Trends in Endocrinology and Metabolism 13 pages 35-43

Mendelsohn, Robert S., M.D. *Confessions of a Medical Heretic.* New York: Warner Books Inc., 1979.

Michalak, Patricia S. *Rodale's Successful Organic Gardening, Herbs.* Emmaus, PA: Rodale Press, 1993.

Mindell, Earl L., R.Ph.D, Ph.D., et al. *Dr. Earl Mindell's Secrets of Natural Health.* Illinois: Keats Publishing, 2000.

Mokken FC, et. Al. (1992) the clinical importance of erythrocyte deformability, a hemorheologically parameter. Annals of Hematology Volume 64 Issue 3

Morales, AJ. et al. *The Effects of Six Months Treatment with a 100 mg Daily Dose of Dehyroepiamdrosterone (DHEA) on Circulating Sex Steroids, Body Composition and Muscle Strength in Age-Advanced Men and Women.* Clinical Endocrinology (Oxf), October, Vol. 49, No. 4, 1998.

Morin, Laurie C., (2000) Endocrine and Metabolic Effects of Metaformin vs. Ethinyl-Cyproterone acetate in Obese Women with Polycystic Ovary Syndrome: A Randomized Study. The Journal of Clinical Endocrinology and Metabolism. Vol. 85 No. 9 pages 3161-3168

Morley J.E., et al. *Potentially Predictive and Manipulable Blood Serum Correlatives of Aging in the Healthy Human Male: Progressive Decreases in Bioavailable Testosterone, Dehydroepiamdrosterone Sulfate, and the Ratio of Insulin-Like Growth Factor 1 to Growth Hormone.* Pro Natl Acad Sci USA, July, Vol. 94, No.14, 1997.

Moss, Ralph W. *The Cancer Industry*. New York: Paragon House, 1989.

Monte, Tom, et al. *World Medicine*. New York: F.P. Putnam's Sons, 1993.

Mullenix, Phyllis J., *Neurotoxicity of Sodium Fluoride in Rats.* Neurotoxicology and Teratology, Vol. 17, No. 2, 1995.

Munzer, T., et al. *Effects of GF and/or Sex Steroid Administration on Abdominal Subcutaneous and Visceral Fat in Healthy Aged Women and Men.* J Clin Endocirinol Metab, August, Vol. 86, No. 8, 2001.

Muramoto, Naboru. *Healing Ourselves*. New York: Avon Books, 1973.

Murray, Michael, N.D., et al. *Encyclopedia of Natural Medicine.* California: Prima Health, 1998.

Myss, Caroline, PhD, et al. *Creation of Health*. New York: Three Rivers Press, 1993.

Nam, S.Y., et al. *Low-Dose Growth Hormone Treatment Combined with Diet Restriction Decreases Insulin Resistance by Reducing Visceral Fat and Increasing Muscle Mass in Obese Type 2 Diabetic Patients.* Int J Obes Relat Metab Disord, August, Vol. 25, No. 8, 2001.

Nelson, David L., et al. *Lehninger Principles of Biochemistry*. 3rd ed. New York: Worth Publishers, 2000.

Netzer, Corinne T. *Encyclopedia of Food Values.* New York: Dell Publishing, 1992.

Nicklas, B.J., et al. *Testosterone, Growth Hormone and IGF-I Response to Acute and Chronic Resistive Exercise in Men Aged 55-70 Years.* Int. Journal of Sports Medicine, October, Vol. 16, No. 7, 1995.

Nitenberg A. Acetylcholine induced coronary vasoconstriction in young, heavy smokers with normal coronary arteriographic findings. Service d'Explorations Fonctionnelles, Unite 251, France.

Ody, Penelope. *The Complete Medicinal Herbal.* New York: Dorling Kindersley Inc, 1993.

Okada, Hidetaka, et. al. (2000) Progesterone Enhances Interleukin-15 Production in Human Endometrial Stromal Cells in Vitro. Journal of Clinical Endocrinology and Metabolism. Volume 85. No. 12 pages 4765-4770

Ornstein, Robert, et al. *The Amazing Brain.* Boston: Houghton Mifflin Company, 1984.

O'Rourke, P.J. *Parliament of Whores.* New York: The Atlantic Monthly Press, 1991.

Paolisso G., et al. *Insulin Resistance and Advancing Age: What Role For Dehydroepiandrosterone Sulfate?* Metabolism, November, Vol.46, No.11, 1997.

Pascal, Alana. *DHEA the Fountain of Youth Discovered?* California: Ben-Wal Printing, 1996.

Peeke, Pamela, MD, MPH. *Fight Fat After Forty.* New York: Penguin Group, 2000.

Persson SU (1996) Correlations between fatty acid composition of the erythrocyte membrane and blood rheology data. Scandinavian Journal of Clinical Laboratory Investigation. April 96 vol. 56 Issue 2

Pert, Candace B., PhD. *The Molecules of Emotion.* New York: Simon and Schuster, Inc, 1997

Petersdorf, Robert G., M.D., et al. *Harrison's Principles of Internal Medicine tenth edition.* McGraw-Hill Book Company, 1983.

Pinchera, Aldo, MD, ed. *Endocrinology and Metabolism*. London: McGraw-Hill International(UK) Ltd., 2001.

Pino, Ana M. et. al. (2000) Dietary Isoflavones Affect Sex Hormone Globulin levels in Postmenopausal Women. The Journal of Clinical Endocrinology and Metabolism. Vol 85. No.8 pages 2797-2800

Porkert, Manfred, M.D., et al. *Chinese Medicine*. New York: Henry Holt and Company, 1982.

Pries, Axel R., et al. *Structural Autoregulation of Terminal Vascular Beds*. Hypertension, 1999.

Quillin, Patrick, PhD, RD, CNS, et al. *Beating Cancer with Nutrition*. Rev ed. Tulsa, OK: Nutrition Times Press, Inc, 2001.

Ravaglia, G., et al. *Regular Moderate Intensity Physical Activity and Blood Concentrations of Endogenous Anabolic Hormones and Thyroid Hormones in Aging Men*. Mech Aging Dev, February, Vol. 122, No. 2, 2001.

Rath, Matthias, MD. *Eradicating Heart Disease*. San Francisco: Health Now, 1993.

Ravel, Richard, MD. *Clinical Laboratory Medicine*. 6th ed. St Louis: Mosby-Year Book, Inc, 1995.

Raynaud-Simon, A., et al. *Plasma Insulin-Like Growth Factor I Levels in the Elderly: Relation to Plasma Dehydroepiandrosterone Sulfate Levels, Nutritional Status, Health and Mortality*. J Gerontology, July-August, Vol.47, No. 4, 2001.

Reaven, Gerald, M.D., et al. *Syndrome X*. New York: Simon & Schuster, 2000.

Reid, Daniel. *The Complete Book of Chinese Health & Healing*. Massachusetts: Shambhala Publications, Inc. 1994.

Reiss, Uzzi, M.D., et al. *Natural Hormone Balance for Woman*. New York: Pocket Books, 2001.

Remington, Dennis, M.D., et al. *Back to Health*. Utah: Publishers Press, 1986.

Rifkind, Richard, et al. *Fundamentals of Hematology*. 2nd ed. Illinois: Year Book Medical Publishers, Inc. 1980.

Robbins, John. *Reclaiming Our Health: Exploding the Myth and Embracing the Source of True Healing*. Tiburon, CA: HJ Kramer Inc, 1998.

Robbins, Stanley L., MD, et al. *Pathologic Basis of Disease*. 2nd ed. Philadelphia: W.B. Saunders Company, 1979.

Rodale, J.I., et al. *The Health Seeker*. Emmaus, PA: Rodale Books, Inc. 1972.

Rodale, J.I., ed. *Health Builder*. Pennsylvania: Rodale Press, Inc., 1971.

Roggenkamp HG (1986) Erythrocyte rigidity in healthy patients and patients with cardiovascualr disease risk factors. KWH Oct 1986 64: 1091-6

Rojo ND, Ruth (2001) Why is it harder to lose weight as we age? Journal of Longevity Vol 7 No 9

Rosedale MD, Ron Presentation at the Health Institute's boulder-Fest, August 1999 seminar

Rosenfeld, Isadore, M.D. *The Complete Medical Exam*. New York: Simon & Schuster, 1978.

Rosmond, Roland, et al. *Stress-Related Cortisol Secretion in Men: Relationships with Abdominal Obesity and Endocrine, Metabolic and Hemodynamic Abnormalities*. Journal of Clinical Endocrinology and Metabolism, February, Vol. 83, No. 6, 1998.

Rosmond, R, Bjortorp, P. *The Interactions Between Hypothalamic-Pituitary-Adrenal Axis Activity, Testosterone, Insulin-Like Growth Factor I and Abdominal Obesity with Metabolism and Blood Pressure in Men*. Int Journal Obes Relat Metab Disord, December, Vol. 22, No. 12, 1998.

Ross, A.C. Gordon, M.B., ChB, MFHom.

Ross, A.C. Gordon, M.B., Chb, MFHom. *Homeopathy An Introductory Guide*. Northamptonshire: Thorsons Publishers Limited: 1976.

Rubin, Philip, ed. *Clinical Oncology sixth edition*. American Cancer Society, 1983.

Ruiz, Gomez F. (1998) Treatments with progesterone analogues decreases macrophage Fcgamma receptors expression. Clinical Immunopathology Dec; 89(3): 231-9

Russell, A.L. *Glycoaminoglycan (GAG) Deficiency in Protective Barrier as an Underlying, Primary Cause of Ulcerative Colitis, Crohn's Disease, Interstitial Cystitis and Possibly Reiter's Syndrome.* Medical Hypotheses, Vol. 52, No. 4, 1999.

Ryan, Graeme B., MB, BS, PhD, et al. *Inflamation.* Kalamazoo, MI: The Upjohn Company, 1977.

Sapolsky, Robert M. *Stress, the Aging Brain, and the Mechanisms of Neuron Death.* Cambridge, MA: The MIT Press, 1992.

_____. *The Trouble with Testosterone.* New York: Simon and Shuster, Inc, 1997.

Sarno, John E., MD. *The Mindbody Prescription.* New York: Warner Books, Inc, 1998.

Schofield, Janice F. *Discovering Wild Plants.* Bothell, WA: Alaska Northwest Books, 1989.

Simpson, Leslie O. (1987) Red cell and hemorheological changes in multiple sclerosis. Pathology, 19 pp51-55

Secomb, T. W. (1998) A model for red cell motion in glycocalyx-lined capillaries. American Journal of Physiology 274 H1016-H1022

Sahelian MD, Ray (October 1996) DHEA Youth in a Bottle? Lets Live

Schechter M. D., Michael, et. Al. (2000) Oral Magnesium Therapy Improves Endothelial Function in Patients with Coronary Artery Disease. Circulation Nov. 7 2000. Pages 2353-2358

Scholl, B.F., PhG, MD, ed. *Library of Health.* Philadelphia: Historical Publishing, Inc, 1932.

Schwarzbein, Nancy, MD, et al. *The Schwarzbein Principle.* Deerfield Beach, FL: Health Communications, Inc, 1999.

Sears, Barry, PhD, et al. *Enter the Zone.* New York: HarperCollins Publishers, Inc, 1995.

Sheally, C.N., MD, PhD, ed. *The Complete Family Guide to Alternative Medicine.* New York: Barnes&Noble, Inc, 1996.

Shippen, Eugene, MD, et al. *The Testosterone Syndrome*. New York: M.Evans and Company, Inc, 1998.

Signorello, LB., et al. *Hormones and Hair Patterning In Men: A Role for Insulin-Like Growth Factor 1?* Journal of the American Academy of Dermatology, February, Vol. 40, No. 2, 1999.

Sobel, David S., MD, et al. *The People's Book of Medical Tests*. New York: Simon and Schuster, 1985.

Solerte, Sebastiano Bruno, et al. *Dehydroepiandrosterone Sulfate Enhances Natural Killer Cell Cytotoxicity in Humans Via Locally Generated Immunoreactive Insulin-Like Growth Factor I*. The Journal of Clinical Endocrinology & Metabolism, Vol. 84, No. 9, 1999.

Song, Linda Z.Y.X., M.D. et al. *Heart-Focused Attention and Heart-Brain Synchronization: Energetic and Physiological Mechanisms*. Alternative Therapies, September, Vol. 4, No. 5, 1998.

Spector, Walter G. *An Introduction to General Pathology*. 2nd ed. Edinburgh, Scotland: Churchill Livingstone, 1980.

Stelfox, Henry Thomas, M.D., et al. *Conflict of Interest in the Debate Over Calcium-Channel Antagonists*. The New England Journal of Medicine, January 8, 1998.

Stewart, Paul M. and Tomlison, Jeremy W. (April 2002) cortisol, 11B-hydroxysteroid dehydrogenase type 1 and central obesity. Trends in Endocrinology and Metabolism pgs.94-96

Stites, Daniel P., MD, et al., eds. *Medical Immunology*. 9th ed. Stamford, CT: Appleton&Lange, 1997.

Stuart, J. (1985) Erythrocyte rheology. J Clinical Pathology Vol. 38 Issue 9

Study Links high Carb to Cancer, Associated Press (April 2002)

Takaya, Kazuhiko, et. al. (2000) Ghrelin Strongly Stimulates Growth Hormone (GH) Release in Humans. The Journal of Clinical Endocrinology and Metabolism. Vol. 85. No. 12 pages 4908-4911

Theodosakis, Jason, MD, MS, MPH, et al. *The Arthritis Cure*. New York: Affinity Communications Corporation, 1998.

Thomas, Lewis, *The Lives of a Cell*. New York: Bantam Books, 1974.

Thrailkill, K.M. *Insulin-Like Growth Factor-I in Diabetes Mellitus: its Physiologic, Metabolic Effects, and Potential Clinical Utility.* Diabetes Technol Ther, Spring, Vol. 2, No. 1, 2000.

Tilford, Gregory L. *Edible and Medicinal Plants of the West.* Missoula: Mountain Press Publishing Company, 1997.

_____. *From Earth to Herbalist.* Missoula: Mountain Press Publishing Company, 1998.

Tiller, William A. (1996) Cardiac Coherence: A New, Noninvasive Measure of Autonomic Nervous System Order. Alternative Therapies Jan 96, Vol. 2, No 1

Tissandier, O., et al. *Testosterone, Dehydroepiandrosterone, Insulin-Like Growth Factor 1, and Insulin in Sedentary and Physically Trained Aged Men.* Eur J Appl Physiol, July, Vol.85, No. 1-2, 2001.

Tsuda K et al (2001) Electron paramagnetic resonance investigation on modulatory effect of 17 Beta-estradiol on membrane fluidity of erythrocytes in postmenopausal women. Arteriosclerosis Thromb Vasc Biol Aug:21(8):1306-12

Tsuji, K. *Specific Binding and Effects of Dehroepiandrosterone Sulfate (DHEA-S) on Skeletal Muscle Cells: Possible Implication for DHEA-S Replacement Therapy in Patients With Myotonic Dystrophy.* Life Science, Vol. 65, No.1, 1999.

Tyler, Varro E., PhD, ScD. *Herbs of Choice.* New York: Pharmaceutical Products Press, 1994.

VanHaaften, M., et al. *Identification of 16-alpha Hydroxyestrone as a Metabolite of Estriol.* Gynecol, Endorinol 2, 1988.

Veldhuis, Johannes D., et al. *Estrogen and Testosterone, But Not a Nonaromatizable Androgen, Direct Network Integration of the Hypothalamo-Somatotrope (Growth Hormone)-Insulin-Like Growth Factor I Axis in the Human: Evidence from Pubertal Pathophysioogy and Sex-Steroid Hormone Replacement.* Journal of Clinical Endocrinology and Metabolism, Vol. 82, No.10, 1997.

Vendola, K., et al. *Androgens Promote Insulin-Like Growth Factor-I and Insulin-Like Growth Factor-I Receptor Gene Expression in the Primate Ovary.* Hum Reprod, September, Vol. 1, No. 9, 1999.

Viveiros, M.M., Liptrap, R.M. *ACTH Treatment Disrupts Ovarian IGF-I and Steroid Hormone Production.* Journal of Endocrinology, 164, 2000.

Volek J.S., et al. *Body Composition and Hormonal Responses to a Carbohydrate Restricted Diet.* Metabolism, July, Vol. 51, No. 7, 2002.

Vondra, K., et al. *Role of the Steroids, SHBG, IGF-I, IGF BP-3 and Growth Hormone in Glucose Metabolism Disorders During Long-Term Treatment with Low Doses of Glucocorticoids.* Cas Lek Cesk, February, Vol. 141, No. 3, 2002.

Wallach, Jacques, MD. *Interpretation of Diagnostic Tests.* 6th ed. New York: Little, Brown and Company, 1996.

Warrier, Gopi. *The Complete Illustrated Guide to Ayurveda.* New York: Barnes&Noble, 1997.

Watkins, Alan D., et al. *The Impact of a New Emotional Self-Management Program on Stress, Emotions, Heart Rate Variability, DHEA and Cortisol.* Integrative Physiological and Behavioral Science, April-June, Vol. 33 No. 2, 1998.

Weast, Robert C., PhD. *Handbook of Chemistry and Physics.* 56th ed. Cleveland, OH: CRC Press, Inc, 1975.

Weil, Andrew, MD. *Natural Health, Natural Medicine.* Boston: Houghton Mifflin Company, 1990.

_____. *Health and Healing.* New York: Houghton Mifflin Company, 1995.

_____. *Spontaneous Healing.* New York: Alfred A. Knopf, Inc, 1995.

_____. *Eating Well for Optimum Health.* New York: Alfred A Knopf, 2000.

Wheelwright, Edith G. *Medicinal Plants and their History.* New York: Dover Publications, Inc, 1974.

Whitaker, Julian MD. *Dr Whitaker's Guide to Natural Healing.* Rocklin, CA: Prima Publishing, 1995.

Whitaker MD, Julian (September 1998) DHEA helps regulate the immune system. Health and Healing Vol 8 No 9

Wild, Russell, ed. *The Complete Book of Natural and Medicinal Cures.* Emmaus, PA: Rodale Press, 1994.

Wilson, Helen E and Ann White (1998) Prohormone: their Clinical Relevance. Trends in Endocrinology and Metabolism 9:396-402

Golden GA et al (1999) rapid and opposite effects of cortisol and estradiol on human erythrocyte Na+, K+-ATPase activity: relationship to steroid intercalation into the cell membrane. Life Science 65(12):1247-55

Wood, D.& J. *The Incredible Healing Needles.* New York: Samuel Weiser Inc., 1974.

Wood, Ian (2002) Pro-inflammatory mechanisms of a nonsteroidal anti-inflammatory drug. Trends in Endocrinology Vol 13 No. 2 March 2002

Wright, Jonathan V., MD, et al. *Natural Hormone Replacement for Women Over 45.* Petaluma, CA: Smart Publications, 1997.

_____, et al. *Natural Hormone Replacement.* California: Smart Publications, 1997.

_____, et al. *The patient's Book of Natural Healing.* California: Prima Health, 1999.

Wright MD, Jonathan and Alan Gaby MD (October 16-19) Nutrional Therapy in Medical Practice, Doubletree Seattle Airport Hotel

Yen, SS, Laughlin GA. *Aging and the Adrenal Cortex.* Exp. Gerontol, Nov-Dec, Vol. 33, No. 7-8, 1998.

Youl, Kang H., et al. *Effects of Ginseng Ingestion on Growth Hormone, Testosterone, Cortisol, and Insulin-Like Growth Factor I Responses to Acute Resistance Exercise.* J Strength Cond Res, May, Vol. 16, No. 2, 2002.

Zachrisson, I., et al. *Determinants of Growth in Diabetic Pubertal Subjects.* Diabetes Care, August, Vol. 20, No. 8, 1997.

Zager PG et Al. (1986) Distribution of 18-hydroxycorticosterone between red blood cells and plasma. J Clin Endocrinology Metab Jan 62: 84-9

Zborowski, Jeanne V., et. Al. (2000) bone Mineral Density, Androgens, and the Polycystic Ovary: The Complex and Controversial Issue of Androgenic Influence in the Female Bone. Vol. 85 No. 10 pages 3496-3506

INDEX

Absorption, 106, 137, 192, 287, 288, 322, 337, 349, 443
Acetate, 40, 135, 136, 153, 292, 335, 336, 338, 340, 341, 342, 395, 430, 445
Acetylcholine, 101, 135, 446
ACTH, 71, 72, 91, 239, 250, 280, 366, 391, 392, 441, 452
Acupuncture, xx, 24, 30, 31, 118
Acute phase reactants, x, xi, xiii, 213, 219, 322, 323, 324, 325, 372
Adrenal cortex, 59, 175, 277, 280
Adrenal insufficiency, 175, 229, 240, 367
Adrenal medulla, 59, 60, 61, 62, 63, 64, 67
Adrenaline, 58, 84, 142, 175, 176, 177, 206, 261, 264, 277
Aging, 32, 37, 38, 56, 66, 95, 109, 114, 122, 146, 149, 159, 164, 167, 265, 268, 269, 279, 285, 323, 331, 356, 357, 394, 423, 437, 438, 442, 445, 447, 449, 453
Aldosterone, xiv, 42, 66, 71, 72, 110, 123, 127, 128, 148, 185, 186, 200, 201, 202, 225, 226, 234, 251, 253, 254, 266, 268, 271, 272, 276, 277, 279, 280, 284, 285, 286, 362, 386, 391, 432

Alkaline, 349
Alternative treatment modalities, xviii, 24, 28
Amino acids, 43, 84, 132, 146, 173, 176, 177, 232, 266, 292, 293, 294, 297, 342, 351, 374, 397, 417, 423, 424, 430, 431
Anabolic, 66, 77, 109, 110, 111, 165, 171, 215, 226, 228, 266, 267, 268, 269, 271, 279, 281, 282, 288, 324, 325, 447
Anaerobic metabolism, 409, 410
Androgen, 96, 97, 98, 109, 110, 148, 157, 163, 165, 166, 167, 168, 172, 173, 174, 181, 182, 185, 188, 190, 192, 206, 208, 209, 213, 226, 227, 228, 249, 250, 252, 259, 264, 267, 271, 272, 273, 275, 276, 279, 281, 283, 295, 300, 314, 315, 325, 328, 360, 369, 370, 374, 381, 385, 386, 437, 439, 451
Androstenedione, 110, 225, 226, 227, 228, 234, 250, 255, 267, 272, 276, 362
Angiotensin converting enzyme, 70, 71, 349, 390
Angiotensin type two, 71, 280
Antibiotics, 82
Antioxidants, 40, 41, 288, 324, 429, 430
Anxiety, 105, 110, 129, 146, 196, 226

Appetite, 144, 188, 189, 199, 207, 355
Arachidonic acid, 426
Arginine, 69, 73, 374, 428, 430, 432
Aromatase, 282, 437, 440
Arthritis, xiv, xix, 39, 151, 231, 379, 395, 421, 426, 450
Asthma, viii, xiv, xix, 39, 92, 93, 231, 236, 364, 395, 421, 425
ATP, 153, 337, 339, 410
Autoimmune disease, xi, 72, 92, 278, 391
Bile, 430
Biogenic amines, 84, 89, 425
Birth control pills, xv, 180, 181, 182, 252, 359, 368, 369
Blood vessels, xvi, xx, 39, 44, 59, 60, 61, 63, 64, 66, 68, 70, 73, 74, 77, 78, 105, 106, 127, 197, 198, 211, 213, 216, 219, 220, 277, 281, 290, 301, 309, 310, 314, 316, 318, 320, 324, 325, 326, 327, 335, 370, 377, 390, 395, 397, 406, 425
Bone marrow, 415, 416
Bones, 145, 150, 157, 171, 172, 199, 267
Bradykinin, 70, 71, 73, 349, 390, 391
Brain, v, ix, xiii, xiv, 59, 60, 63, 64, 66, 82, 83, 84, 85, 86, 87, 88, 89, 90, 91, 93, 94, 95, 96, 98, 99, 100, 101, 102, 103, 104, 105, 106, 107, 108, 109, 110, 112, 114, 115, 119, 120, 121, 126, 128, 131, 132, 135, 137, 138, 139, 140, 144, 164, 189, 207, 226, 227, 228, 236, 280, 282, 305, 337, 373, 393, 398, 406, 412, 414, 416, 417, 440, 441, 444, 446, 449, 450
Breast cancer, 183, 243, 247, 248, 259, 382, 384, 387
Bronchial tone, 262
Calcium, 48, 49, 50, 51, 52, 53, 55, 56, 73, 74, 106, 112, 122, 123, 125, 134, 186, 194, 204, 254, 407, 409, 410, 411, 414, 450
Capillaries, 70, 390, 407, 414, 449
Carbohydrates, 104, 135, 144, 187, 199, 204, 207, 208, 318, 340, 352, 353
Carbon dioxide, 335, 336, 338, 341, 412
Carbon monoxide, 326
Carnitine, xi, 336, 337, 338
Cartilage, 38, 39, 96, 351, 395, 419
Catabolic, 77, 109, 158, 165, 166, 171, 172, 173, 174, 215, 216, 225, 226, 266, 268, 269, 279, 281, 310, 324, 424
Catalase, 119, 416
Cell charge, 55, 106, 125, 127, 128
Cell membrane, 55, 56, 110, 122, 123, 127, 135, 153, 154, 201, 255, 265, 311, 326, 409, 410, 411, 415, 418, 453
Cell power plants, 147, 154, 191, 311, 337, 339
Chelation, xiii, 69, 322
Chi, 31, 32

Chiropractic, xx, 24, 118, 403
Choline, 101, 102, 135, 138, 417
Chronic fatigue, 168, 341
Coenzyme Q10, 339, 340, 429
Colon, xix, 312, 314, 418, 428, 430
Coronary arteries, 35, 61, 319
Cortisol, x, xiv, 59, 71, 72, 75, 77, 78, 79, 80, 104, 108, 109, 110, 125, 128, 143, 152, 161, 168, 172, 173, 174, 175, 181, 189, 191, 192, 202, 205, 206, 208, 211, 215, 216, 217, 221, 222, 223, 225, 226, 227, 228, 229, 230, 232, 233, 234, 237, 238, 239, 240, 247, 252, 264, 266, 268, 270, 272, 276, 277, 278, 279, 281, 284, 291, 293, 294, 296, 297, 298, 299, 300, 309, 310, 312, 323, 324, 325, 328, 336, 342, 351, 355, 356, 357, 360, 361, 362, 364, 365, 366, 367, 369, 373, 375, 376, 381, 388, 391, 392, 415, 432, 440, 441, 448, 450, 452, 453
C-reactive protein, 219, 322, 323, 372
Cytoskeleton, 39, 395
DHEA, 42, 71, 73, 74, 110, 157, 163, 165, 167, 174, 175, 178, 180, 206, 208, 221, 225, 226, 227, 228, 234, 267, 268, 272, 276, 281, 282, 294, 295, 309, 362, 375, 391, 443, 445, 446, 449, 451, 452, 453
DHT, 282, 443

Diabetes, vi, xi, xix, 36, 39, 76, 95, 145, 151, 163, 179, 187, 196, 197, 214, 290, 293, 295, 299, 300, 301, 303, 304, 307, 308, 309, 312, 314, 356, 357, 374, 377, 385, 386, 395, 400, 406, 413, 421, 432, 433, 434, 435, 436, 440, 442, 451, 453
Diseases of middle age, xix
DNA, ix, xiv, 26, 31, 66, 74, 106, 107, 109, 121, 127, 131, 149, 150, 151, 152, 154, 155, 157, 165, 167, 168, 169, 170, 178, 185, 234, 235, 236, 237, 238, 239, 241, 242, 243, 247, 249, 251, 253, 255, 256, 257, 258, 260, 261, 264, 266, 267, 268, 270, 275, 278, 280, 294, 296, 297, 309, 311, 325, 349, 359, 363, 365, 366, 375, 382, 415, 422, 423, 424, 437
Dopamine, 64, 82, 84, 85, 91, 92, 94, 95, 98, 132, 133, 177, 356
Emotions, iii, 111, 220, 322, 452
Endoplasmic reticulum, 264
Endothelin, 68, 78, 216, 425
Entropy, 29
Enzymes, 36, 44, 106, 119, 134, 139, 165, 201, 226, 228, 261, 264, 265, 269, 286, 287, 356, 415, 416, 419, 423, 425
Eosinphils, xiv, 240, 367
Epinephrine, ix, xi, xiii, 58, 59, 60, 61, 62, 63, 64, 65, 66, 67, 68, 79, 80, 84, 85, 92,

93, 94, 104, 132, 133, 143, 148, 152, 161, 172, 174, 175, 176, 189, 192, 205, 217, 222, 223, 225, 226, 278, 291, 293, 297, 298, 299, 336, 342, 347, 348, 351, 355, 356, 357, 373, 376, 425

Essential fatty acids, 102, 138, 426, 427

Estrogen, xv, 111, 143, 148, 152, 166, 167, 179, 180, 181, 182, 183, 184, 189, 191, 192, 205, 209, 234, 242, 243, 244, 245, 246, 247, 248, 249, 250, 252, 253, 255, 257, 258, 273, 274, 276, 277, 282, 294, 295, 300, 313, 328, 336, 344, 349, 359, 360, 362, 367, 368, 369, 370, 375, 381, 387, 415, 440, 441, 443, 451

Exercise, xii, 49, 57, 104, 111, 142, 159, 164, 169, 173, 181, 188, 190, 191, 205, 206, 207, 209, 219, 221, 292, 293, 304, 305, 306, 309, 319, 320, 328, 329, 331, 336, 354, 356, 357, 372, 375, 384, 386, 400, 446, 453

Ferririn, 219, 220, 322

Ferritin, 322

Fibrinogen, 213, 219, 220, 322, 432

Fibrocystic breast disease, 183, 243, 247, 248, 259

Fibroids, 183, 243, 247, 248, 259

Fibromyalgia, 231, 406, 436, 443

Fluoride, 77, 113, 114, 115, 121, 216, 326, 411, 420, 429, 441, 445

Folate, 64, 65, 69, 70, 73, 85, 86, 88, 94, 102, 132, 139, 177, 286, 287, 337, 379, 428

GABA, 110, 133, 134, 226

GAG, 40, 42, 43, 44, 265, 314, 394, 395, 396, 397, 419, 449

Galactosamine, 40, 41, 395, 409, 418

Genetic program, 107, 149, 169, 170, 234, 235, 349, 363, 416

Ginger, 41

Ginseng, 283, 289, 453

Glucosamine, 40, 41, 395, 409, 418

Glutathione, 112, 120, 409, 413, 417, 419, 430

Glycogen, 34, 127, 147, 156, 197, 198, 291, 292, 293, 294, 306, 311, 317, 349, 351, 353, 372, 424

Glycogen storage, 198

Glycosaminoglycans, 39, 40, 42, 43, 44, 265, 314, 394, 395, 396, 397, 419, 449

Gonads, 91, 97, 99, 107, 109, 110, 127, 128, 142, 165, 166, 171, 182, 201, 205, 207, 208, 220, 228, 233, 264, 271, 272, 276, 277, 280, 281, 282, 283, 284, 288, 324, 328, 333, 361, 386

Growth hormone, xiii, xiv, xv, xvi, 42, 78, 79, 80, 95, 96, 97, 98, 99, 104, 105, 143, 148, 152, 157, 158, 159,

160, 161, 163, 164, 173,
174, 175, 178, 179, 180,
181, 188, 190, 191, 205,
206, 209, 213, 216, 217,
220, 221, 222, 223, 230,
232, 233, 234, 258, 278,
291, 293, 294, 295, 297,
299, 300, 304, 307, 308,
309, 311, 312, 313, 342,
344, 350, 351, 352, 353,
354, 355, 356, 357, 358,
360, 361, 368, 369, 373,
374, 375, 376, 381, 384,
385, 386, 388, 440
Gynecomastia, xi
HDL cholesterol, 437
Heart, iii, vi, viii, xi, xiii, xvi,
xix, 34, 35, 36, 39, 44, 54,
56, 58, 59, 60, 61, 63, 64,
66, 72, 96, 97, 98, 106, 108,
114, 129, 145, 151, 179,
186, 187, 218, 254, 262,
282, 290, 292, 293, 299,
300, 301, 304, 307, 310,
313, 314, 316, 317, 319,
320, 321, 322, 325, 337,
339, 340, 367, 377, 378,
379, 386, 392, 395, 397,
400, 406, 407, 421, 426,
439, 440, 447, 450, 452
Heart disease, vi, viii, xi, xiii,
xvi, xix, 34, 35, 36, 39, 44,
58, 59, 61, 66, 145, 151,
187, 218, 290, 293, 299,
300, 301, 304, 307, 310,
313, 314, 316, 317, 319,
320, 321, 322, 325, 340,
367, 378, 379, 386, 395,
397, 400, 421, 426, 439
Heartburn, 92
Hemoglobin, xii, 386, 387,
409, 411, 413, 417

Hierarchy of hormones, 422
Histamine, xi, 70, 71, 72, 84,
85, 90, 91, 93, 95, 133, 349,
390, 392
HMG Co A reductase, xvi,
303, 305, 323, 324, 380
Homeopathy, xx, 24, 448
Homocysteine, 62, 63, 65, 66,
94, 133, 148, 177, 344, 377,
378, 379, 387, 439
Hormonal fats, 425, 426, 427
Hormone imbalances, 96, 190,
193, 394, 422
Hormone mimics, xviii, 182,
183, 184, 382
Hormones, viii, ix, xii, xiii, xx,
32, 34, 38, 40, 42, 43, 44,
49, 59, 60, 63, 66, 67, 75,
79, 80, 83, 84, 91, 95, 98,
99, 100, 103, 104, 106, 107,
108, 109, 111, 121, 123,
143, 144, 147, 148, 149,
151, 152, 153, 155, 156,
157, 158, 159, 161, 162,
163, 165, 166, 167, 168,
169, 170, 171, 172, 173,
174, 175, 179, 181, 182,
185, 187, 188, 189, 190,
192, 195, 205, 206, 208,
212, 218, 221, 223, 225,
226, 227, 228, 229, 230,
232, 234, 235, 236, 241,
242, 243, 244, 245, 246,
247, 248, 249, 250, 253,
254, 255, 257, 258, 259,
260, 261, 262, 264, 265,
267, 268, 269, 270, 274,
279, 282, 291, 292, 293,
294, 297, 298, 299, 309,
320, 321, 328, 329, 330,
331, 342, 349, 351, 352,
356, 357, 360, 362, 363,

369, 370, 372, 374, 375, 376, 381, 382, 383, 384, 385, 386, 387, 388, 389, 396, 397, 399, 415, 420, 421, 422, 423, 424, 425, 426, 427, 428, 432, 439, 447, 450

Hypertension, 46, 57, 58, 444, 447

Hypoglycemia, 230, 232, 278, 298, 360, 414

Hypothalamus, 91, 95, 236, 248, 249, 250, 252, 356, 360

Informational substance, ix, x, 32, 33, 61, 68, 84, 86, 91, 92, 100, 101, 106, 108, 120, 259, 260, 261, 262, 263, 264, 265, 266, 267, 329, 421

Insulin, viii, x, xi, xii, xiii, xv, xvi, 34, 35, 36, 42, 43, 46, 47, 49, 57, 58, 68, 73, 74, 75, 76, 77, 78, 79, 80, 81, 103, 104, 105, 126, 127, 133, 143, 144, 145, 148, 152, 155, 156, 157, 158, 159, 160, 161, 162, 163, 164, 168, 172, 173, 175, 178, 179, 180, 181, 186, 188, 189, 190, 191, 192, 193, 195, 196, 197, 198, 199, 202, 204, 205, 206, 207, 208, 209, 210, 211, 212, 213, 214, 215, 216, 217, 220, 221, 222, 223, 226, 227, 228, 229, 230, 232, 233, 234, 243, 254, 258, 261, 270, 278, 281, 291, 292, 293, 294, 295, 296, 297, 298, 299, 300, 301, 302, 303, 304, 305, 306, 307, 308, 309, 310, 311, 312, 313, 314, 316, 317, 318, 319, 320, 321, 323, 324, 325, 327, 328, 330, 333, 336, 342, 344, 347, 349, 350, 351, 352, 353, 354, 355, 356, 357, 358, 361, 362, 368, 369, 371, 372, 373, 375, 376, 377, 380, 381, 384, 385, 386, 396, 397, 398, 400, 411, 419, 423, 424, 426, 427, 435, 436, 437, 438, 439, 440, 443, 444, 445, 446, 447, 448, 450, 451, 453

Insulin receptor, 160, 352, 384

Insulin resistance, xii, xiii, xv, 47, 75, 76, 126, 158, 159, 160, 190, 191, 192, 195, 196, 197, 198, 214, 215, 230, 233, 254, 278, 293, 299, 300, 302, 305, 313, 353, 354, 356, 357, 362, 373

Insulin-like growth factor type 1, 75, 148, 155, 156, 351

Intelligent energy, 24, 28, 30, 32

Iron, 77, 216, 308, 312, 322, 393, 413, 417

Joints, 38

Kidneys, 49, 56, 89, 126, 128, 201, 342, 349, 412, 430

Lactic acid, ix, xvi, 288, 303, 304, 340, 341, 408

LDL cholesterol, xv, 34, 74, 127, 164, 198, 199, 206, 207, 211, 233, 290, 291, 294, 296, 300, 302, 314, 318, 319, 320, 326, 336,

353, 355, 357, 361, 369, 372, 377, 406, 424
Leukotrienes, 425
Licorice root, 92
Life field, 24, 26, 27, 28
Ligaments, 270
Linoleic acid, 426
Linolenic, 426
Lipids, 443
Lipoic acid, 120, 136, 287, 341, 429, 430
Liver, x, xi, xii, xv, xvi, 34, 35, 43, 47, 54, 59, 60, 61, 63, 64, 75, 76, 79, 80, 81, 95, 103, 104, 126, 127, 138, 139, 142, 147, 150, 155, 156, 157, 158, 159, 160, 161, 162, 163, 167, 168, 174, 178, 179, 180, 181, 184, 190, 191, 192, 195, 197, 198, 199, 206, 207, 208, 213, 214, 215, 220, 221, 222, 223, 232, 243, 255, 256, 258, 278, 288, 290, 291, 292, 293, 294, 295, 296, 297, 299, 300, 302, 303, 304, 305, 306, 307, 308, 309, 310, 311, 312, 313, 314, 316, 317, 318, 319, 320, 321, 324, 333, 337, 341, 342, 348, 350, 351, 352, 353, 354, 355, 356, 357, 361, 368, 369, 372, 373, 374, 375, 376, 377, 379, 380, 384, 385, 397, 417, 418, 419, 421, 423, 428, 429, 430
Lungs, 70, 108, 150, 390
Lymphatics, 317
Lymphocytes, 240, 278, 367
Macrophages, 35, 127, 164, 291, 293, 300, 302, 318, 319, 320, 326, 353, 372, 377
Mast cells, 71, 91, 390
McKenzie Jefferies, MD, William, 237
Melatonin, 84, 86, 88, 89
Mercury, 116, 117, 138, 398, 399
Message content, viii, x, xi, xii, xiv, 34, 35, 42, 47, 58, 59, 60, 63, 64, 67, 68, 71, 75, 76, 77, 80, 96, 97, 98, 103, 108, 109, 128, 147, 149, 150, 151, 152, 154, 155, 156, 159, 160, 161, 162, 164, 165, 166, 167, 168, 169, 170, 171, 172, 173, 175, 179, 180, 181, 182, 183, 184, 186, 187, 190, 192, 198, 199, 201, 202, 206, 208, 214, 215, 218, 219, 223, 226, 228, 229, 232, 235, 237, 238, 241, 242, 243, 244, 245, 246, 247, 250, 253, 254, 255, 256, 257, 258, 261, 264, 265, 266, 267, 268, 269, 270, 273, 274, 275, 276, 278, 280, 282, 283, 284, 291, 292, 293, 294, 295, 296, 297, 299, 300, 302, 303, 304, 306, 309, 310, 311, 313, 314, 317, 324, 325, 328, 331, 334, 347, 351, 352, 353, 361, 363, 365, 366, 368, 369, 372, 373, 374, 377, 380, 382, 383, 390, 396, 415, 418, 422, 423, 424, 425, 426, 427

Methionine, 62, 65, 70, 102, 132, 139, 177, 337, 379, 433
Methyl donor system, xii, 58, 62, 63, 65, 66, 86, 88, 92, 102, 121, 132, 135, 139, 177, 337, 348, 379, 409, 413, 414, 416, 417
Mitochondria, xvi, 69, 111, 113, 119, 122, 257, 264, 283, 284, 291, 292, 311, 312, 336, 337, 338, 339, 341, 408, 414
Mucous, 39, 44, 395, 397
Muscles, 34, 59, 61, 63, 81, 145, 157, 161, 173, 175, 199, 200, 226, 230, 231, 267, 270, 288, 292, 293, 294, 297, 303, 305, 306, 308, 322, 341, 350, 351, 353, 354, 355, 358, 372, 373, 375, 376
Muses, Carl, 29
Myelin, 100, 101, 110
Myelin sheath, 101
Naturopathy, 118
Neutrophils, 240, 367
Niacin, 89, 335, 336, 337, 339, 341
Nitric oxide, x, 68, 69, 70, 71, 73, 74, 78, 216, 389, 390, 391, 394, 400, 425, 427
Nitric oxide synthase, 68, 69
Noradrenaline, 58, 177
Norepinephrine, ix, 58, 60, 61, 62, 63, 64, 66, 67, 68, 84, 93, 94, 132, 133, 177, 299, 348
Nutrition, iv, v, 45, 69, 76, 78, 79, 126, 130, 131, 134, 138, 146, 158, 159, 160, 162, 175, 178, 179, 181, 185, 189, 197, 198, 222, 223, 242, 253, 283, 296, 308, 312, 318, 331, 334, 354, 355, 371, 373, 384, 428, 434, 435, 447
Osteoporosis, 168, 171, 248, 259, 273
Ovary chain of health, 242, 250
Oxidants, 105, 112, 120, 121, 288, 409, 417, 419, 420, 429, 430
Pancreas, viii, 36, 75, 76, 80, 81, 91, 126, 142, 155, 158, 159, 161, 162, 163, 179, 181, 195, 197, 214, 220, 223, 232, 292, 296, 300, 301, 305, 307, 308, 309, 310, 313, 314, 333, 349, 350, 356, 361, 372, 376, 412
pH, 303, 349, 413
Phenylalanine, 62, 132, 133, 176, 177
Phosphate, 64, 132, 133, 134
Phospholipids, 430
Pituitary gland, 91, 95, 96, 157, 180, 368
Placenta, xiii, xv, 91, 95, 181, 182, 192, 251, 252, 358, 359, 369
Portal vein, 75, 76, 80, 158, 161, 162, 214, 223, 232, 306, 310, 318, 324, 350, 361, 372, 376
Potassium, viii, ix, 41, 47, 48, 49, 55, 56, 57, 58, 71, 72, 76, 112, 124, 125, 126, 127, 128, 129, 134, 139, 144, 185, 186, 194, 195, 196, 197, 198, 199, 200, 201, 202, 203, 206, 209, 215,

239, 253, 254, 280, 285, 292, 293, 300, 301, 305, 306, 320, 349, 354, 367, 372, 381, 391, 398, 400, 409, 410, 411, 412
Prana, 31, 32
Pregnenolone, 127, 185, 253, 283, 284
Progesterone, 73, 74, 101, 110, 111, 118, 134, 182, 183, 184, 225, 226, 234, 242, 243, 244, 246, 247, 248, 249, 250, 252, 255, 257, 267, 268, 271, 272, 273, 274, 275, 276, 277, 282, 289, 360, 362, 370, 388, 442, 443, 446, 448
Prolactin, xiii, 90, 91, 95, 96, 97, 98, 103, 143, 148, 152, 181, 182, 233, 251, 252, 344, 358, 359, 360, 361, 369, 387
Prostaglandins, 425
Protein, xii, xiii, 26, 31, 79, 80, 81, 107, 129, 132, 134, 135, 143, 144, 153, 159, 161, 165, 173, 174, 176, 182, 190, 193, 195, 199, 200, 201, 205, 207, 217, 219, 222, 223, 225, 226, 230, 233, 235, 236, 254, 255, 256, 257, 260, 268, 294, 297, 299, 303, 305, 306, 310, 316, 317, 318, 319, 322, 323, 328, 336, 338, 344, 349, 351, 355, 356, 357, 358, 361, 363, 370, 372, 373, 374, 376, 380, 411, 414, 415, 419, 426, 435, 436, 438, 443
PSA, 386, 387
Pulse diagnosis, 31

Reis, MD, Uzzi, 273
Retrolental fibroplasia, 120
Reverse T3, 386
Rhythm, 56, 100
SAMe, 62, 63, 64, 65, 85, 86, 88, 94, 101, 102, 132, 177, 337, 379
Saxon Burr, Harold, 26
Selenium, 41, 139, 429
Serotonin, xv, 84, 86, 87, 88, 89, 90, 91, 95, 96, 97, 116, 132, 251, 252, 356, 359, 360, 436, 444
Sex hormone binding globulin, xv, 255, 272
Skin, ix, 39, 43, 74, 145, 146, 150, 171, 172, 199, 200, 211, 212, 281, 283, 334, 358, 395, 396, 397, 418
Sodium, x, 46, 47, 48, 49, 50, 51, 52, 53, 55, 56, 57, 58, 71, 72, 77, 78, 112, 125, 128, 129, 134, 144, 186, 190, 194, 195, 196, 197, 201, 202, 203, 206, 215, 226, 254, 280, 285, 305, 306, 320, 391, 398, 400, 409, 410, 412, 441, 445
Steroid pressure, 107, 128, 171, 172
Steroid tone, 95, 127, 170, 171, 172, 250, 267, 268, 269, 270, 271, 272, 273, 274, 275, 276, 277, 278, 279, 280, 281, 282, 283, 284, 285, 286, 288
Steroids, viii, ix, xiv, 59, 66, 73, 74, 90, 106, 107, 109, 110, 111, 127, 129, 148, 149, 163, 165, 166, 167, 168, 170, 171, 172, 174, 175, 186, 201, 208, 226,

229, 234, 235, 237, 238, 243, 247, 249, 251, 252, 253, 254, 255, 256, 257, 258, 266, 267, 268, 269, 270, 271, 272, 274, 275, 276, 280, 281, 282, 283, 284, 286, 288, 298, 323, 325, 328, 344, 349, 358, 359, 360, 362, 363, 365, 386, 409, 415, 422, 431, 436, 438, 442, 445, 452
Stomach, viii, 132, 176, 288, 314, 349, 412
Stress hormones, 49, 108, 109, 168, 172, 269
Sulfation factor, 42, 43, 160, 314, 371, 396, 419
Survival response, 108, 220, 225, 266
T3, xiv, 148, 152, 386
T4, xiv, 152
Temperature, 98, 152
Thiols, 428, 429
Third law of thermodynamics, 28, 29
Torture chamber, 142, 143, 144, 146, 159, 187, 188, 190, 191, 204, 205, 207, 208
Toxins, xii, 40, 41, 119, 138, 139, 263, 331, 428, 429, 430, 439
Triglycerides, xv, 198, 207, 212, 314, 424
Twenty-four hour urine, 90, 99, 168, 171, 190, 238, 239, 245, 256, 275, 283, 298, 309, 325, 328, 329, 330, 365, 366, 367
Tyrosine, 62, 84, 85
Ulcerative colitis, 231, 421

Urine, viii, 63, 86, 90, 99, 166, 168, 171, 190, 191, 238, 239, 243, 245, 246, 256, 257, 259, 272, 273, 275, 283, 298, 309, 323, 325, 328, 329, 330, 349, 365, 366, 367, 432
Uterine cancer, 243, 247, 259
Vitamin A, viii, 106, 107, 111, 138, 142, 149, 150, 151, 155, 169, 171, 234, 235, 257, 258, 261, 267, 269, 286, 349, 362, 363, 422, 429
Vitamin B1, 65, 86, 88, 94, 102, 132, 139, 177, 337, 379, 430
Vitamin B12, 65, 86, 88, 94, 102, 132, 139, 177, 337, 379
Vitamin B2, 69, 73, 337, 430
Vitamin B3, 89, 337, 430
Vitamin B6, 64, 65, 85, 86, 87, 88, 92, 94, 102, 132, 133, 134, 139, 177, 337, 379, 430
Vitamin C, ix, 27, 41, 64, 65, 67, 85, 92, 94, 120, 132, 138, 177, 253, 286, 337, 348, 409, 413, 417, 429
Vitamin E, 120, 138, 429
Water, xx, 37, 39, 40, 42, 43, 48, 72, 77, 78, 112, 123, 225, 226, 266, 272, 280, 327, 328, 335, 336, 338, 341, 342, 394, 395, 396, 397, 408, 419, 420, 428, 429, 430
Wheezing, 347, 348
Whitaker MD, Julian, 453

Zinc, viii, 41, 138, 139, 185, 253, 257, 282, 288, 349, 409, 412, 429

Let your patients discover how holistic medicine provides affordable, effective, and healing treatment. To order copies of this book or *The Body Heals,* fill out and send the following order form.

Name_____

Address_____

City_____State_____Zip_____

Phone_____

Quantity

____ *Why is My Doctor So Dumb?* x $40.

____ *Glandular Failure-Caused Obesity* x $30.

____ *The Body Heals* x $50.

Shipping ($7. per book) $ _____

Purchase all three books for $75.

Total $_____

We accept checks, credit cards, or money orders.

Send to:
The Bridge Medical Publishers
P.O. Box 324
Whitefish, MT 59937

Orders only - Toll free 866 675-5714
www.thebodyheals.com   info@thebodyheals.com